ON CALL
OBSTETRICS AND GYNECOLOGY

Be ON CALL with confidence!

Successfully managing on-call situations requires a masterful combination of speed, skill, and knowledge. Rise to the occasion with **W.B. SAUNDERS' On Call Series!** These pocket-size resources provide you with immediate access to the vital, step-by-step information you need to succeed!

Other Titles in the On Call Series

Adams & Bresnick: *On Call Surgery,* 2nd Edition

Bernstein et al: *On Call Psychiatry,* 2nd Edition

Bresnick & Adams: *On Call Procedures*

Dirschl & LeCroy: *On Call Orthopedics*

Henry & Mathur: *On Call Laboratory Medicine and Pathology*

Khan: *On Call Cardiology,* 2nd Edition

Lewis & Nocton: *On Call Pediatrics,* 2nd Edition

Marshall & Mayer: *On Call Neurology,* 2nd Edition

Marshall & Ruedy: *On Call Principles and Protocols,* 3rd Edition

ON CALL

OBSTETRICS AND GYNECOLOGY

Second Edition

Homer G. Chin, MD, FACOG

Professor and Vice Chairman
Director, Division of Obstetrics and Gynecology
Department of Reproductive Medicine
University of California, San Diego, School of Medicine
San Diego, California

W.B. SAUNDERS COMPANY

A Harcourt Health Sciences Company
Philadelphia   London   New York   St. Louis   Sydney   Toronto

. SAUNDERS COMPANY
arcourt Health Sciences Company

· Curtis Center
'ependence Square West
dladelphia, Pennsylvania 19106

Library of Congress Cataloging-in-Publication Data

Chin, Homer G.
On call obstetrics and gynecology / Homer G. Chin.—2nd ed.

   p.;   cm.—(On call series)
title: Obstetrics and gynecology.
Includes index.

ISBN 0–7216–9254–0

1. Obstetrical emergencies. 2. Gynecologic emergencies. I. Title:
  Obstetrics and gynecology.   II. Title.   III. Series. [DNLM:
  1. Pregnancy Complications.   2. Genital Diseases, Female. WQ 240
  C539o 2001]

RG571.C46 2001   618'.0425—dc21   00–053801

Acquisitions Editor: William Schmitt
Manuscript Editor: Amy Norwitz
Production Manager: Norm Stellander
Illustration Specialist: John Needles
Book Designer: Matt Andrews

ON CALL OBSTETRICS AND GYNECOLOGY   ISBN 0–7216–9254–0

Printed in the United States of America

Last digit is the print number: 9   8   7   6   5   4   3   2   1

To Vicki, Stephanie, and Meredith

PREFACE

The second edition of *On Call Obstetrics and Gynecology* was written in an effort to ensure that this book continues to be a valuable aid to residents, medical students, and other health care providers who care for obstetrical and gynecological patients with urgent problems while on call. Since the publication of the first edition of this book in 1997, there have been significant advances in the specialty of obstetrics and gynecology. For example, new diagnostic tests are available to aid in identifying pregnant women at risk for preterm labor. Because the care of patients with obstetrical complications might involve the decision to induce labor with or without prior cervical ripening, a new chapter was added on induction of labor and the use of agents currently available for cervical ripening. All chapters have undergone revisions, and many chapters have undergone major revisions to make this book current and therefore clinically relevant and useful. New management plans for certain conditions have been added to this edition. As was true with the first edition of this book, the management plans presented do not define the standard of care but rather present the reader with the management strategies that are commonly used. Information concerning the use of drugs in lactating mothers was added to the on call formulary.

The care of patients while on call is and will continue to be a critical aspect of the clinical practice of obstetrics and gynecology and an essential part of the training in this specialty. It is hoped that this edition of *On Call Obstetrics and Gynecology* will serve as a useful and practical aid to all who are engaged in these endeavors. The author wishes to thank W.B. Saunders Company for continuing to support this book.

Homer G. Chin

NOTICE

Obstetrics & Gynecology is an ever-changing field. Standard safety precautions must be followed, but as new research and clinical experience broaden our knowledge, changes in treatment and drug therapy may become necessary or appropriate. Readers are advised to check the most current product information provided by the manufacturer of each drug to be administered to verify the recommended dose, the method and duration of administration, and the contraindications. It is the responsibility of the treating physician, relying on experience and knowledge of the patient, to determine dosages and the best treatment for each individual patient. Neither the publisher nor the editor assumes any liability for any injury and/or damage to persons or property arising from this publication.

THE PUBLISHER

COMMONLY USED ABBREVIATIONS

AB	abortus
ABG	arterial blood gas
AC	before meals
ACTH	adrenocorticotropic hormone
AFI	amniotic fluid index
AFP	alpha-fetoprotein
AIDS	acquired immunodeficiency syndrome
ALT	alanine aminotransferase
ARDS	adult respiratory distress syndrome
AROM	artificial rupture of membranes
ART	artificial reproductive technologies
AST	aspartate transaminase
BE	barium enema
BID	two times per day
BP	blood pressure
BPP	biophysical profile
BSO	bilateral salpingo-oophorectomy
BST	breast stimulation test
BTL	bilateral tubal ligation
BUN	blood urea nitrogen
CA-125	cancer antigen-125
CBC	complete blood count
CHF	congestive heart failure
CIN	cervical intraepithelial neoplasia
CLE	continuous lumbar epidural
CIS	carcinoma in situ
CMV	cytomegalovirus

CNS	central nervous system
CO	cardiac output
CPD	cephalopelvic disproportion
CrCL	creatinine clearance
C&S	culture and sensitivity
CSF	cerebrospinal fluid
CST	contraction stress test
CT	computed tomography
CVA	costovertebral angle
CVS	chorionic villus sampling
CXR	chest x-ray
D&C	dilatation and curettage
D5LR	5% dextrose in lactated Ringer's
D5NS	5% dextrose in normal saline
D5 ½ NS	5% dextrose and 0.5 normal saline
D5W	5% dextrose in water
DES	diethylstilbestrol
DIC	disseminated intravascular coagulation
DUB	dysfunctional uterine bleeding
DVT	deep vein thrombosis
E_1	estrone
E_2	estradiol
E_3	estriol
EBL	estimated blood loss
ECG	electrocardiogram
EDC	estimated date of confinement
ELISA	enzyme-linked immunosorbent assay
EMB	endometrial biopsy
ESR	erythrocyte sedimentation rate
FCA	fetal cardiac activity
FFP	fresh frozen plasma
FHR	fetal heart rate

FSE	fetal scalp electrode
FSH	follicle-stimulating hormone
FSP	fibrin split products
FTA-ABS	fluorescent treponemal antibody absorption
G	gravida
CC	gonorrhea
GFR	glomerular filtration rate
GI	gastrointestinal
GIFT	gamete intrafallopian tube transfer
GnRH	gonadotropin-releasing hormone
GTN	gestational trophoblastic neoplasia
GTT	glucose tolerance test
hCG	human chorionic gonadotropin
hCS	human chorionic somatomammotropin
HDL	high-density lipoprotein
HIV	human immunodeficiency virus
HPV	human papillomavirus
HSG	hysterosalpingogram
HSV	herpes simplex virus
IGF-I	insulin-like growth factor-I
IM	intramuscular
IRP	International Reference Preparation
ITP	idiopathic thrombocytopenic purpura
IUD	intrauterine device
IUFD	intrauterine fetal demise
IUP	intrauterine pregnancy
IUPC	intrauterine pressure catheter
IV	intravenous
IVF	in vitro fertilization
IVH	intraventricular hemorrhage
IVP	intravenous pyelogram
LAVH	laparoscopically assisted vaginal hysterectomy

LC	living children
L&D	labor and delivery
LDL	low-density lipoprotein
LEEP	loop electrosurgical excision procedure
LGV	lymphogranuloma venereum
LH	luteinizing hormone
LLETZ	large loop excision of the transformation zone
LMP	last menstrual period
L/S	lecithin/sphingomyelin
LT C/S	low transverse cesarean section
MHA	microhemagglutination assay
MLE	midline episiotomy
MMK	Marshall-Marchetti-Kranz retropubic urethropexy
MRI	magnetic resonance imaging
MVP	mitral valve prolapse
NG	nasogastric
NPO	nothing by mouth
NS	normal saline
NSAID	nonsteroidal anti-inflammatory drug
NST	nonstress test
NSVD	normal spontaneous vaginal delivery
OA	occiput anterior
OP	occiput posterior
OT	occiput transverse
P	parity or para
PC	after meals
Pco_2	partial pressure of carbon dioxide
PDA	patent ductus arteriosus
PG	phosphatidylglycerol
PGE$_2$	prostaglandin E$_2$
PI	phosphatidylinositol
PID	pelvic inflammatory disease

PIH	pregnancy-induced hypertension
PMN	polymorphonuclear cell
PMS	premenstrual syndrome
PO	per os
Po_2	partial pressure of oxygen
PR	per rectum
PRL	prolactin
PRN	as necessary
PROM	premature rupture of membranes
PT	prothrombin time
PTL	preterm labor
PTT	partial thromboplastin time
PTU	propylthiouracil
PVC	premature ventricular contraction
QHS	each bedtime
QID	four times per day
RBC	red blood cell
RDS	respiratory distress syndrome
RPF	renal plasma flow
RPR	rapid plasma reagin
RR	respiratory rate
SAB	spontaneous abortion
SC	subcutaneous
SIL	squamous intraepithelial lesion
SL	sublingual
SLE	systemic lupus erythematosus
SO	salpingo-oophorectomy
S/P	status post
SROM	spontaneous rupture of membranes
STD	sexually transmitted disease
SVR	systemic vascular resistance
T	testosterone

T_3	triiodothyronine
T_4	thyroxine
TAB	therapeutic abortion
TAH	total abdominal hysterectomy
TB	tuberculosis
TBG	thyroid hormone–binding globulin
TID	three times per day
TPI	*Treponema pallidum* immobilization (test)
TOA	tubo-ovarian abscess
TPN	total parenteral nutrition
T_3RU	triiodothyronine resin uptake
TSH	thyroid-stimulating hormone
TSS	toxic shock syndrome
TVH	total vaginal hysterectomy
UTI	urinary tract infection
VDRL	Venereal Disease Research Laboratory
VTX	vertex
WBC	white blood cell

CONTENTS

INTRODUCTION

1. Approach to On-Call Obstetrical and
   Gynecological Problems 3
2. The Female Reproductive System:
   Conception to Menopause 7
3. Maternal Physiological Changes in
   Pregnancy 19

PATIENT-RELATED OBSTETRICAL
PROBLEMS: THE COMMON CALLS

4. Abnormal Fetal Heart Rate Patterns 33
5. Abnormal Labor 46
6. Amniotic Fluid Embolism 57
7. Fetal Death 63
8. Hypertensive Disorders 69
9. Incompetent Cervix 85
10. Induction of Labor and Cervical Ripening 90
11. Malpresentation 99
12. Mastitis 112
13. Meconium Passage 116
14. Multiple Gestation 120
15. Placenta Previa 130
16. Placental Abruption 137
17. Postpartum Depression 146
18. Postpartum Fever 151
19. Postpartum Hemorrhage 158
20. Premature Rupture of Membranes 168
21. Preterm Labor 183

22. Shoulder Dystocia 201

23. Trauma in Pregnancy 207

PATIENT-RELATED GYNECOLOGICAL PROBLEMS: THE COMMON CALLS

24. Abnormal Uterine Bleeding ...,, ... 217

25. Bartholin's Abscess 225

26. Ectopic Pregnancy 230

27. Gonorrhea and Chlamydial Infection 244

28. Molar Pregnancy 251

29. Pelvic Inflammatory Disease 261

30. Pelvic Mass 270

31. Pelvic Pain 281

32. Sexual Assault 289

33. Spontaneous Abortion 297

34. Toxic Shock Syndrome 308

35. Vulvar Lesions and Ulcers 315

36. Vulvovaginitis 331

APPENDICES

A. Guidelines, Illustrations, and Tables for Obstetrics 343

B. Guidelines, Illustrations, and Tables for Gynecology 360

C. On Call Formulary for Obstetrics and Gynecology 368

INDEX 407

INTRODUCTION

1 | Approach to On-Call Obstetrical and Gynecological Problems

There is a vast array of clinical problems that are unique to women. A comprehensive understanding of the female reproductive system is critical in order to make the correct diagnosis and properly manage these problems. Knowledge of the profound physiological, anatomical, and endocrinological maternal adaptations to pregnancy is crucial for the management of obstetrical disorders. Furthermore, because obstetrical disorders affect two patients concurrently, the mother and the fetus, the welfare of both must be considered. The optimal management of an obstetrical problem might favor one but be detrimental to the other. Many obstetrical and gynecological problems present acutely in a labor and delivery suite, emergency room, or urgent care clinic. In this book, acute and urgent obstetrical and gynecological problems are presented in a concise format that will aid those who are on call. Each chapter is divided into sections as described below.

■ BACKGROUND AND DEFINITIONS

Although this book is not intended to be a comprehensive reference book, the knowledge of key background information and the understanding of terminologies and definitions are essential to the understanding and management of these disease processes.

■ CLINICAL PRESENTATION

This section describes the presenting signs and symptoms of each clinical problem.

■ PHONE CALL

The on-call physician will most likely be contacted initially by telephone. This section is intended to aid in quickly obtaining important information about the patient. This section is divided into two parts.

Questions

Questions that should be asked initially over the telephone are listed.

Degree of Urgency

This part addresses how quickly the patient should be seen.

■ ELEVATOR THOUGHTS

This section consists of information that should be reviewed while on the way to see the patient. This includes the differential diagnosis as well as other key information that might help in confirming the diagnosis and in treating the patient. This section is presented as lists to allow for a quick review.

■ MAJOR THREAT TO LIFE

This section lists the means by which a patient's life is threatened by a clinical problem. With obstetrical problems, the lives of the mother and fetus are addressed separately.

■ BEDSIDE

Assessment of the patient and the medical chart should be performed in a careful and yet timely and efficient manner. This section deals with the key elements in assessing a patient in an urgent and acute situation. After the initial evaluation, orders can be given for both diagnostic and therapeutic purposes. There are five parts to this section.

Quick Look Test

This is the initial part of the patient assessment in which a quick evaluation is performed to determine the severity of the patient's condition. The severity will often dictate how the patient managed.

Vital Signs

Many of the clinical problems presented in this book are associated with abnormal vital signs, especially those consistent with shock from hemorrhage.

Selective History and Chart Review

This section lists the key information that should be obtained when taking the patient's history and when reviewing her medical record and hospital chart. This information will assist in confirming the diagnosis and will affect the management of the patient.

Selective Physical Examination

This section lists the findings on physical examination that are consistent with and sometimes pathognomonic of the diagnosis.

Orders

Orders that can be given to initiate patient care and laboratory studies are enumerated.

■ DIAGNOSTIC TESTING

Because there are many diagnostic tests that are unique to obstetrics and gynecology, a separate section listing all the pertinent diagnostic tests and the information they provide is included. These tests might help in confirming the diagnosis or determining the appropriate management for a patient. These tests include laboratory tests, radiographic studies, and diagnostic procedures. Inclusion of a test or procedure in this section should not imply that the test must always be ordered. Decisions as to which tests should be ordered and which procedures performed depend on the individual patient's condition and the clinical judgment and experience of the health care provider.

■ MANAGEMENT

This section covers the management of the patient once the diagnosis has been confirmed. Often, there are many management strategies that can be used. In such cases, several management plans are listed and discussed. Which management plan is chosen depends on the individual patient's condition and needs and also on the health care provider's personal experience, training, and clinical judgment.

At the end of the book, the following three appendices are included:

■ **APPENDIX A: GUIDELINES, ILLUSTRATIONS, AND TABLES FOR OBSTETRICS**

■ **APPENDIX B: GUIDELINES, ILLUSTRATIONS, AND TABLES FOR GYNECOLOGY**

These appendices contain guidelines, illustrations, and tables that are pertinent to both normal and abnormal conditions. These appendices can be used for quick reference as well as for rapid review in preparation for rounds or examinations.

■ **APPENDIX C: ON CALL FORMULARY FOR OBSTETRICS AND GYNECOLOGY**

This formulary contains drugs commonly prescribed to obstetrical and gynecological patients, including drugs recommended in this book for the treatment of clinical problems. Information concerning use of the drug in pregnant and lactating women is included when it is available.

2 | The Female Reproductive System: Conception to Menopause

■ SEXUAL DIFFERENTIATION AND ENDOCRINOLOGY IN THE FETUS

Even though genetic gender is determined at the time of conception, the fetal gonads remain undifferentiated until 4 to 5 weeks of gestation. At this time, testicular development is initiated in males, under the influence of the Y chromosome. A plasma membrane histocompatibility antigen known as the H-Y antigen appears to be the testes-determining factor. In the absence of the Y chromosome and H-Y antigen, the ovaries and müllerian duct system develop in females. Ovarian differentiation begins at 6 to 8 weeks of gestation with the multiplication of germ cells. The number of oocytes reaches a peak of 6 to 7 million at approximately 20 weeks of gestation. This represents the maximum egg content of the ovaries. At the same time, there is an elevation in the gonadotropins, luteinizing hormone (LH), and follicle-stimulating hormone (FSH) (Fig. 2–1). This elevation in gonadotropins results in varying degrees of oocyte maturation. Furthermore, there is ovarian estrogen production, although the amount is minor when compared with placental estrogen. Over the next 50 years of life, eggs are gradually depleted, with the nadir reached at menopause. The process of egg atresia and depletion begins as early as 15 weeks of gestation. The major mechanism

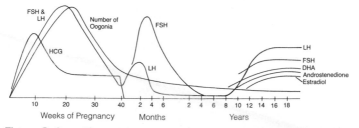

Figure 2–1 □ Changes in gonadotropins and oocytes from fetal life to puberty. (Adapted from Speroff L, Glass RH, Kase NG: Neuroendocrinology. In: Clinical Gynecologic Endocrinology and Infertility, 6th ed. Baltimore, Williams & Wilkins, 1999, p 193, © 1999, the Williams & Wilkins Co, Baltimore.)

for egg depletion in the fetus is loss through the ovarian capsule into the peritoneal cavity.

■ NEONATAL PERIOD AND CHILDHOOD

At birth, the number of oocytes has fallen to approximately 2 million. The ovary is appproximately 1 cm in diameter, and varying degrees of oocyte maturation are present. After birth, the loss of exposure to placental and maternal estrogens results in a rise in gonadotropins, which peak at 3 months of age and then gradually fall to a plateau at 2 to 4 years of age. LH and FSH remain suppressed between the ages of 4 and 10 years.

■ PUBERTY

At the beginning of puberty, the number of oocytes remaining is approximately 300,000. Puberty represents a transition between the immature reproductive system of childhood and the mature reproductive system of adulthood. It is characterized by a reactivation of the hypothalamic-pituitary axis, which was active in the fetal period and suppressed in the childhood period. As a result, puberty is associated with the appearance of pulsatile gonadotropin-releasing hormone (GnRH) and episodic LH secretion during sleep. In puberty, secondary sexual characteristics develop and fertility is achieved.

The stages of pubertal development require an average of 4.5 years with a range of 1.5 to 6 years and consist of the following events (Table 2–1):

1. **Thelarche (breast budding)**—occurs at a mean age of 9.8 years with a range of 8 to 13 years and is usually the first physical sign of puberty. The stages of breast development can be defined by Tanner stages (Fig. 2–2).

Table 2–1 □ STAGES OF PUBERTAL DEVELOPMENT

Stage	Mean Age (yr)	Age Range (yr)
Thelarche (breast budding)	9.8	8–13
Adrenarche (pubic or axillary hair)	11	8–14
Peak height velocity (maximal growth)	11.5	10–14
Menarche	13	9–16
Mature pubic hair	14	12–18
Mature breasts	14.5	12–18

Figure 2–2 □ Tanner stages of breast development. Stage 1: Preadolescent—elevation of the papilla only. Stage 2: Breast bud stage—elevation of the breast and papilla with enlargement of the areolar region. Stage 3: Further enlargement of the breast and areola without separation of their contours. Stage 4: Projection of the areola and papilla to form a secondary mound above the level of the breast. Stage 5: Mature stage—projection of the papilla only, resulting from recession of the areola to the general contour of the breast. (From Hacker NF, Moore JG: Essentials of Obstetrics and Gynecology, 3rd ed. Philadelphia, WB Saunders Co, 1998, p 570.)

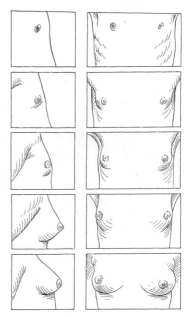

2. **Adrenarche or pubarche (pubic or axillary hair)**—occurs at a mean age of 11 years with a range of 8 to 14 years. In approximately 20% of girls, the appearance of pubic hair is the first sign of puberty. Pubic hair usually appears first, with axillary hair appearing about 2 years later. The stages of female pubic hair development can be defined by Tanner stages (Fig. 2–3).

3. **Peak height velocity or maximal growth**—occurs at a mean age of 11.5 years with a range of 10 to 14 years; it usually occurs 2 years after thelarche and 1 year before menarche. It occurs in females approximately 2 years earlier than in males. The average patient increases her height between 2 and 4 inches in 1 year. This accelerated growth is mediated by growth hormone, estradiol, and insulin-like growth factor-I (IGF-I) or somatomedin-C. Very low levels of estrogen are required to stimulate long-bone cortical growth.

4. **Menarche (beginning of menses)**—occurs at a mean age of 13 years with a range of 9 to 16 years; first menses are typically anovulatory and therefore irregular and often heavy and prolonged (see Chapter 24). Adolescents can have anovulatory cycles for as long as 12 months.

5. **Mature pubic hair**—usually achieved by 14 years of age with a range of 12 to 18 years.

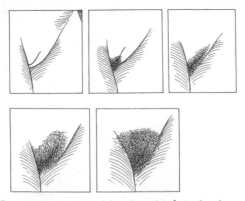

Figure 2-3 □ Tanner stages of female pubic hair development. Stage 1: Preadolescent—absence of pubic hair. Stage 2: Sparse hair along the labia. Stage 3: Hair sparsely over the junction of the pubes. Hair is darker and coarser. Stage 4: Adult-type hair without spread to the medial surface of the thighs. Stage 5: Adult-type hair with spread to the medial thighs. (From Hacker NF, Moore JG: Essentials of Obstetrics and Gynecology, 3rd ed. Philadelphia, WB Saunders Co, 1998, p 571.)

   6. **Mature breasts**—usually achieved by 14.5 years of age with a range of 12 to 18 years.

Precocious puberty is defined as the appearance of pubertal changes before 8 years of age, which represents 2.5 standard deviations below the expected age of pubertal development. Maximal growth is often the first sign of precocious puberty.

The final milestone in puberty is development of positive feedback by estrogen on the hypothalamus and pituitary. This results in estrogen stimulation of the LH surge, which in turn stimulates ovulation and the regular menses that are associated with ovulatory cycles.

■ ADULTHOOD: REPRODUCTIVE MATURITY

Reproductive maturity in women is characterized by regular menstrual cycles of follicular maturation, ovulation, and corpus luteum formation during the next 30 to 40 years after puberty. The normal menstrual cycle is characterized by an intricate coordination of gonadotropin release, ovarian steroidogenesis, follicular maturation and ovulation, and histophysiological changes in the uterine endometrium (Fig. 2-4).

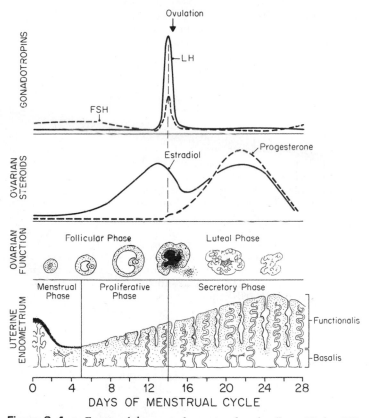

Figure 2–4 □ Events of the normal menstrual cycle. (From Hacker NF, Moore JG: Essentials of Obstetrics and Gynecology, 3rd ed. Philadelphia, WB Saunders Co, 1998, p 61.)

The Normal Menstrual Cycle

The normal ovulatory menstrual cycle begins with the first day of menstrual bleeding, which by convention is referred to as "day 1." The average length of the menstrual cycle is 28 days with a normal range of 21 to 35 days. The normal duration of bleeding is 4 to 5 days with a normal range of 3 to 7 days. The average blood loss during menses is 35 ml with a normal range of 20 to 80 ml. The normal menstrual cycle can be divided into the follicular or proliferative phase and the luteal or secretory phase. The luteal phase is the more constant phase, with a mean duration of 14 days and a range of 12 to 16 days; the follicular phase has a range of 7 to more than 21 days.

1. **Follicular or proliferative phase**

   This phase begins with the onset of menses and concludes with the preovulatory LH surge. Folliculogenesis and an increase in FSH actually begin in the last few days of the luteal phase of the previous cycle. The initial rise in FSH is the result of escape of FSH secretion from the negative feedback provided by estrogen and progesterone when levels of these steroids decrease secondary to the regression of the corpus luteum from the preceding cycle. Rising FSH initiates recruitment and growth of a cohort of 3 to 30 follicles, from which a single dominant follicle is chosen for ovulation. After the selection of the dominant follicle, the remaining follicles of the cohort undergo atresia or degeneration. LH begins to rise several days after the rise in FSH. LH continues to increase slowly in the follicular phase secondary to positive feedback from rising estradiol produced in the granulosa cells of the enlarging follicle. In contrast, FSH begins to decrease in the late follicular phase due to negative feedback from rising estradiol. Rising estrogen levels result in proliferation of the endometrium (hence the term "proliferative phase"). There are also increased cervical vascularity and edema. Furthermore, the amount of cervical mucus is increased, as is the elasticity of the mucus, referred to as "spinnbarkeit." The LH surge immediately precedes ovulation and marks the end of the follicular or proliferative phase.

2. **Ovulation (midcycle)**

   Ovulation, the release of the ovum from the mature dominant follicle, occurs 32 to 34 hours after the onset of the LH surge or the peak of estradiol. The site of ovulation is random and does not necessarily alternate between the two ovaries. If one ovary is removed, every ovulation will occur in the remaining ovary, and the number of ovulatory cycles in the woman's reproductive life will not be decreased.

3. **Luteal or secretory phase**

   The luteal phase begins after ovulation and is characterized by suppression of both LH and FSH secondary to negative feedback from rising levels of estrogen and progesterone. In the luteal phase, the corpus luteum develops from the luteinized granulosa and theca cells of the ovary. The corpus luteum secretes progesterone, which supports the ovum and induces histological changes of the endometrium that prepare it for implantation of the fertilized ovum. In response to progesterone, endometrial glands become coiled and secretory with increased vascularity (hence the term "secretory phase"). Progesterone peaks at a level > 10 ng/ml approximately 7 days after the LH surge. Progesterone increases the morning basal body temperature, and a rise of

0.3°C or greater over the nadir is presumptive evidence of ovulation. If fertilization does not occur, progesterone decreases and the corpus luteum regresses through a process referred to as luteolysis. This results in a fall in estrogen and progesterone, which causes endometrial edema, necrosis, and finally, bleeding that represents menses. Furthermore, this fall in estrogen and progesterone releases FSH from negative feedback. FSH begins to rise, and this rise continues into the follicular phase of the next menstrual cycle.

Fertilization and Implantation

After ovulation, the ovum can be fertilized for 12 to 24 hours. After ejaculation, sperm can fertilize an egg for up to 48 hours. Even though several hundred million sperm are ejaculated into the vagina, fewer than 200 actually reach the egg, and usually only one fertilizes the egg. The zona pellucida that surrounds the egg contains species-specific sperm receptors and undergoes zona reaction, which makes the zona impervious to other sperm once fertilization has occurred. Fertilization occurs in the ampullary portion of the fallopian tube. The fertilized ovum reaches the uterine cavity approximately 2 to 3 days after fertilization. Implantation begins 2 to 3 days after the fertilized ovum enters the uterine cavity. At the time of implantation, the zona pellucida is shed and the conceptus is in the blastocyst stage. Human chorionic gonadotropin (hCG) is produced by the conceptus at about the time of implantation. The blastocyst has an outer mass of cells that become trophoblasts and an inner cell mass that becomes the embryo. The trophoblasts proliferate and invade the decidua. Maternal blood vessels are trapped to form lacunae, which are filled with maternal blood. At approximately 12 days after fertilization, primitive villi are present traversing the lacunae. The primitive villi eventually develop into the placenta.

The endometrium undergoes changes referred to as decidual changes under the influence of progesterone. Endometrial stroma cells develop into enlarged, round decidual cells, and, during pregnancy, the decidua reaches a thickness of 5 to 10 mm. Decidual basalis refers to the decidua at the implantation site, and decidua capsularis refers to the decidua overlying the conceptus (Fig. 2–5). Decidual parietalis or vera lines the remaining uterine cavity. The decidua capsularis and decidua parietalis fuse at 14 to 16 weeks of gestation, and the uterine cavity becomes obliterated by the conceptus.

■ CLIMACTERIC AND MENOPAUSE

Climacteric refers to the period of decreasing ovarian function that begins as early as 40 years of age. It is characterized by

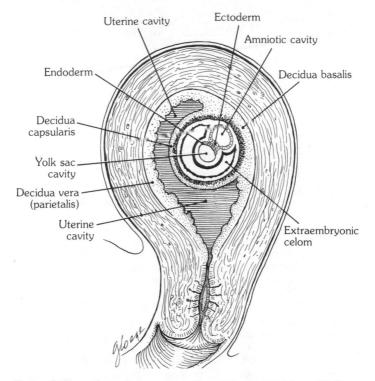

Figure 2–5 □ The early conceptus. (From Hacker NF, Moore JG: Essentials of Obstetrics and Gynecology, 3rd ed. Philadelphia, WB Saunders Co, 1998, p 70.)

decreased fertility and progressive tissue atrophy and aging from decreasing estrogen production. Climacteric culminates in menopause, which is defined as the cessation of menstruation. The median age of menopause in the United States is 51 years with a range of 45 to 55 years. Spontaneous menopause before the age of 40 years is defined as premature ovarian failure. The diagnosis of menopause should be suspected in any patient in this age group who has had 6 to 12 months of amenorrhea. The basic feature of menopause is the depletion of ovarian follicles. This leads to the inability of the ovaries to respond to gonadotropins and a decrease in ovarian production of estrogen, progesterone, and androstenedione. Even in the perimenopausal years preceding menopause, women have lower estradiol levels and higher FSH levels. Women in this age group commonly have anovulation or oligo-ovulation. Even when ovulation occurs, the quality of the ovum decreases as a woman ages. This results in a decrease in the likelihood of fertilization and an increase in the incidence of chromosomal abnormalities in the embryo when fertilization does occur. Furthermore, decreased progesterone production by the ovum results in shorter menstrual cycles and irregular bleeding.

Postmenopausal women have elevated levels of gonadotropins and decreased levels of estrogens, progesterone, and androgens (Table 2–2). FSH is increased by 10- to 20-fold, and a level of >40 mIU/ml is diagnostic of menopause. LH is increased only threefold because it is cleared much faster than FSH. The half-life of LH is approximately 30 minutes, whereas the half-life of FSH is almost 4 hours. Serum estradiol is decreased to 5 to 25 pg/ml, and serum estrone falls to 30 to 70 pg/ml. Serum progesterone falls to <1 ng/ml. Serum testosterone decreases from 20 to 80 ng/dl to 10 to 40 ng/dl. Ovarian production of testosterone remains unchanged when a woman enters menopause, and the decrease in serum testosterone is the result of diminished production from the adrenal glands. Plasma androstenedione decreases from approximately 150 ng/dl to close to 90 ng/dl. This decrease is a result of decreased production from both the adrenal glands and the ovaries. The clinical manifestations of menopause include the following:

1. **Vasomotor symptoms**

   Also referred to as hot flashes or flushes, vasomotor symptoms are experienced by almost 75% of postmenopausal women. Approximately 10% of women experience vasomotor symptoms before menopause. Vasomotor symptoms are caused by a relative decrease in estrogen levels, rather than a specific level of estrogen. Patients with gonadal dystrophy produce no endogenous estrogen and therefore do not experience vasomotor symptoms unless they are given exogenous estrogen and then it is withdrawn. The cause of vasomotor symptoms is an alteration of the central thermoregulatory mechanism.

Table 2–2 □ GONADOTROPIN AND STEROID LEVELS

Hormone	Follicular Phase	Midcycle	Luteal Phase	Postmenopausal
Serum FSH (mIU/ml)	5–20	10–40	5–20	>40
Serum LH (mIU/ml)	5–20	15–60	5–20	>40
Serum estradiol (pg/ml)	25–75	200–600	100–300	5–25
Serum progesterone (ng/ml)	<1	<1	5–20	<1
Serum testosterone (ng/dl)	20–80	20–80	20–80	10–40

2. **Atrophic genital and urological changes**

Vaginal dryness and irritation, dysuria, and atrophic vaginitis are caused by decreased circulating estrogen. Atrophy of the vaginal epithelium can also result in dyspareunia and vaginal bleeding. Furthermore, the support for the uterus and urethra can be weakened, and this can result in uterine descensus and stress urinary incontinence.

3. **Osteoporosis**

Osteoporosis, a reduction in the quantity of bone mass, develops when osteoclastic activity exceeds osteoblastic activity. Estrogen deficiency is the major cause for osteoporosis in postmenopausal women. It has been estimated that at least 75% of bone mass loss in women in the first 20 years of menopause is caused by the loss of estrogen rather than by aging. As a result, women who have been postmenopausal for more than 10 years have a fracture rate that is three to five times greater than that of men of comparable age. High-risk factors for the development of osteoporosis include white or Asian ethnicity, smoking, slender and small body frame, sedentary lifestyle, steroid use, and a diet that is low in calcium and vitamin D and high in alcohol, caffeine, and protein. In women with high-risk factors, approximately 1 to 1.5% of bone mass is lost each year after menopause. Most calcium is lost from trabecular bone, where there may be a loss in bone mass of up to 50%. In contrast, osteoporosis in cortical bone occurs later, and bone mass loss is only approximately 5%. Therefore, the spinal column and femoral neck are the most vulnerable to fracture. The incidence of hip or femur fractures rises from 0.3 in 1000 to 20 in 1000 between the ages of 45 and 85 years. Spinal compression fractures result in loss of height, pain, and postural deformities. Almost one-third of women older than 65 years of age have spinal compression fractures, and the average postmenopausal woman who is not receiving estrogen replacement shrinks 2.5 inches in height. Colles' fractures of the distal forearm increase 10-fold in the postmenopausal years in women who do not take estrogen replacement.

Estrogen replacement protects against osteoporosis probably by decreasing bone resorption. In postmenopausal women who take estrogen, there is a slight increase in the levels of serum calcium and phosphorus and a decrease in the levels of parathyroid hormone and 1,25-dihydroxyvitamin D, the active form of vitamin D. The amount of estrogen necessary to prevent osteoporosis is 0.625 mg of equine estrogen or 1.25 mg of piperazine estrone sulfate. Calcium supplementation is also helpful in preventing osteoporosis, although it is not as critical as estrogen. Estrogen users should take 1000 mg of calcium supplementation per day, whereas nonusers should take 1500 mg/day. The average daily diet contains approximately 800 mg of calcium. The protective effects of estrogen are present only while the patient is taking estrogen. If estrogen is taken initially and then discontinued, osteoporosis will usually occur at an accelerated rate.

4. **Increased cardiovascular disease**

In postmenopausal women in the United States, cardiovascular disease is by far the leading cause of death (Fig. 2–6). Premenopausal women have a significantly lower incidence of cardiovascular disease than men of the same age. However, among postmenopausal women the incidence of heart disease rises, so that 6 to 10 years after the onset of menopause this incidence is the same for both genders. Furthermore, the relative risk of cardiovascular disease increases with earlier age at menopause. Among women who undergo bilateral oophorectomy before the age of 35 years, the relative risk of myocardial infarction is 7.2, almost three times higher than in women between the ages of 35 and 39 years who do not undergo bilateral oophorectomy.

Cholesterol, low-density lipoprotein (LDL), and high-density lipoprotein (HDL) are important in the development of coronary heart disease. High levels of cholesterol and LDL are positively correlated with the risk of coronary heart

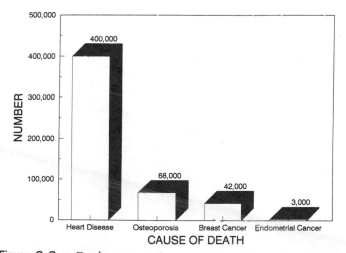

Figure 2–6 □ Deaths per year by cause among women in the United States. (From Copeland LJ: Textbook of Gynecology. Philadelphia, WB Saunders Co, 1993, p 622.)

disease. In contrast, HDL is protective against atherosclerosis, and the level of HDL is inversely related to the risk of heart disease. There is an estimated 3 to 5% decrease in the risk of coronary heart disease for every 1-mg/dl increase in HDL level. There is a 2% decrease in the risk of coronary heart disease for every 1% decrease in total cholesterol level. Among menopausal women who do not take estrogen replacement, lipid changes are atherogenic. Serum cholesterol, LDL, and triglycerides increase, whereas HDL decreases.

It has been estimated that estrogen replacement decreases the risk of cardiovascular disease by 50 to 65% in postmenopausal women. Estrogen use is associated with a slight increase in serum cholesterol, but more importantly, there is an increase in HDL and a decrease in LDL. In addition to its effects on lipid levels, estrogen may have a local effect on arteries and protect against intimal plaque formation. Unfortunately, progestins, which are given along with estrogen to postmenopausal patients who have not had prior hysterectomies, result in a decrease in HDL and therefore blunt the protective effects of estrogen. Micronized progesterone appears to have less of this unfavorable effect than does medroxyprogesterone.

5. **Emotional and psychological changes**

   Menopause is associated with the following emotional and/or psychological changes:

   - Insomnia
   - Poor memory
   - Mental confusion
   - Lethargy
   - Irritability
   - Nervousness
   - Fatigue
   - Dizziness
   - Inability to cope
   - Loss of libido

   These symptoms may be caused by a decrease in estrogen and androgens or, at least partially, by the presence of significant vasomotor symptoms and atrophic genital changes.

3 | Maternal Physiological Changes in Pregnancy

Profound anatomical, endocrinological, and physiological maternal changes occur during pregnancy. These changes adapt the mother to the needs of the fetus. Many of these adaptations begin early in pregnancy. To understand the many pathological conditions encountered in pregnancy, it is necessary first to understand the maternal adaptations that occur during normal pregnancy.

■ HEMATOLOGICAL SYSTEM

Blood Volume—Increased

Maternal blood volume increases by approximately 45% near term because of an increase in plasma volume and a slightly smaller increase in red blood cell mass. This increase begins in the first trimester, reaches the greatest rate of increase in the second trimester, and reaches a plateau near term. Plasma volume begins to increase as early as 6 weeks of gestational age and peaks at a volume of approximately 5 L at term, an increase of 45%. Red blood cell mass increases by 300 to 400 ml by term, an increase of 20 to 30%.

Hematocrit and Hemoglobin—Decreased

Because the increase in plasma volume is usually greater than the increase in red blood cell volume, both hematocrit and hemoglobin concentration decrease despite accelerated erythropoiesis. This dilutional effect can result in a decrease in hemoglobin concentration to 11 g/dl.

White Blood Cell Count—Increased

The normal white blood cell count in pregnancy is 5000 to 12,000/mm^3. However, during labor, the white blood cell count increases to approximately 15,000/mm^3 and can be as high as 25,000/mm^3.

Coagulation Factors

Serum fibrinogen increases to 300 to 600 mg/dl, a 50% rise over normal nonpregnant levels. This increase in fibrinogen results in an increase in erythrocyte sedimentation rate (ESR) in normal pregnancy. Levels of factors II, VII, VIII, IX, and X are also increased in normal pregnancy. Levels of factors XI and XIII are slightly decreased. Platelet count is slightly decreased, to between 150,000 and 400,000/mm³.

Iron Requirements—Increased

The total iron requirement for a normal singleton pregnancy is approximately 1 g. This 1 g consists of 300 mg for the fetus, 500 mg for the increased maternal red blood cell volume, and 200 mg that is lost through normal excretion. The total iron requirement translates to a daily requirement of 6 to 7 mg/day in the second half of pregnancy. The normally low absorption rate of iron through the gastrointestinal tract is only modestly increased in pregnancy. Therefore, the iron absorbed from diet and available from iron stores is not sufficient to meet the requirements imposed by pregnancy, and iron supplementation should be provided.

■ CARDIOVASCULAR SYSTEM

Anatomical Changes

The cardiac apex is displaced upward and to the left by the elevating diaphragm. There is also an increase in the size of the cardiac silhouette.

Heart Rate—Increased

The resting heart rate increases by 10 to 18 beats/min during pregnancy. The heart rate begins to increase late in the first trimester and reaches a plateau in the mid-second trimester (Fig. 3–1).

Stroke Volume—Increased

Cardiac stroke volume increases by 10 to 30%. Stroke volume starts to increase as early as 10 weeks of gestational age, peaks at approximately 20 weeks, and decreases slightly near term (see Fig. 3–1).

Cardiac Output—Increased

Cardiac output, a product of heart rate and stroke volume, increases by 33 to 50%. This increase in cardiac output peaks in the early second trimester.

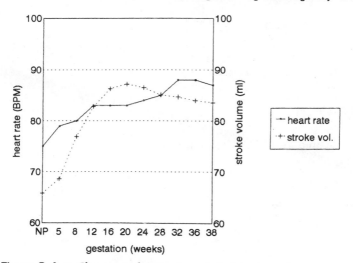

Figure 3–1 □ Changes in heart rate and stroke volume in pregnancy. (Adapted from Robson SC, Hunter S, Boys RJ, et al: Serial study of factors influencing changes in cardiac output during human pregnancy. Am J Physiol 1989;256:H1060–H1065.)

Heart Sound Changes (Fig. 3–2)

1. Exaggerated splitting of S_1 in 88% of patients
2. Systolic murmur in 96% of patients
3. Diastolic murmur in 18% of patients
4. Prominent S_3 in 84% of patients

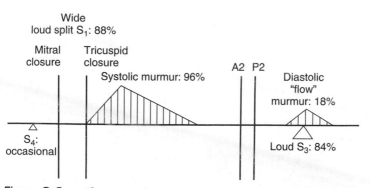

Figure 3–2 □ Changes in heart sounds in pregnancy. (Redrawn from Cutforth R, MacDonald CB: Heart sounds and murmurs in pregnancy. Am Heart J 1966;71:741.)

Blood Pressure

Arterial blood pressure decreases in pregnancy as early as the first trimester. This decrease is caused primarily by a fall in systemic vascular resistance (SVR). Systolic blood pressure decreases by 4 to 6 mm Hg, and diastolic blood pressure decreases by 8 to 15 mm Hg. The nadir is reached between 24 and 32 weeks of gestation.

Systemic Vascular Resistance—Decreased

SVR is decreased in pregnancy due to the low-resistance uteroplacental circulation and the vasodilatatory effect of progesterone. SVR (in dynes $\times$ sec $\times$ cm^{-5}) calculated by the following equation:

$$SVR = \frac{(\text{mean arterial pressure} - \text{central venous pressure}) \times 80}{\text{cardiac output}}$$

The decrease in SVR reaches a nadir between 14 and 24 weeks of gestation.

■ RESPIRATORY SYSTEM

Changes in lung volumes during pregnancy are summarized in Table 3–1.

Tidal Volume—Increased

Tidal volume is increased by close to 40%.

Functional Residual Capacity—Decreased

Functional residual capacity is decreased due to elevation of the diaphragm.

Residual Volume—Decreased

Residual volume is decreased by approximately 20% due to elevation of the diaphragm.

Total Body Oxygen Consumption—Increased

Oxygen consumption is increased by 15 to 20%. About 50% of this increase is used by the uterus, placenta, and fetus. The increased work by the maternal heart, lungs, and kidneys accounts for most of the remaining increase in oxygen consumption.

Table 3-1 □ CHANGES IN PULMONARY VOLUMES AND CAPACITIES IN PREGNANCY

Test	Definition	Change in Pregnancy
Respiratory rate	—	No significant change
Tidal volume	The volume of air inspired and expired at each breath	Progressive rise throughout pregnancy of 0.1–0.2 L
Expiratory reserve volume	The maximum volume of air that can be additionally expired after a normal expiration	Lowered by about 15% (0.55 L in late pregnancy compared with 0.65 L postpartum)
Residual volume	The volume of air remaining in the lungs after a maximum expiration	Falls considerably (0.77 L in late pregnancy compared with 0.96 L postpartum)
Vital capacity	The maximum volume of air that can be forcibly inspired after a maximum expiration	Unchanged, except for possibly a small terminal diminution
Inspiratory capacity	The maximum volume of air that can be inspired from resting expiratory level	Increased by about 5%
Functional residual capacity	The volume of air in lungs at resting expiratory level	Lowered by about 18%
Minute ventilation	The volume of air inspired or expired in 1 minute	Increased by about 40% as a result of the increased tidal volume and unchanged respiratory rate

Adapted from Main DM, Main EK: Obstetrics and Gynecology. A Pocket Reference. Chicago, Year Book, 1984, p 14.

Because the arterial partial pressure of oxygen (PaO_2) is unchanged and the arteriovenous oxygen difference and the difference volume actually decreases, this increased oxygen consumption is accompanied by increased cardiac output and increased tidal volume.

Arterial Carbon Dioxide Tension—Decreased

The arterial partial pressure of carbon dioxide ($PaCO_2$) is decreased because of hyperventilation, which is caused by an increased tidal volume and not by an increased respiratory rate. $PaCO_2$ decreases from a nonpregnant level of 35 to 40 mm Hg to approximately 30 mm Hg during pregnancy.

■ RENAL SYSTEM

Anatomical Changes

Renal dilatation and hydronephrosis are found in 90% of pregnant patients and are most prominent on the right side. The kidneys of a pregnant patient are approximately 1.5 cm longer than those of a nonpregnant patient. These changes are the result of both the relaxation of smooth muscle of the ureters due to progesterone and the obstruction of the ureters at the pelvic brim by the enlarging uterus.

Renal Plasma Flow—Increased

Renal plasma flow (RPF) increases by 60 to 80% by the mid-second trimester and then falls slightly to 50% more than the nonpregnant level in the third trimester (Fig. 3–3).

Glomerular Filtration Rate—Increased

Glomerular filtration rate (GFR) increases beginning as early as 6 weeks of gestational age. It peaks at 50% over the nonpregnant level at 16 to 20 weeks of gestational age (see Fig. 3–3). Creatinine clearance peaks at close to 150 ml/min.

Serum Creatinine and Blood Urea Nitrogen—Decreased

Both serum creatinine and blood urea nitrogen (BUN) are decreased from nonpregnant levels becaused of increased GFR.

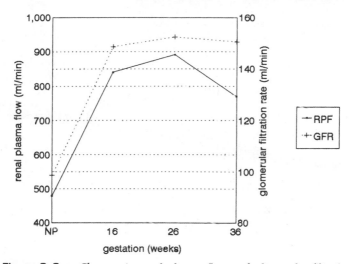

Figure 3–3 □ Changes in renal plasma flow and glomerular filtration rate in pregnancy. (Adapted from Dunlop W: Serial changes in renal hemodynamics during normal human pregnancy. Br J Obstet Gynecol 1981;88:1.)

Urinalysis

Glucosuria in pregnancy is not necessarily abnormal. The increased glomerular filtration rate and impaired tubular reabsorption of glucose result in glucosuria in 15% of normal pregnant women.

■ ENDOCRINE SYSTEM

Pancreas—Insulin and Carbohydrate Metabolism

Fetal growth, development, and maturation require profound changes in maternal metabolic regulation. Pregnancy can be diabetogenic; pre-existing diabetes mellitus may be aggravated or new-onset diabetes may appear. Approximately 2 to 3% of pregnancies are complicated by diabetes, and 90% of these cases are caused by gestational diabetes. The following are usually found in normal pregnancy:

- Hyperinsulinemia and pancreatic beta-cell hypertrophy
- Progressive insulin resistance
- Mild fasting hypoglycemia
- Postprandial hyperglycemia

Rising estrogen and progesterone levels result in pancreatic beta-cell hypertrophy and hyperinsulinemia as early as 10 weeks of gestation. This results in a mean decrease in fasting serum glucose of approximately 10 mg/dl in pregnancy when compared with the nonpregnant state. In the second half of pregnancy, progressive insulin resistance develops as a result of rising levels of human chorionic somatomammotropin (hCS) and prolactin from the placenta as well as maternal cortisol and glucagon (Table 3–2).

Thyroid Gland

The thyroid gland is moderately enlarged during normal pregnancy. Rising levels of estrogen result in higher levels of thyroxine-binding globulin (TBG). Increased TBG results in a decrease in the level of triiodothyronine resin uptake (T_3RU) and increases in the levels of total thyroxine (T_4) and triiodothyronine (T_3). Total T_4 begins to increase in the first trimester and eventually reaches levels of 9 to 16 μg/dl compared with 5 to 12 μg/dl in the nonpregnant woman. Although total T_3 and T_4 are elevated, free T_3 and T_4 as well as TSH are in the normal nonpregnant range, and pregnant patients are usually euthyroid.

Pituitary Gland

The pituitary gland is enlarged to approximately 135% during pregnancy. The anterior lobe may increase to two to three times the size in nonpregnant women. This is due primarily to hyperplasia and hypertrophy of prolactin-secreting cells. Serum prolactin increases in pregnancy to a mean level of 150 ng/ml, or almost 10 times greater than in the normal nonpregnant woman.

Adrenal Glands

Levels of corticosteroid-binding globulin or transcortin are increased threefold in pregnancy secondary to rising estrogen levels. Both adrenocorticotropic hormone (ACTH) and cortisol are elevated beginning in the late first trimester. Free cortisol, aldosterone, and deoxycorticosterone are also elevated in pregnancy.

■ GASTROINTESTINAL SYSTEM

Anatomical Changes

The stomach and intestines are displaced upward by the enlarging uterus. The appendix is displaced upward and laterally, sometimes reaching the right flank (Fig. 3–4). This results in a change

Table 3-2 □ CARBOHYDRATE METABOLISM IN LATE PREGNANCY

Hormonal Change	Effect	Metabolic Changes
↑ Human somatomammotropin	"Diabetogenic" ↓ glucose tolerance	Facilitated anabolism during feeding and
↑ Prolactin	Insulin resistance	Accelerated starvation during fasting ↓
↑ Bound and free cortisol	↓ Hepatic glycogen stores ↑ Hepatic glucose production	Ensures glucose and amino acids to fetus

From Creasy RK, Resnik R: Maternal-Fetal Medicine: Principles and Practice, 4th ed. Philadelphia, WB Saunders Co, 1999, p 965.

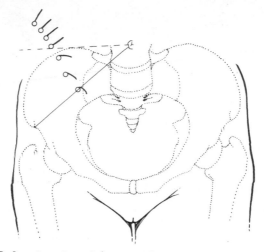

Figure 3–4 □ Location of the appendix in pregnancy. (From Plauche WC, Morrison JC, O'Sullivan M: Surgical Obstetrics, Philadelphia, WB Saunders Co, 1992, p 236.)

in the clinical presentation of appendicitis in pregnant patients. The change in the position of the stomach also contributes to the higher incidence of esophageal reflux and pyrosis or heartburn. Intragastric pressures are increased and intraesophageal pressures are decreased in pregnancy.

Gastric Emptying

Gastric emptying and intestinal transit time are delayed in pregnancy. This delay is caused by the effects of progesterone on the relaxation of smooth muscle and by the mechanical effects of the enlarging pregnant uterus on the gastrointestinal tract.

Liver

No morphological changes in the liver are associated with normal pregnancy. Furthermore, liver size and hepatic blood flow do not change significantly in pregnancy. However, the levels of some liver function tests are altered in normal pregnancy (Table 3–3). Total serum alkaline phosphatase is normally elevated al-

Table 3–3 □ LIVER FUNCTION TESTS IN NORMAL PREGNANCY

Serum Test	Level in Pregnancy
No Change	
Prothrombin time	
Total bilirubin	
AST	May be lower than normal reference limits
ALT	May be lower than normal reference limits
Alkaline phosphatase (liver)	
Gamma GT	
5-Nucleotidase	
Rise	
Total alkaline phosphatase	Accelerated in third trimester*
Globulins alpha and beta	Progressive to term
Lipids	Progressive to term
Fibrinogen	Progressive to term
Ceruloplasmin	
Transferrin	
Fall	
Albumin	20% first trimester
Globulins: gamma	Minor or unchanged

*Placental and skeletal isoenzymes only.
AST = aspartate aminotransferase; ALT = alanine aminotransferase; gamma GT = gamma glutamyl transpeptidase.
From Creasy RK, Resnick R: Maternal-Fetal Medicine: Principles and Practice, 4th ed. Philadelphia, WB Saunders Co, 1999, p 1055.

most twofold due to placental production of alkaline phosphatase. Albumin is normally decreased by approximately 20%.

Gallbladder

Gallbladder contractility is decreased and there is an increase in residual volume. This effect is probably due to increased levels of progesterone and its effect on the relaxation of smooth muscle. The end result is increased stasis, which in turn increases the risk of gallstones.

PATIENT-RELATED OBSTETRICAL PROBLEMS: THE COMMON CALLS

4 | Abnormal Fetal Heart Rate Patterns

■ BACKGROUND AND DEFINITIONS

Intrapartum fetal heart rate monitoring is used to detect abnormal fetal heart rate patterns that may be associated with hypoxia, acidosis, and fetal asphyxia. Episodes of hypoxia and acidosis are commonly encountered in normal labor. These episodes are usually tolerated well by the fetus. Long-term neurological damage to the fetus is a concern only when these episodes of hypoxia and acidosis are extreme and persistent. Fetal heart rate patterns can be described as "reassuring" or "nonreassuring."

Acidosis: Decreased pH in tissue

Acidemia: Decreased pH in blood

Hypoxia: Decreased oxygen level in tissue

Hypoxemia: Decreased oxygen level in blood

Fetal asphyxia: Hypoxia with metabolic acidosis

Baseline fetal heart activity: Baseline characteristics of the fetal heart rate

Periodic fetal heart rate activity: Characteristics of the fetal heart rate that are associated with uterine contractions or fetal movements. Periodic changes in fetal heart rate are extremely common.

Abnormal fetal heart rate patterns can consist of abnormalities of baseline fetal heart rate activity, abnormalities of periodic fetal heart rate activity, or both. Abnormalities of baseline fetal heart activity include the following:

1. **Abnormal rate.** The normal baseline fetal heart rate in the third trimester is 120 to 160 beats/min. Occasional accelerations are associated with a normal fetal heart rate pattern (Fig. 4–1). Deceleration of the fetal heart rate is the initial response to hypoxia. If hypoxia is persistent, a baseline tachycardia often develops. Other causes of tachycardia are maternal fever and chorioamnionitis.

   Mild bradycardia: Baseline rate of 100 to 119 beats/min

   Moderate bradycardia: Baseline rate of 80 to 99 beats/min for at least 3 minutes (Fig. 4–2)

   Severe bradycardia: Baseline rate of <80 beats/min for at least 3 minutes

   Mild tachycardia: Baseline rate of 161 to 180 beats/min

   Severe tachycardia: Baseline rate of >180 beats/min

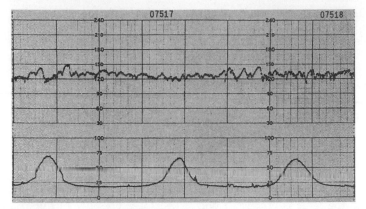

Figure 4–1 □ Normal fetal heart rate with accelerations. (From Creasy RK, Resnik R: Maternal-Fetal Medicine: Principles and Practice, 4th ed. Philadelphia, WB Saunders Co, 1999, p 277.)

2. **Abnormal beat-to-beat variability.** Variability is the oscillatory appearance of the fetal heart rate when recorded on graph paper. It is regulated by the fetal autonomic nervous system and is an indicator of the integrity of the fetal central nervous system. Decreased variability usually precedes decelerations of the fetal heart rate. In fact, decreased variability in the absence of fetal heart rate deceleration can result from causes other than hypoxia. Administration of certain drugs such as magnesium sulfate to the mother and the natural fetal sleep cycle can be causes of decreased variability.

Short-term variability: Instantaneous change in fetal heart rate from one beat to the next. Short-term variability can be detected only by internal electronic fetal monitoring.

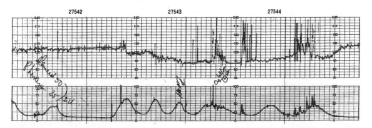

Figure 4–2 □ Prolonged fetal bradycardia. (From Creasy RK, Resnik R: Maternal-Fetal Medicine: Principles and Practice, 4th ed. Philadelphia, WB Saunders Co, 1999, p 278.)

Normal short-term variability is a beat-to-beat change of 3 to 7 beats/min, and increased short-term variability is a beat-to-beat change of >7 beats/min. Both are reassuring of fetal well-being. Decreased or absent short-term variability can be an indication of fetal compromise, especially if it is persistent (Fig. 4–3).

Long-term variability: Oscillatory changes in fetal heart rate over 1 minute, resulting in a wavy baseline. The normal frequency of the "waves" or cycle changes is 3 to 5/min. Decreased long-term variability is defined as <2 cycle changes/min. Decreased or absent long-term variability, if persistent, can indicate fetal compromise.

3. **Cardiac arrhythmia.** Found in approximately 1% of patients monitored and can be detected only by electronic monitoring. Most arrhythmias are supraventricular and resolve spontaneously in the neonatal period. Ventricular arrhythmias are infrequent in fetuses. Most fetal cardiac arrhythmias are of little clinical significance if fetal cardiac failure, manifested by the presence of hydrops, is absent. However, the presence of cardiac arrhythmias can make interpretation of fetal heart rate patterns difficult.

4. **Sinusoidal heart rate pattern.** A distinct pattern consisting of regular, smooth oscillations resembling a sine wave with a frequency of 3 to 5 cycles/min, amplitude of 5 to 15 beats/min, absence of short-term variability, and duration of at least 10 minutes (Fig. 4–4). When this pattern is persistent, it is usually associated with fetal acidosis and hypoxia. However, a sinusoidal heart rate pattern can also be associated with severe and chronic fetal anemia and the administration of alphaprodine. Unfortunately, frequent low-amplitude accelerations of the fetal heart rate can appear like a sinusoidal

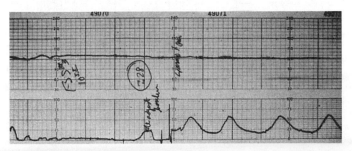

Figure 4–3 □ Absence of variability. (From Creasy RK, Resnik R: Maternal-Fetal Medicine: Principles and Practice, 4th ed. Philadelphia, WB Saunders Co, 1999, p 279.)

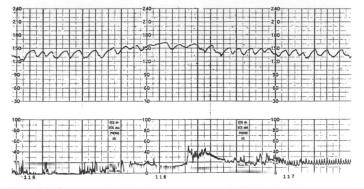

Figure 4–4 □ Sinusoidal pattern. (From Creasy RK, Resnik R: Maternal-Fetal Medicine: Principles and Practice, 4th ed. Philadelphia, WB Saunders Co, 1999, p 289.)

pattern even though these accelerations are reassuring of fetal well-being.

Abnormalities of periodic fetal heart rate activity include the following:

1. **Early deceleration.** A smooth, shallow, and symmetrical fall in fetal heart rate, beginning and ending with the uterine contraction and resembling a mirror image of the contraction (Fig. 4–5). Rarely does the absolute heart rate fall to <100 beats/min or >30 beats below the baseline. Early decelera-

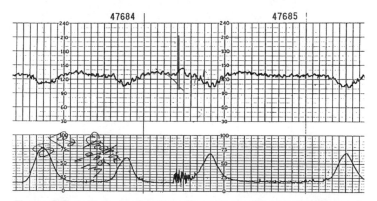

Figure 4–5 □ Early decelerations. (From Creasy RK, Resnik R: Maternal-Fetal Medicine: Principles and Practice, 4th ed. Philadelphia, WB Saunders Co, 1999, p 281.)

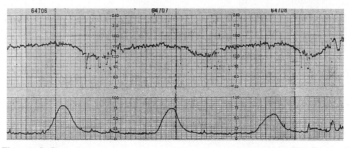

Figure 4–6 □ Late decelerations. (From Creasy RK, Resnik R: Maternal-Fetal Medicine: Principles and Practice, 4th ed. Philadelphia, WB Saunders Co, 1999, p 280.)

tions are caused by fetal head compression during active labor and do not indicate fetal compromise.

2. **Late deceleration.** A uniform, smooth fall in the fetal heart rate, beginning at or after the peak of the uterine contraction and returning to baseline after the end of the contraction (Figs. 4–6 and 4–7). The nadir of a late deceleration is

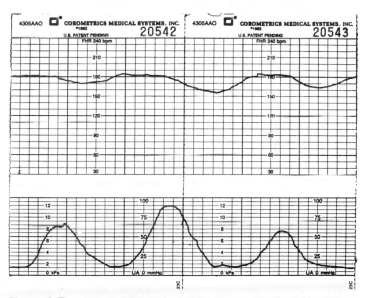

Figure 4–7 □ Late decelerations with loss of variability. (From Newton M, Newton ER: Complications of Gynecologic and Obstetric Management. Philadelphia, WB Saunders Co, 1988, p 273.)

reached after the peak of the uterine contraction. Late decelerations can be subtle, with a fall of only 10 to 30 beats below baseline. The heart rate rarely falls more than 30 to 40 beats below baseline. Occasional late decelerations are of no clinical significance. They may be secondary to transient hypoxia caused by decreased uteroplacental blood flow during a uterine contraction. However, repetitive late decelerations can be an indication of central nervous system hypoxia and even myocardial depression. The depth of the late deceleration does not correlate with the degree of hypoxia.

3. **Variable deceleration.** A rapid fall in fetal heart rate, with a steep downslope and a rapid return to baseline. A variable deceleration resembles the shape of the letter U or the letter V and can be variable in duration, depth, and shape from one contraction to the next (Fig. 4–8). Each deceleration may be preceded or followed by an acceleration. This type of deceleration is the most common type detected in labor. It is caused by umbilical cord compression and is present frequently in the second stage of labor. These decelerations usually are coincident with uterine contractions or pushing efforts on the part of the woman. Variable decelerations are rarely indicative of fetal asphyxia unless they are severe and repetitive. Severe variable decelerations are defined by the "rule of 60s," as follows: (1) the rate falls to <60 beats/min, (2) the rate falls ≥60 beats below the baseline, or (3) the duration of the deceleration is >60 seconds. Variable decelerations with slow return to baseline are also of concern.

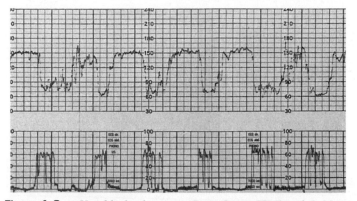

Figure 4–8 □ Variable decelerations. (From Creasy RK, Resnik R: Maternal-Fetal Medicine: Principles and Practice, 4th ed. Philadelphia, WB Saunders Co, 1999, p 283.)

■ CLINICAL PRESENTATION

Abnormal fetal heart rate patterns are not necessarily associated with any specific symptoms. Patients with intrauterine growth restriction and premature labor are more likely to have abnormal fetal heart rate patterns. Patients in whom fetal compromise is caused by placental abruption might have symptoms of abruption such as vaginal bleeding, uterine pain, or uterine tenderness. Likewise, patients with uterine hypertonus, excessive uterine contractions, or uterine rupture might have increased uterine pain. In many situations, conduction analgesia can mask these symptoms of uterine pain.

■ PHONE CALL

Questions

1. **What are the patient's vital signs?**

   Maternal hypotension can result in abnormal fetal heart rate patterns.

2. **Does the patient appear to be in hypovolemic shock?**

   Hypovolemic shock caused by placental abruption or uterine rupture can cause abnormal fetal heart rate patterns.

3. **Does the patient appear to be in an excessive amount of pain?**

   Excessive pain can result from hyperstimulation of the uterus, caused by oxytocin administration, placental abruption, or uterine rupture. These are all potential causes of abnormal fetal heart rate patterns.

Degree of Urgency

A patient whose fetus has abnormal heart rate patterns should be seen immediately.

■ ELEVATOR THOUGHTS

What are the causes of abnormal fetal heart rate patterns?
1. Maternal hypoperfusion
   - Hypotension from the use of conduction analgesia
   - Decreased blood return due to uterine compression of the vena cava in the supine position
2. Excessive uterine activity, usually from oxytocin administration
   - Hypertonus with elevated resting uterine tone

- Excessively frequent uterine contractions with inadequate rest periods (lasting <1 minute) between contractions
- Prolonged uterine contractions (lasting >90 seconds)
3. Uterine rupture
4. Decreased umbilical cord blood flow
    - Umbilical cord compression
    - Umbilical cord knot
    - Umbilical cord prolapse
5. Placental dysfunction
    - Maternal hypertension
    - Maternal diabetes mellitus
    - Maternal autoimmune disorders
    - Placental abruption

■ MAJOR THREAT TO FETAL LIFE

- Fetal asphyxia
    Abnormal fetal heart rate patterns can indicate fetal asphyxia with possible neonatal morbidity and mortality.

■ BEDSIDE

Quick Look Test

What types of abnormal fetal heart rate patterns are present?
Certain fetal heart rate patterns, such as early decelerations and mild, variable decelerations, can be detected in normal pregnancies and are not worrisome. Other patterns, such as recurrent late decelerations and sinusoidal patterns, may be suggestive of fetal compromise.

How long have the abnormal fetal heart rate patterns been present?
Occasional isolated abnormal heart rate patterns are usually of no significance, whereas recurrent abnormal patterns can be more ominous.

Is the patient in labor? If so, what is the quality and frequency of her contractions?
Hyperstimulation of the uterus by oxytocin administration can cause abnormal heart rate patterns. Excessively frequent contractions (occurring more frequently than every 3 minutes), prolonged contractions (lasting >90 seconds), and an elevated uterine resting tone are indicative of hyperstimulation.

How much is the patient's cervix dilated and how close is the patient to delivery?
If the fetus has a nonreassuring heart rate pattern and is also

close to delivery, facilitation of delivery by forceps or by vacuum should be considered.

Vital Signs

Hypotension caused by poor blood return in a supine position, placental abruption, and uterine rupture can result in abnormal heart rate patterns.

Selective History and Chart Review

1. Does the patient have any medical conditions such as hypertension, diabetes mellitus, or collagen-vascular disorders that cause chronic placental dysfunction?
2. Has there been evidence of intrauterine growth restriction?
   Intrauterine growth restriction can result from chronic placental dysfunction, which may in turn be associated with a higher incidence of abnormal fetal heart rate patterns.

Selective Physical Examination

Abdominal	Tender in placental abruption
Pelvic	
External genitalia and vagina	Normal unless there is excessive vaginal bleeding or meconium passage
Cervix	Usually normal
Uterus and adnexa	Normal unless there is uterine tenderness, irritability, or hypertonus caused by placental abruption, hyperstimulation, or uterine rupture

Orders

1. Start an intravenous (IV) fluid infusion if the patient does not already have one.
2. Turn the patient on her side to increase blood return through the inferior vena cava.
3. Administer supplemental oxygen to the mother, with a face mask and at an oxygen flow rate of 8 to 10 L/min.
4. Have available a fetal scalp electrode for internal fetal heart rate monitoring.

■ DIAGNOSTIC TESTING

1. Electronic fetal heart rate monitoring

Fetal heart rate can be monitored either with continuous electronic monitoring or with intermittent auscultation. When there is a 1:1 nurse-to-patient ratio, there is no difference between intermittent auscultation and continuous electronic monitoring as far as neonatal morbidity is concerned. In low-risk patients, the fetal heart rate tracing should be evaluated every 30 minutes in the first stage of labor and every 15 minutes in the second stage of labor. If intermittent auscultation is used, the fetal heart rate should be auscultated and recorded every 30 minutes in the first stage of labor and every 15 minutes in the second stage of labor. If the presence of high-risk factors makes intensified monitoring necessary, the fetal heart rate should be evaluated every 15 minutes in the first stage of labor and every 5 minutes in the second stage of labor. When auscultation of the heart rate is nonreassuring and abnormalities are suspected, fetal heart rate should be monitored electronically. Furthermore, if external electronic fetal heart rate monitoring is not adequate or if abnormal heart rate patterns are suspected, internal electronic monitoring by a fetal scalp electrode can be used.

■ MANAGEMENT OF NONREASSURING FETAL HEART RATE PATTERN

Nonreassuring fetal heart rate patterns can be caused by factors other than fetal compromise. These patterns cannot be used to reliably predict fetal well-being versus fetal compromise. If nonreassuring fetal heart rate patterns are present, the following conservative steps should first be taken:

1. **Place the patient in the lateral position**
   Placement of the patient in the lateral position displaces the uterus from the midline and relieves compression of the vena cava, resulting in increased blood return to the heart.
2. **Perform pelvic examination**
   Digital examination can rule out prolapse of the umbilical cord or rapid descent of the presenting part of the fetus, both of which can be associated with nonreassuring fetal heart rate patterns.
3. **Administer supplemental oxygen**
   Oxygen should be administered at a flow rate of 8 to 10 L/min via a tight-fitting face mask. Although arterial partial pressure of oxygen (PaO_2) in the fetus is approximately one-fourth of the PaO_2 in the mother, fetal blood can deliver a large amount of oxygen from the placenta because of the high concentration of fetal hemoglobin and its high oxygen affinity. Supplemental oxygen will increase total blood oxygen content in the fetus by at least 30 to 40%.
4. **Decrease uterine contractions**
   a. **Discontinue oxytocin**
      Every uterine contraction is associated with a transient

decrease in blood flow to the placenta, and subsequently to the fetus. Therefore, if the patient is receiving oxytocin, discontinuation of the infusion will decrease both the intensity and the frequency of uterine contractions and increase uterine blood flow. Discontinuation of oxytocin is also the best treatment for uterine hyperstimulation and uterine hypertonus. After resolution of the hyperstimulation and/ or improvement in the fetal heart rate pattern, oxytocin can be restarted at a lower infusion rate.

b. Administer a tocolytic agent

Tocolytic drugs such as terbutaline sulfate or magnesium sulfate can be administered to decrease both the intensity and the frequency of uterine contractions, regardless of whether the patient is receiving oxytocin.

(1) **Terbutaline sulfate 0.25 mg subcutaneously (SC) or 0.125 to 0.25 mg IV**

If a decrease in uterine activity is not achieved in 15 to 30 minutes, a second dose can be administered.

(2) **Magnesium sulfate 2.0 g IV over 10 minutes**

5. Correct maternal hypotension

Maternal hypotension can decrease uterine blood flow, which in turn can cause abnormal fetal heart rate patterns. Hypotension is often the result of conduction analgesia used during labor, occurring in 5 to 25% of epidural procedures.

a. Increase IV infusion rate or give IV bolus of 500–1000 ml lactated Ringer's solution.

b. Administer ephedrine sulfate 10 to 25 mg intramuscularly (IM) or IV

c. Displace the uterus to the left to increase blood flow back to the heart

6. Amnioinfusion

Amnioinfusion can cause a decrease in both the frequency and the severity of variable decelerations, especially in a patient with decreased amniotic fluid. Amnioinfusion is performed through an intrauterine catheter and can be performed as a bolus or a continuous infusion. Bolus infusion of 500 to 800 ml of room-temperature normal saline is administered at a rate of 10 to 15 ml/min. The bolus infusion of a similar or smaller amount can be repeated depending on the response of the fetal heart rate pattern, sonographic assessment of intra-amniotic fluid, and ongoing loss of fluid as labor progresses. Continuous infusion is initiated by infusing 10 ml/min of room-temperature normal saline for 1 hour followed by a maintenance infusion of 3 ml/min. Improvement in the fetal heart rate pattern usually occurs no sooner than 20 to 30 minutes after amnioinfusion is begun. Overdistention of the uterine cavity should be avoided because it can result in in-

Table 4–1 □ **INDICATIONS FOR FETAL SCALP BLOOD SAMPLING**

Absent or decreased short-term variability
Persistent late decelerations
Persistent, severe variable decelerations
Sinusoidal heart rate pattern
Heart rate patterns nonreassuring due to difficulties in interpretation

creased uterine tone and also deterioration of the fetal heart rate pattern.

If the above steps do not resolve the abnormal fetal heart rate patterns, then the fetal status should be ascertained, as follows:

1. Fetal scalp blood sampling

Measurement of capillary blood pH can be used to identify a fetus with acidosis (Table 4–1). The cervix must be dilated at least 2 to 3 cm, and the membranes must be ruptured, to perform fetal scalp blood sampling. An endoscope with a light source is inserted into the vagina and is placed against the fetal scalp. The scalp is then wiped clean and coated with a silicone gel, which causes the fetal blood to form into globules. With a special blade, a punch incision is made into the fetal scalp to a depth of approximately 2 mm, and the blood is collected with a heparinized glass capillary tube. If fetal capillary blood pH is >7.25, it is reassuring, and labor is allowed to proceed with continuous electronic monitoring of the fetal heart rate (Table 4–2). If the pH range is 7.20 to 7.25, the fetal scalp blood sampling should be repeated within approximately 30 minutes, depending on the subsequent fetal heart rate tracing. If the fetal heart rate pattern becomes more ominous, then

Table 4–2 □ **FETAL SCALP BLOOD VALUES IN LABOR***

	Early First Stage	Late First Stage	Second Stage
pH	7.33 ± 0.03	7.32 ± 0.02	7.29 ± 0.04
P_{CO_2} (mm Hg)	44 ± 4.05	42 ± 5.1	46.3 ± 4.2
P_{O_2} (mm Hg)	21.8 ± 2.6	21.3 ± 2.1	16.5 ± 1.4
Bicarbonate (mmol/L)	20.1 ± 1.2	19.1 ± 2.1	17 ± 2
Base excess (mmol/L)	3.9 ± 1.9	4.1 ± 2.5	6.4 ± 1.8

*Mean ± standard deviation.
From Creasy RK, Resnik R: Maternal-Fetal Medicine: Principles and Practice, 4th ed. Philadelphia, WB Saunders Co, 1999, p 333. Abstracted from Huch R, Huch A: In: Beard RW, Nathanielsz PW, eds: Fetal Physiology and Medicine. New York, Marcel Dekker Inc, 1984.

fetal scalp sampling should be repeated sooner. If the fetal heart rate pattern becomes normal, then fetal scalp sampling can be delayed. If the pH is <7.20, the fetus should be delivered either immediately or after a repeated fetal scalp sampling performed immediately shows that acidemia is still present.

2. **Fetal scalp stimulation test**

   If fetal scalp sampling is not possible, fetal scalp stimulation can be performed instead. Acceleration of the fetal heart rate, in response to pinching of the fetal scalp with a surgical instrument such as an Allis clamp, is almost always associated with a normal scalp blood pH. However, the converse is not always true. Absence of acceleration is associated with fetal acidosis only in approximately 50% of patients.

   If nonreassuring fetal heart rate patterns are noted and there is evidence of fetal acidemia, the fetus should be delivered immediately. This can be done by either cesarean delivery or, when possible, vaginal delivery assisted by forceps or vacuum extraction if the patient is in the second stage of labor.

5 | Abnormal Labor

■ BACKGROUND AND DEFINITIONS

Basic Labor

Labor: Uterine contractions with adequate frequency, strength, and duration to result in progressive effacement and dilatation of the cervix

First stage of labor: From the onset of labor to full cervical dilatation or 10 cm of cervical dilatation; consists of the latent phase and the active phase

    Latent phase of labor: In this phase, uterine contractions are irregular and infrequent although they can be uncomfortable. These contractions result in softening and effacement of the cervix but only modest dilatation.

    Active phase of labor: This phase usually begins when the cervix reaches 3 to 4 cm of dilatation. In this phase, there is an increased rate of cervical dilatation and effacement when compared to the latent phase of labor.

Second stage of labor: From full cervical dilatation to delivery of the infant

Third stage of labor: From delivery of the infant to delivery of the placenta

In the active phase of labor, nulliparous patients should dilate at the rate of $\geq$1.2 cm/hr, and multiparous patients should dilate at the rate of $\geq$1.5 cm/hr (Table 5–1). The duration of the second stage of labor varies from 20 minutes in multiparous patients to several hours in nulliparous patients. Even though prolonged second stage is commonly defined as a second stage of >2 hours, nulliparous patients can have second stages of up to 3 hours

Table 5–1 □ NORMAL DURATION OF THE STAGES OF LABOR

Stages of Labor	Nullipara	Multipara
First stage		
Latent phase	$\leq$20 hr	$\leq$14 hr
Active phase	5–8 hr	2–5 hr
Rate of dilatation	$\geq$1.2 cm/hr	$\geq$1.5 cm/hr
Second stage	$\leq$2 hr	$\leq$1 hr
Third stage	$\leq$30 min	$\leq$30 min

if epidural anesthesia is used. Furthermore, in the absence of nonreassuring fetal heart rate patterns, the duration of the second stage of labor is not related to perinatal outcome. The third stage of labor can last 30 minutes in both nulliparous and multiparous patients.

Abnormal Labor

Dystocia: Abnormally slow or difficult delivery

Cephalopelvic disproportion (CPD): Disproportion between the size of the fetal head and maternal pelvis

Failure to progress: General term used to refer to lack of progressive dilatation and/or descent of the fetal presenting part

Prolonged latent phase of labor: Latent phase that lasts >20 hours in a nulliparous patient or >14 hours in a parous patient

Protracted active phase dilatation: Rate of cervical dilatation is <1.2 cm/hr in a nulliparous patient or <1.5 cm/hr in a parous patient

Arrest of dilatation: No cervical dilatation in 2 hours in the active phase of labor

Protracted descent: Rate of descent of the fetus is <1 cm/hr in a nulliparous patient or <2 cm/hr in a parous patient

Arrest of descent: No descent of the fetus in 1 hour

Abnormal labor is the most common indication for three times as many cesarean sections as either abnormal fetal heart rate patterns or malpresentation. Prolonged latent phase of labor is encountered in approximately 3 to 4% of patients and is not usually associated with an increase in maternal or fetal morbidity or mortality. Abnormalities in the active phase of labor are the most common types of labor abnormalities. Approximately 25% of nulliparous labors and 15% of multiparous labors are complicated by an abnormality in the active phase of labor.

■ CLINICAL PRESENTATION

Patients with abnormal labor cannot be distinguished from patients with normal labor based on clinical findings. They can be distinguished only by differences in their labor curves. A labor curve can be drawn by simply plotting cervical dilatation and descent of the fetal presenting part against time. Figure 5–1 shows a normal labor curve.

■ PHONE CALL

Questions

1. **What type or types of labor abnormality does the patient exhibit on her labor curve?**

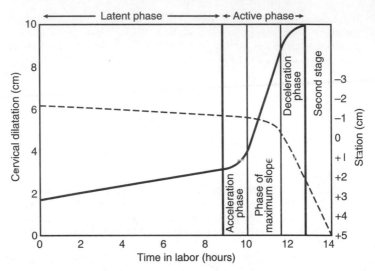

Figure 5-1 □ Normal labor curves. Solid line, cervical dilatation; dashed line, station. (Redrawn from Cohen WR, Friedman EA: Management of Labor. Gaithersburg, MD, Aspen Publishers, Inc, 1983, p 13.)

2. Is epidural analgesia being administered?

The use of lumbar epidural anesthesia can prolong the latent phase of labor. It can also cause protracted descent because both the sensory and the motor blocks of epidural analgesia may interfere with the patient's ability to push in the second stage of labor.

Degree of Urgency

The patient and her labor curve should be evaluated as soon as possible, but the patient does not need to be seen immediately if she is stable and the fetal heart rate pattern is reassuring.

■ ELEVATOR THOUGHTS

What factors are associated with the prolonged latent phase of labor?
- Excessive sedation
- Excessive or early administration of epidural anesthesia
- Unfavorable cervical status: cervix is undilated, uneffaced, and firm

What are the causes of abnormal labor?

- Abnormalities of the fetus
    Macrosomia
    Malpresentation
    Congenital anomalies
- Abnormalities of the maternal pelvis
    An abnormally small or contracted pelvis can result in CPD, which in turn causes abnormal labor. The same is true with a normal pelvis when the fetus is macrosomic.
- Abnormalities of the expulsive forces
    Inadequate uterine contractions
        Contractions of inadequate strength
        Contractions of inadequate frequency
    Inadequate pushing effort in the second stage of labor
- Abnormalities of the uterus, cervix, vagina, or vulva
    Uterine leiomyomata (fibroids)
    Cervical stenosis
    Vaginal septum
    Extensive vulvar condylomata acuminata

Abnormal labor is most often caused by one of three "Ps": power, passage, and passenger. Power refers to the adequacy of uterine contractions. Passage refers to the adequacy of the bony maternal pelvis as well as abnormalities of the uterus, cervix, vagina, and vulva. Passenger refers to the fetus. Not only is the size of the fetus a factor, but so are malpresentations of the fetus. These may include extension or asynclitism of the fetal head.

■ MAJOR THREAT TO FETAL LIFE

- Fetal asphyxia
    In rare cases, prolonged or arrested labor is associated with fetal compromise.

■ MAJOR THREAT TO MATERNAL LIFE

- Hemorrhage and hypovolemic shock
    If abnormal labor is ignored, uterine rupture can occur, resulting in hemorrhage and in significant maternal and fetal morbidity. Prolonged labor is associated with an increased risk of postpartum uterine atony, resulting in postpartum hemorrhage and, possibly, hypovolemic shock.

■ BEDSIDE

Quick Look Test

Does the patient appear to be having adequate uterine contractions?

If the patient has not already received analgesia, her level of discomfort is often a good indicator of the quality of her uterine contractions. Although it is not as helpful as internal uterine pressure monitoring, external uterine monitor tracing can also be used to evaluate quickly the quality, duration, and frequency of a patient's uterine contractions.

What is the estimated fetal weight?
Patients with large fetuses are at greater risk for CPD, which is manifested by abnormal labor.

If the patient is pushing in the second stage of labor, is she pushing with adequate effort?
A patient who is exhausted or has excessive sensory and motor nerve block from epidural anesthesia will often not push adequately.

Are there any abnormal fetal heart rate patterns that suggest fetal compromise?
Management of some types of abnormal labor is expectant as long as fetal compromise is not suspected.

Vital Signs

Vital signs are usually normal.

Selective History and Chart Review

1. Has the patient given birth previously, and if so, what was that infant's birth weight and method of delivery?
   The birth weights of previous infants delivered vaginally can provide information concerning the adequacy of the patient's pelvis. Previous abnormal labor resulting in cesarean delivery of an infant with a low birth weight suggests a small maternal pelvis.
2. Was the patient's prior pregnancy complicated by abnormal labor?
   Certain causes of abnormal labor, such as small pelvis and poor expulsive forces due to either inadequate uterine contractions or poor pushing in the second stage of labor, may exist in subsequent pregnancies.
3. Does the patient have diabetes mellitus?
   Diabetes mellitus and gestational diabetes can cause fetal macrosomia.
4. Does the patient have an abnormality of the birth canal that predisposes to abnormal labor, such as cervical stenosis, uterine leiomyomata, or a vaginal septum?

Selective Physical Examination

Abdominal	The fetus should be palpated for estimated birth weight.
Pelvic	
External genitalia and vagina	Vaginal and vulvar lesions, such as vaginal septum and extensive condylomata acuminata, can cause abnormal labor by obstructing descent of the fetus.
Cervix	**Cervical dilatation** (cm), **effacement** (%), and the **station** of the presenting fetal part, in relation to the ischial spine of the maternal pelvis (" $-x$ " or " $+x$ "), should be determined by digital examination. A station of $-x$ means that the presenting fetal part is x cm above the level of the ischial spine, and $+x$ means that the presenting fetal part is x cm below the level of the ischial spine. **Fetal position**, which refers to the relationship between a point on the fetal presenting part and the maternal pelvis, should also be determined. This point is the fetal occiput, chin, and sacrum, for vertex, face, and breech presentations, respectively. Figure 5–2 illustrates fetal positions for vertex, face, and breech presentations.
Uterus and adnexa	Palpation of the uterus should be performed to determine the strength and the frequency of uterine contractions. Examination will also reveal uterine leiomyomata and ovarian masses, which might cause abnormal labor by obstructing descent of the fetus.

Orders

1. Start intravenous (IV) oxytocin infusion if the uterine contractions are clearly inadequate.
2. Prepare the patient for placement of an intrauterine pressure monitor if suboptimal uterine contractions are suspected.
3. Type and crossmatch for 2 units of blood if cesarean section is anticipated.

■ DIAGNOSTIC TESTING

The diagnosis of abnormal labor is based on an abnormal labor curve. Diagnostic tests may help in determining the cause or causes of abnormal labor.

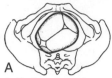
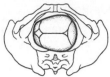
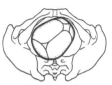

Left Occipito-Anterior   Left Occipito-Transverse   Left Occipito-Posterior

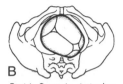
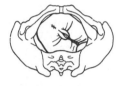
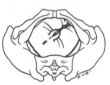

Right Occipito-Anterior   Right Occipito-Transverse   Right Occipito-Posterior

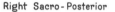

Left Sacro-Anterior   Right Sacro-Anterior   Right Sacro-Posterior

Figure 5–2 □ Fetal positions. *A*, Left positions in occiput presentations, with the fetal head viewed from below. *B*, Right positions in occiput presentations. *C*, Left and right positions in breech presentations. (From Pritchard JA, MacDonald PC: Williams' Obstetrics, 16th ed. East Norwalk, CT, Appleton-Century-Crofts, 1980, p 297. Reproduced with permission of The McGraw-Hill Companies.)

1. **Ultrasound examination**
   Ultrasound examination can be used to diagnose some of the fetal causes of dystocia. Fetal measurements can provide an estimated fetal weight and can thereby help in diagnosis of macrosomia. Unfortunately, ultrasound examination at term is not always accurate in predicting fetal weight. Abnormal fetal presentation and congenital anomalies can also be diagnosed by ultrasound, as can some uterine and ovarian causes of abnormal labor, such as leiomyomata and ovarian masses.
2. **Internal uterine pressure monitor**
   Manual palpation of the uterus and external uterine monitoring can help determine the adequacy of uterine contractions. However, internal uterine pressure monitoring is superior, because it provides quantitative measurements of both the strength and the frequency of uterine contractions (Fig. 5–3).

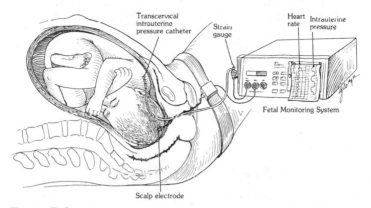

Figure 5–3 □ Intrauterine pressure monitoring. (From Hacker NF, Moore JG: Essentials of Obstetrics and Gynecology, 3rd ed. Philadelphia, WB Saunders Co, 1998, p 291.)

Adequate uterine contractions reach an amplitude at least 25 mm Hg above the resting or baseline pressure and occur at a frequency of not less than three contractions every 10 minutes.

An alternative means of measuring uterine contractions is by Montevideo units. Montevideo units are calculated by subtracting the baseline uterine pressure from the peak uterine pressure, for each contraction in a 10-minute period as measured by an internal uterine pressure catheter, and by adding these pressure differences (Fig. 5–4). Adequate labor usually generates 95 to 395 Montevideo units.

The following two criteria should be met before arrest of dilatation can be diagnosed: (1) The patient should have completed the latent phase of labor and have cervical dilatation ≥4 cm, and (2) a uterine contraction pattern attaining ≥200

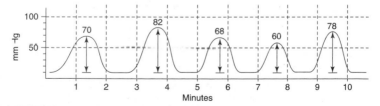

Figure 5–4 □ Calculation of Montevideo units. The term "Montevideo units" was coined by Caldeyro-Barcia and Alvarez in 1960. Montevideo units are calculated by summing the intensity (mm Hg) of all uterine contractions in a 10-minute period. In this example, the sum of all contractions yielded 358 Montevideo units.

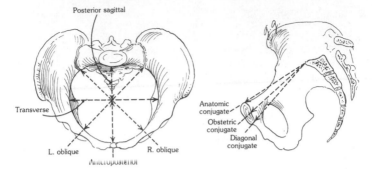

Figure 5–5 □ Pelvic inlet diameters. (From Hacker NF, Moore JG: Essentials of Obstetrics and Gynecology, 3rd ed. Philadelphia, WB Saunders Co, 1998, p 143.)

Montevideo units should be present for ≥2 hours without change in cervical dilatation.
3. **Pelvimetry**
    Radiographic pelvimetry can be performed by either conventional x-ray or computed tomography (CT) scan to determine adequacy of the bony pelvis. The anterior-posterior and transverse diameters of the pelvic inlet and of the midpelvis are measured (Fig. 5–5). The minimum diameters are listed in Table 5–2. Pelvimetry is currently used in patients with breech presentations of the fetus, but it is of limited value in patients with vertex presentations of the fetus. For vertex presentations, adequacy of the patient's pelvis is determined by allowing labor to proceed and by ruling out other causes of abnormal labor if such labor is encountered. Radiographic pelvimetry provides no measurement of soft tissue resistance from the vagina or perineum.

Table 5–2 □ **NORMAL PELVIMETRY MEASUREMENTS**

	Anterior-Posterior Diameter (cm)	Transverse Diameter (cm)
Pelvic inlet	≥10.5	≥11.5
Midpelvis	≥11.5	≥10.0

■ MANAGEMENT

1. Prolonged latent phase of labor
a. Rest and sedation

Because most patients with prolonged latent phases are exhausted and frustrated, rest and sedation can be therapeutic. Most patients will wake up refreshed and in active labor. This conservative management is appropriate only if the fetal heart rate pattern is reassuring. One of the following regimens can be used:

(1) **Morphine sulfate 10 to 15 mg intramuscularly (IM) every 4 hours** or

(2) **Meperidine hydrochloride (Demerol) 50 to 100 mg IM every 4 hours** or

(3) **Pentobarbital sodium (Nembutal) 100 mg capsule by mouth**

b. Oxytocin IV infusion

An alternative to rest and sedation is IV infusion of oxytocin to induce labor. This management has been called "active management of labor" and can be used in any patient, but it is absolutely indicated for a patient with a nonreassuring fetal heart rate pattern.

2. Protracted active phase dilatation or protracted descent

Protracted labor abnormalities can be managed expectantly if the patient is stable and there is no evidence of fetal compromise. Uterine contractions should be optimized.

a. Oxytocin IV infusion

Oxytocin should be infused if uterine contractions have an amplitude of less than 25 mm Hg above the resting pressure, if they occur at a frequency of less than three contractions every 10 minutes, or if the Montevideo units measure < 95 units. A solution of **10 IU oxytocin in 1000 ml of 5% dextrose and lactated Ringer's solution**, or **in 1000 ml of 5% dextrose and 0.5 normal saline**, is used. This solution has an oxytocin concentration of 10 mIU/ml and is infused intravenously by an infusion pump. There are several dose regimens that can be used.

(1) **Low-dose regimens** begin with a starting dose of 0.5 to 2.0 mIU/min and increase in increments of 1 to 2 mIU/min every 15 to 40 minutes. A commonly used regimen starts with a dose of 1 mIU/min. The dose is then increased by 1 mIU/min every 20 to 30 minutes up to a dose of 8 mIU/min. Thereafter the dose is increased by 2 mIU/min every 20 to 30 minutes up to a dose of 20 mIU/min.

(2) **High-dose regimens** begin with a dose of 6 mIU/min and increase in increments of 1 mIU/min, 3 mIU/min, or 6 mIU/min every 20 to 40 minutes up to a maximum

dose of 42 mIU/min. Increments of 6 mIU/min are normally used. If hyperstimulation is encountered, increments of 3 mIU/ml are used, and if hyperstimulation is recurrent, increments of 1 mIU/min are used. Hyperstimulation is defined as the presence of more than five contractions in a 10-minute period, contractions lasting 2 minutes or longer, or contractions occurring within 1 minute of each other.

If high doses (>40 mIU/min) are required for prolonged periods, it should be remembered that oxytocin has an antidiuretic effect. High doses given over a prolonged period can cause water intoxication. These patients should have fluids restricted, and oxytocin should be administered in a more concentrated solution to restrict fluids further.

3. Arrest of dilatation or arrest of descent

When protracted labor abnormalities are encountered, uterine contractions should be optimized if they are inadequate.

a. Oxytocin IV infusion

The oxytocin infusion described above should be administered if uterine contractions are inadequate.

b. Cesarean section

If a patient has arrest of dilatation or arrest of descent, despite the presence of adequate uterine contractions, a cesarean section should be considered. Operative vaginal delivery can be attempted in patients with complete cervical dilatation.

c. Operative vaginal delivery

If the patient has reached complete cervical dilatation but has arrest of descent, despite the presence of adequate uterine contractions, operative vaginal delivery with forceps or with vacuum assistance should be considered if it can be performed safely. The safety of operative vaginal delivery depends on estimated fetal size, station of the vertex, position, skill of the operator, and fetal status. If operative vaginal delivery cannot be done safely, then a cesarean section should be performed.

6 | Amniotic Fluid Embolism

■ BACKGROUND AND DEFINITIONS

Amniotic fluid embolism: Entrance of amniotic fluid into the maternal circulation, resulting in hypoxemia, cardiovascular collapse, and disseminated intravascular coagulation (DIC)

Although it is a rare complication, with an incidence rate of 1 in 7000 to 1 in 30,000 deliveries, amniotic fluid embolism is the cause of 4 to 10% of all maternal deaths. Amniotic fluid embolism usually occurs in the third trimester of pregnancy either during delivery or during the immediate postpartum period. However, it has also been encountered as early as in the first trimester, during suction curettage for pregnancy termination, and as late as several days postpartum. For amniotic fluid embolism to develop, there must first exist open endocervical or uterine veins, a tear through the fetal membranes, and enough of a pressure gradient to force amniotic fluid into the maternal circulation. The severity of this complication is directly related to the amount of debris and other particulate matter in the fluid, such as meconium, fetal lanugo, and fetal squamous cells.

Amniotic fluid embolism results in a biphasic pattern of hemodynamic abnormalities. The first phase consists of **vasospasm of the pulmonary vasculature**, resulting in pulmonary hypertension, hypoxia, and right-sided heart failure. In this initial phase, pulmonary hypertension develops from the shower of occlusive emboli that causes increased pulmonary vascular resistance. Pulmonary hypertension may also result from pulmonary vasoconstriction caused by a vasoactive substance in the amniotic fluid. This initial phase accounts for 50% of maternal deaths in the first hour. The second phase consists of **left-sided heart failure** with mild to moderate elevation of pulmonary arterial pressure. Coagulopathy occurs in up to 40% of patients and is caused by the thromboplastic effects of trophoblasts in the maternal circulation.

■ CLINICAL PRESENTATION

Sudden onset of dyspnea
Cyanosis
Hypotension out of proportion to blood loss
Seizures
Hemorrhage
Often, the patient states that she feels she is going to die

■ PHONE CALL

Questions

1. How ill does the patient appear?

Although severe cases are often lethal, milder and suble-thal cases have been reported. In these cases, the patient's symptoms are self-limiting, and with supportive care, survival is the rule.

Degree of Urgency

Amniotic fluid embolism is one of the most catastrophic conditions encountered in obstetrics. Patients should be seen immediately.

■ ELEVATOR THOUGHTS

What factors predispose for amniotic fluid embolism?
- Tumultuous labor
- Use of oxytocin
- Advanced maternal age
- Multiparity

What other obstetrical complications can mimic amniotic fluid embolism?
- Placental abruption
- Preeclampsia

Placental abruption can also result in hypovolemic shock out of proportion to the amount of visible bleeding. Preeclampsia can lead to eclampsia or seizures. Both placental abruption and severe preeclampsia can cause DIC.

■ MAJOR THREAT TO FETAL LIFE

- Fetal asphyxia

    If amniotic fluid embolism occurs before delivery, maternal hypoxia and cardiovascular collapse can result in fetal asphyxia and fetal death.

■ MAJOR THREAT TO MATERNAL LIFE

- Hypoxia
- Hypovolemic shock
- Cardiac failure
- DIC

Overall, amniotic fluid embolism has a maternal mortality rate of approximately 85%.

■ BEDSIDE

Quick Look Test

Has the patient suffered cardiorespiratory arrest?
Cardiopulmonary resuscitation (CPR) should be initiated immediately in patients who have had cardiorespiratory arrest.

Vital Signs

Hypotension out of proportion to bleeding may occur. Cardiorespiratory arrest may be encountered.

Selective History and Chart Review

1. Does the patient have any other obstetrical complications, such as placental abruption and severe preeclampsia, that might mimic amniotic fluid embolism?
2. Has the patient's labor been complicated by meconium passage?
    Amniotic fluid embolism is much more catastrophic in the presence of thick meconium.

Selective Physical Examination

General	Cyanotic, often unconscious and unresponsive. Patients will almost always experience cardiorespiratory arrest.
	Bleeding from IV and venipuncture sites if DIC has developed
Abdominal	Normal
Pelvic	
External genitalia and vagina	Bleeding may be present if the patient has developed DIC
Cervix	Normal for the intrapartum or postpartum period. Heavy bleeding from the cervix may be present if the patient has developed DIC.
Uterus and adnexa	Normal for the intrapartum or postpartum period.

Orders

1. Order complete blood count (CBC).
2. Order platelet count.
3. Order serum fibrinogen level.

4. Order fibrin split products.
5. Prepare for placement of a pulmonary artery catheter (Swan-Ganz catheter).
6. Begin oxygen supplementation at a flow rate of 8 to 10 L/min via a face mask.
7. Insert a Foley catheter.
8. Type and crossmatch for whole blood or packed red blood cells.
9. Order fresh frozen plasma.

■ DIAGNOSTIC TESTING

The diagnosis of amniotic fluid embolism is made by the patient's clinical presentation. The diagnosis can often be confirmed retrospectively in two ways.

1. **Smear of buffy coat suspension of central blood**
   Blood should be obtained from the pulmonary artery via the Swan-Ganz catheter, and a smear of the buffy coat of the aspirated blood should be made. Special stains can be used to help identify fetal squamous cells and fat cells. Standard staining with hematoxylin and eosin may not reveal these diagnostic findings. Instead, special stains, such as Alcian blue stain and others that stain for acid mucopolysaccharide, keratin, and fat, must be used.
2. **Autopsy**
   In women who die from amniotic fluid embolism, fetal squamous cells and fat cells can be found on autopsy not only in the lungs but also in the vascular systems of the uterus, heart, brain, kidneys, and ovaries. As is true with blood smears, hematoxylin and eosin stains may be insufficient for diagnosis.

■ MANAGEMENT

Treatment of a patient with amniotic fluid embolism has the following three general goals: oxygenation of the patient, maintenance of cardiac output and blood pressure, and treatment of coagulopathy.

1. **Perform cardiopulmonary resuscitation.**
   CPR should be initiated immediately if the patient has suffered cardiorespiratory arrest.
2. **Intubate and oxygenate the patient.**
   The patient should be intubated and given 100% oxygen if she has had respiratory arrest.
3. **Place pulmonary artery catheter (Swan-Ganz catheter).**
   A pulmonary artery catheter provides the intensive hemody-

namic monitoring necessary for maintenance of cardiac output and blood pressure. In amniotic fluid embolism, pulmonary capillary wedge pressure is commonly elevated. Normal hemodynamic measurements obtained by pulmonary artery catheter are listed in Table 6–1.

4. **Treat cardiogenic shock.**
   a. **Infusion of IV fluids**
      Fluid resuscitation will improve cardiac output by increasing preload.
   b. **Dopamine 5 μg/kg/min by IV infusion, with dose increases of 5 μg/kg/min to a maximum of 50 μg/kg/min**
      Dopamine, a vasoactive amine, has a positive inotropic effect and increases both myocardial contractility and heart rate. Dopamine also increases organ perfusion by vasodilation of renal, mesenteric, coronary, and cerebral vasculatures. The dose is monitored by Swan-Ganz catheter measurements of pulmonary artery and capillary wedge pressures.

5. **Treat coagulopathy and blood loss.**
   a. **Red blood cells**
      Red blood cells (RBCs) increase oxygen-carrying capacity in anemic patients. Each unit of packed red blood cells has a volume of 250 ml, and 1 unit of whole blood has a volume of 450 ml. Each unit of RBCs should increase the hematocrit by 3% and the hemoglobin by 1 g/dl. Coagulation studies

Table 6–1 □ **NORMAL CENTRAL HEMODYNAMIC MEASUREMENTS IN NONPREGNANT AND PREGNANT PATIENTS**

Parameter	Nonpregnant	Pregnant
Cardiac output (L/min)	4.3 ± 0.9	6.2 ± 1.0
Heart rate (beats/min)	71 ± 10.0	83 ± 10.0
Systemic vascular resistance (dyne $\times$ cm $\times$ sec^{-5})	1530 ± 520	1210 ± 266
Pulmonary vascular resistance (dyne $\times$ cm $\times$ sec^{-5})	119 ± 47.0	78 ± 22
Colloid oncotic pressure (mm Hg)	20.8 ± 1.0	18.0 ± 1.5
Colloid oncotic pressure–pulmonary capillary wedge pressure (mm Hg)	14.5 ± 2.5	10.5 ± 2.7
Mean arterial pressure (mm Hg)	86.4 ± 7.5	90.3 ± 5.8
Pulmonary capillary wedge pressure (mm Hg)	6.3 ± 2.1	7.5 ± 1.8
Central venous pressure (mm Hg)	3.7 ± 2.6	3.6 ± 2.5
Left ventricular stroke work index (g $\times$ m $\times$ m^{-2})	41 ± 8	48 ± 6

From Clark SL, Cotton DB, Lee W, et al: Central hemodynamic assessment of normal term pregnancy. Am J Obstet Gynecol 1989;161:1439.

should be obtained after every 5 to 10 units of RBCs transfused.

b. **Platelets**

Platelets should be transfused for a patient with a platelet count of <20,000/mm^3 or for a patient with a platelet count of <50,000/mm^3 in whom a cesarean section is planned. Each unit of platelets should increase the platelet count by 5000 to 10,000/mm^3.

c. **Fresh frozen plasma**

Fresh frozen plasma should be transfused for coagulopathy due to a deficiency of clotting factors, usually manifested by a prothrombin time (PT) or partial thromboplastin time (PTT) that is >1.5 times normal. Each unit of fresh frozen plasma will increase any clotting factor by 2 to 3%. The usual initial dose is 2 units, and each unit has a volume of 200 to 250 ml.

d. **Cryoprecipitate**

Cryoprecipitate should be transfused for coagulopathy due to deficiency of factor VIII, von Willebrand's factor, factor XIII, fibrinogen, and/or fibronectin. Cryoprecipitate is concentrated from fresh frozen plasma, and each bag has a volume of 10 to 15 ml. Each bag contains at least 150 mg of fibrinogen.

6. **Perform electronic fetal monitoring.**

Amniotic fluid embolism is often accompanied by fetal compromise, and therefore continuous electronic fetal monitoring should be used to follow the fetal status. If the patient has attained complete cervical dilatation, operative vaginal delivery should be performed if it can be accomplished quickly and safely. Delivery will benefit the fetus and will furthermore facilitate efforts to resuscitate the mother. If the cervix is not completely dilated and delivery can be accomplished only by cesarean section, the gestational age and the status of the fetus, the condition of the mother, and the effects of the cesarean section on the mother must all be considered in making the decision to perform surgery.

7 | Fetal Death

■ BACKGROUND AND DEFINITIONS

Fetal death, intrauterine fetal demise (IUFD), or stillbirth: No signs of life present at birth in fetuses beyond 20 weeks of gestational age

Neonatal death: The death of a live-born infant after birth and before 28 days of life

Perinatal mortality rate: The sum of fetal and neonatal deaths per 1000 total births

The fetal death rate in the United States in 1992 was 7.4 per 1000 total births, representing more than half of the perinatal mortality rate, which was 12.8 per 1000 total births. Most states require the reporting of fetal death after 20 weeks of gestation, and many states require the recording of birth weight. The major risk of fetal demise for the mother is consumptive coagulopathy, presumably caused by release of thromboplastin from the dead fetus and the placenta. This complication occurs rarely before 1 month after fetal death, and even then, the incidence of coagulopathy is only approximately 25%.

■ CLINICAL PRESENTATION

Absence of fetal movement detected by the patient
Absence of fetal cardiac activity as recorded by auscultation with a fetoscope or by Doppler monitoring

■ PHONE CALL

Questions

1. What attempts have been made to document fetal viability?

Fetal cardiac activity is not usually detected by auscultation with a fetoscope until after 20 weeks of gestational age, but with a Doppler monitor, fetal cardiac activity is usually detected after 10 weeks of gestation. Fetal movement is not usually felt by the mother until after 20 weeks, but ultrasound examination can usually detect a fetal heart beat at 6 to 7 weeks of gestation.

2. **Was the patient being monitored while in active labor when fetal heart tones were lost?**

   The loss of fetal heart tones during labor is usually caused by movement of the patient that displaces the monitoring device, rather than by fetal death, especially in the absence of abnormal fetal heart rate patterns.

3. **Does the patient have any bleeding suggesting the presence of coagulopathy?**

Degree of Urgency

Fetal death is not life threatening to the patient unless she has disseminated intravascular coagulation (DIC). Nevertheless, because patients are extremely anxious when confronted with the possibility of fetal demise, the patient should be seen as soon as possible.

■ ELEVATOR THOUGHTS

What characteristics of the patient and the pregnancy are associated with an increased risk of fetal death?
- Multiple gestation
- Young maternal age
- Advanced maternal age
- Unmarried status
- Male fetal gender

What are the most common causes of fetal death?
1. Maternal conditions
   - Diabetes mellitus
   - Chronic hypertension
   - Pregnancy-induced hypertension
   - Viral and bacterial infections
      Cytomegalovirus
      Listeria monocytogenes
      Syphilis
   - Rh isoimmunization
   - Antiphospholipid syndrome

      This syndrome is an autoimmune disorder characterized by increased levels of circulating antiphospholipid antibodies. Two such antibodies are lupus anticoagulant antibodies and anticardiolipin antibodies. Patients with this syndrome are at risk for fetal loss, arterial and venous thrombotic events, autoimmune thrombocytopenia, transient ischemic attacks, Coombs'-positive hemolytic anemia, and livedo reticularis of the skin.
   - Thyroid disease

2. Fetal disease
   - Congenital abnormalities
      As many as 35% of fetal deaths are associated with congenital abnormalities.
3. Placental, umbilical cord, and uterine complications
   - Placenta previa
   - Placental abruption
   - Prolapsed umbilical cord
   - Umbilical cord knot
   - Uterine rupture
4. Fetal–maternal hemorrhage

■ MAJOR THREAT TO MATERNAL LIFE

- Hemorrhage secondary to DIC

■ BEDSIDE

Quick Look Test

Does the patient appear to be bleeding?
   Bleeding may be a result of placental abruption, placenta previa, uterine rupture, or DIC.

Is the patient having pelvic pain consistent with placental abruption or uterine rupture?

Does the patient appear to be ill from a systemic infection?

Vital Signs

Vital signs are usually normal unless the patient has developed hypovolemic shock with hypotension and tachycardia from blood loss secondary to coagulopathy, placental abruption, or placenta previa.

Selective History and Chart Review

1. What is the gestational age?
   The gestational age will determine the management and method of delivery.
2. Does the patient have any of the medical conditions that are associated with an increased risk of fetal death?
3. Does the patient have a history of fetal losses?
   Patients with multiple pregnancy losses are more likely to have a recurrent cause. Causes of recurrent pregnancy loss include chromosomal abnormalities in the mother or the

father or both, chronic medical conditions such as diabetes and hypertension, and antiphospholipid syndrome.

Selective Physical Examination

Fetal death is often asymptomatic.

Abdominal	Usually negative
	Tenderness with placental abruption or uterine rupture
Pelvic	Usually negative
External genitalia, vagina, and cervix	Bleeding from placental abruption, placenta previa, or uterine rupture
Uterus and adnexa	Usually normal
	Uterine tenderness with placental abruption or uterine rupture

Orders

1. Obtain a complete blood count (CBC) with differential.
2. Obtain coagulation studies: prothrombin time (PT), partial thromboplastin time (PTT), platelet count, fibrinogen, fibrin split products.
3. Obtain a Kleihauer–Betke stain of maternal blood.
4. Obtain blood type and Rh.
5. Obtain antibody screen.

■ DIAGNOSTIC TESTING

1. Ultrasound examination

Ultrasound examination is used to detect fetal cardiac activity. The absence of cardiac activity is diagnostic of fetal death.

■ MANAGEMENT

Management of a patient with fetal death has three goals. First is safe and timely delivery of the fetus. Timely delivery is especially important because of the emotional trauma associated with fetal death. Second is appropriate support throughout the grieving process for the patient and family. And third is an investigation to attempt to determine the cause of fetal death.

1. Delivery of the fetus

Approximately 80 to 90% of patients who have suffered a fetal death begin spontaneous labor within 2 weeks. The time between fetal death and onset of labor increases proportionately with the degree of prematurity of the fetus.

a. **Prostaglandin E₂ suppository (Prostin) intravaginally every 4 hours**

In pregnancies of <28 weeks' duration, delivery can be facilitated by PGE_2 20-mg suppositories inserted into the vagina every 4 hours until the patient begins to labor. Side effects of PGE_2 include diarrhea, fever, and vomiting; therefore, administration of prophylactic medications should be considered.

b. **Misoprostol (Cytotec) 200 to 800 µg tablets intravaginally every 12 hours**

Misoprostol is contraindicated in advanced pregnancies if the mother has had a prior cesarean delivery.

c. **Oxytocin intravenous infusion**

Intravenous infusion of dilute oxytocin is a well-established and safe method for inducing labor, although it is less successful the more premature the fetus. A solution of **10 IU of oxytocin in 1000 ml of 5% dextrose and lactated Ringer's solution or in 1000 ml of 5% dextrose and 0.5 normal saline** is used. This solution has an oxytocin concentration of 10 mIU/ml; it is infused, starting at a rate of 0.1 ml/min or 1 mIU/min, and is increased until regular uterine contractions are achieved. The infusion rate is increased by 1 mIU/min every 20 to 30 minutes, to a dose of 8 mIU/min. After this dose, the rate can be increased, in increments of 2 mIU/min every 20 to 30 minutes, to a dose of 20 mIU/min. Alternatively, a high-dose regimen can be used. This regimen consists of a starting dose of 6 mIU/min followed by incremental increases of 1 to 6 mIU/min every 20 to 40 minutes to a maximum dose of 42 mIU/min. If higher doses are required, patients should have their fluid intake restricted, and the oxytocin solution should be concentrated. These precautions should be taken because high doses of oxytocin can result in water intoxication due to the antidiuretic effect of oxytocin.

If cervical dilatation and delivery are not accomplished despite the prolonged use of PGE_2 suppositories, misoprostol, or IV oxytocin, ectopic pregnancy and especially abdominal pregnancy should be considered.

2. **Grief and emotional support**

The classic grief reaction to a fetal death includes shock, guilt, anger, disorientation, and reorganization. All health care providers must recognize and meet the emotional needs of the parents and family members going through the grieving process. It should be emphasized to patients that neither they nor their health care providers are to blame for most cases of fetal death. After delivery of the fetus, the parents and family members should be given the opportunity to hold the infant, to name the infant, and to take something as a keepsake, such as a lock of hair or the blanket with which the infant was wrapped. The parents should be given the opportunity to arrange for a funeral service. At the time of discharge from the hospital, patients should be given the telephone numbers of support groups that provide ongoing help.

3. **Investigation of the cause or causes of the fetal death**

    The following tests should be ordered in an attempt to determine the cause of fetal death:

    a. **Blood antibody screen**—Maternal blood group antibodies can cause hemolytic disease of the fetus.

    b. **Kleihauer-Betke stain of maternal blood**—Significant fetal-maternal hemorrhage is a cause of fetal death even in the absence of trauma. Fetal–maternal hemorrhage is detected in 3 to 5% of all fetal deaths. It is detected by a Kleihauer-Betke stain of a blood smear of peripheral maternal blood. After acid-elution treatment, fetal red blood cells, which contain high concentrations of hemoglobin F, stain darkly. In contrast, maternal red blood cells, which contain low concentrations of hemoglobin F, do not stain and therefore appear ghostly.

    c. **VDRL**—Congenital syphilis can result in fetal death.

    d. **Serum glucose**—Poorly controlled diabetes mellitus can be complicated by fetal death.

    e. **Urine toxicology screen**—Illicit drug use can be associated with fetal death.

    Depending on the patient's history and the findings of the physical examination, some of the following tests might be indicated:

    f. **Cytomegalovirus acute and convalescent titers (immunoglobulins M and G)**

    g. **Karyotype of fetal tissue**—A normal karyotype rules out a chromosomal abnormality and makes karyotyping of the parents unnecessary.

    h. **Lupus anticoagulant and anticardiolipin antibody**

    i. **Thyroid function tests**—Both hypothyroidism and hyperthyroidism have been associated with fetal death.

    j. **Cultures for *Listeria monocytogenes***—Maternal blood and placental cultures are the best tests for ruling out listeriosis.

8 | Hypertensive Disorders

■ BACKGROUND AND DEFINITIONS

Hypertensive disorders are encountered in 6 to 8% of pregnancies and are responsible for approximately 12% of all maternal mortality. The classification of hypertensive disorders associated with pregnancy is confusing and not standardized; furthermore, terms used historically add to the confusion. Hypertensive disorders in pregnancy can be classified under two broad categories: **pregnancy-induced hypertension (PIH)**, which refers to hypertensive disorders that are encountered after 20 weeks of gestation, and **chronic hypertension**, which refers to hypertension encountered before 20 weeks of gestation. PIH usually occurs before labor but can also occur in the intrapartum or postpartum period.

The predominant component of PIH is vasospasm. Because vasospasm has numerous end-organ effects, PIH is a disease that can affect many organ systems. PIH can result in impaired perfusion of the kidneys, liver, brain, and placenta. Depending on the specific end-organ effects, several clinical scenarios or syndromes have been identified. The following clinical scenarios or syndromes all fall under the broader and more general heading of PIH:

Preeclampsia: This clinical scenario is one of PIH and renal involvement resulting in proteinuria. The classic triad of clinical findings associated with preeclampsia consists of edema, hypertension, and proteinuria. This triad represents common signs of preeclampsia, not the causes of preeclampsia. Preeclampsia can be present in either a mild form or a severe form.

Eclampsia: In this clinical scenario, central nervous system involvement results in seizures in a patient with preeclampsia and no other condition that causes seizures. As with preeclampsia, eclampsia can occur in the prepartum, intrapartum, or postpartum period.

HELLP syndrome: *H*emolysis, *e*levated *l*iver enzymes, and *l*ow *p*latelet count (HELLP) syndrome is a rare but morbid variant of preeclampsia and of eclampsia. It is usually found in multiparous patients in whom the gestational age of the fetus is less than 36 weeks. HELLP syndrome can be found in as many as 15% of all patients with preeclampsia or eclampsia. Conversely, approximately 50% of the patients with HELLP syndrome have severe preeclampsia, 30% have mild preeclampsia, and 20% are normotensive.

Preeclampsia superimposed on chronic hypertension: In this condition, preeclampsia that develops in a patient with chronic or pre-existent hypertension. The prognosis for patients with pre-eclampsia superimposed on chronic hypertension is often worse than the prognosis for patients with preeclampsia or chronic hypertension alone.

Toxemia of pregnancy: This is an older term used for hypertensive disorders of pregnancy as well as other obstetrical disorders including liver disease and hyperemesis gravidarum. The term toxemia reflects the mistaken belief that these conditions were caused by toxins. The term toxemia of pregnancy is not commonly used today.

■ CLINICAL PRESENTATION

1. **Mild preeclampsia**
   a. **Hypertension**
      (1) Blood pressure (BP) $\geq 140/90$ or
      (2) Mean arterial pressure (MAP) ≥ 105 if prior blood pressure is unknown
      Either of these elevations in blood pressure must be recorded on at least two measurements taken at least 6 hours apart. MAP can be calculated from the BP by the following formula:

   $$MAP = diastolic\ BP + (1/3 \times pulse\ pressure)$$

   where

   $$Pulse\ pressure = systolic\ BP - diastolic\ BP$$

   b. **Edema**
      Edema of the face and hands is more commonly associated with sodium retention and is therefore a more reliable indicator of preeclampsia than edema of the lower extremities, which is more commonly influenced by gravity. A weight gain of ≥ 5 lb in 1 week may also be a sign of impending preeclampsia. The presence of edema cannot be used alone as a diagnostic indicator of preeclampsia because 10 to 15% of normal pregnant women have edema of the face and hands.
   c. **Impaired renal function**
      (1) Proteinuria secondary to glomerular damage
         (a) Urine protein ≥ 0.1 g/L in a random specimen
         (b) Urine protein ≥ 0.3 g/L in a 24-hour urine collection
      (2) Sodium retention
      (3) Decreased glomerular filtration rate
      (4) Decreased clearance of uric acid

(5) Oliguria or anuria

(6) Hematuria

d. Hematological changes

(1) Contraction of volume resulting in hemoconcentration

(2) Thrombocytopenia

e. Central nervous system (CNS) symptoms

(1) Headache, usually frontal and not relieved by analgesics

(2) Mental confusion

(3) Dizziness

(4) Drowsiness

(5) Blurred vision

(6) Scotomata

(7) Diplopia

(8) Flashes of light in the visual field

(9) Blindness

f. Gastrointestinal symptoms

(1) Epigastric pain from distention of the hepatic capsule

(2) Nausea

(3) Vomiting

(4) Hematemesis

2. Severe preeclampsia

a. Hypertension

Systolic blood pressure ≥160 or diastolic blood pressure ≥110 recorded on at least two occasions at least 6 hours apart

b. Proteinuria

Urine protein ≥5 g in a 24-hour collection. This usually correlates with $3+$ or $4+$ on qualitative dipstick test.

c. Oliguria

Urine output ≤500 ml in 24 hours

d. Elevated serum creatinine

e. CNS symptoms

These include signs of CNS involvement such as headaches, scotomata, blurred vision, and seizures.

f. Visual symptoms

g. Epigastric pain

h. Hepatocellular injury

This is manifested by elevated liver enzymes, alanine aminotransferase (ALT) and aspartase aminotransferase (AST).

i. Pulmonary edema

j. Thrombocytopenia

Platelet count $<100,000/mm^3$

k. Microangiopathic hemolysis

l. Intrauterine growth restriction or oligohydramnios

This is manifested by low estimated fetal weight, abnormally low interval growth, or decreased amniotic fluid.

3. Eclampsia
   a. Signs and symptoms of either mild or severe eclampsia
   b. Seizures
   c. Convulsions
   d. Common symptoms that precede eclampsia are listed in Table 8–1.
4. Chronic or pre-existing hypertension
   Blood pressure $\geq 140/90$ recorded before 20 weeks of gestation or after 42 days postpartum or documented before pregnancy.

■ PHONE CALL

Questions

1. **What is the patient's blood pressure?**
2. **What is the result of her urine dipstick test for qualitative protein?**
3. **Does the patient complain of epigastric or right upper quadrant pain?**
   These complaints are ominous because they may be caused by distention of the liver capsule.
4. **Does the patient complain of any neurological or visual symptoms?**
   Severe neurological or visual symptoms are indicative of poor perfusion of the CNS and possibly impending seizures.

Table 8–1 □ FREQUENCY OF SYMPTOMS THAT PRECEDE ECLAMPSIA

Symptom	Patients with Symptom (%)
Headache	83
Hyperreflexia	80
Proteinuria	80
Edema	60
Clonus	46
Visual signs	45
Epigastric pain	20

Adapted from Sibai BM, Lipshitz J, Anderson GD, Dilts PV Jr: Reassessment of intravenous MgSO₄ therapy in preeclampsia-eclampsia. Obstet Gynecol 1981;57:199. Reprinted with permission from the American College of Obstetricians and Gynecologists.

5. **Does the patient have any signs of bleeding from any site?**

Bleeding may be indicative of coagulopathy, which is associated with severe preeclampsia.

Degree of Urgency

Patients with chronic hypertension or mild preeclampsia should be seen as soon as possible. Mild preeclampsia can progress to severe preeclampsia quickly and without warning. Patients with severe preeclampsia or HELLP syndrome must be seen immediately.

■ ELEVATOR THOUGHTS

What factors are associated with an increased risk of pre-eclampsia and eclampsia, and what are the known risk ratios for each risk factor?
- Nulliparity, risk ratio 3:1
- Young maternal age
- Advanced maternal age (>40 years), risk ratio 3:1
- Family history of preeclampsia or eclampsia, risk ratio 5:1
- Antiphospholipid syndrome, risk ratio 10:1
- Lower socioeconomic status, risk ratio 1.5:1

Lower socioeconomic status has not been shown in all studies to be associated with a higher risk of preeclampsia, but it has been clearly shown to be associated with an increased risk of eclampsia.
- Diabetes mellitus, risk ratio 2:1
- Obesity
- Chronic or pre-existent hypertension, risk ratio 10:1
- Chronic renal disease, risk ratio 20:1
- Multiple pregnancy, risk ratio 4:1
- Hydatidiform mole
- Fetal hydrops

What complications can result from preeclampsia?
- Coagulopathy

Thrombocytopenia is probably a result of microangiopathic hemolysis caused by arteriolar spasm. Approximately 10% of patients with either preeclampsia or eclampsia develop disseminated intravascular coagulation (DIC). However, DIC is rare in the absence of placental abruption or severe thrombocytopenia.
- Abnormal renal function

The cause of renal dysfunction in patients with preeclampsia is probably the abnormal renal perfusion that is caused by vasospasm. This results in glomerular damage. Abnormal renal function can progress to renal failure.

- Placental abruption
- Eclampsia
- Hepatic rupture

Distention of the liver capsule, hepatomegaly, liver tenderness, and abnormal liver function tests may be signs of impending hepatic rupture. The maternal mortality rate from hepatic rupture is close to 65%.

■ MAJOR THREAT TO FETAL LIFE

- Fetal compromise from placental insufficiency secondary to vasospasm or placental abruption
- Prematurity

Delivery of the infant is the only true cure for preeclampsia and eclampsia. The severity of preeclampsia and the development of eclampsia are often indications for delivery even at a premature gestational age.

■ MAJOR THREAT TO MATERNAL LIFE

- Hypovolemic shock from hemorrhage due to placental abruption, rupture of the liver, or DIC
- Eclampsia
- Stroke

■ BEDSIDE

Quick Look Test

How ill does the patient appear?

Does the patient have an altered mental status with confusion and drowsiness?

The patient who appears ill or toxemic and who has an altered mental status is at risk for the development of eclampsia.

Does the patient appear to be having abdominal or epigastric pain?

Both placental abruption and distention of the liver capsule can cause abdominal pain.

Vital Signs

The patient is hypertensive but otherwise has normal vital signs, unless rupture of the liver or placental abruption has occurred. These complications usually lead to hypovolemic shock with hypotension and tachycardia.

Selective History and Chart Review

1. Does the patient have a history of chronic hypertension?
2. If the patient has been pregnant before, did she develop preeclampsia or eclampsia during a previous pregnancy?
3. Has the patient had an ultrasound examination during the pregnancy to document gestational age and to rule out multiple gestation or hydatidiform mole?
4. Does the patient have a history of neurological problems including seizures?

Selective Physical Examination

General	Generalized edema including facial and hand edema
	Altered mental status with drowsiness or confusion
	Bleeding from intravenous (IV) and venipuncture sites if DIC develops
Fundoscopic	Narrowing and segmental spasms of the retinal arterioles
Abdominal	Tender if hepatic rupture or placental abruption develops
	Hepatomegaly and liver tenderness may be signs of hepatic capsular distention and impending hepatic rupture
Pelvic	
External genitalia and vagina	Normal
	Vaginal bleeding if placental abruption or DIC develops
Cervix	Normal
Uterus and adnexa	Irritable, tender, and hard if placental abruption develops
Neurological	Hyperactive reflexes
	Clonus
	Seizures if eclampsia develops

Orders

1. Obtain a complete blood count (CBC).
2. Obtain urinalysis.
3. Obtain renal function tests: serum creatinine, serum uric acid, and blood urea nitrogen (BUN).

4. Obtain 24-hour urine collection for protein and creatinine clearance.
5. Obtain liver function tests: AST and ALT.
6. Obtain coagulation studies: platelet count, prothrombin time (PT), partial thromboplastin time (PTT), fibrinogen, fibrin split products.
7. Check the patient's deep tendon reflexes.

■ DIAGNOSTIC TESTING FOR PREGNANCY-INDUCED HYPERTENSION

1. **Ultrasound examination**

   Ultrasound examination should be performed to confirm the gestational age, to determine fetal presentation, and to rule out multiple gestation. Knowing the gestational age of the fetus is important for proper management of the patient with preeclampsia.

2. **Renal function tests**
   a. Serum creatinine: Elevated (normal, 0.5–1.0 mg/dl)
   b. BUN: Elevated (normal, 5–10 mg/dl)
   c. Serum uric acid: Elevated (normal, 3.0–5.5 mg/dl)
   d. 24-hour urine collection for creatinine clearance: Decreased, <100 ml/min (normal, 130–150 ml/min; borderline, 100–129 ml/min)
   e. 24-hour urine collection for total protein: Elevated (≥0.3 g/24 hr is found in mild preeclampsia; >5 g/24 hr is found in severe preeclampsia)
   f. Urinalysis: Proteinuria (3+ or 4+ proteinuria on a qualitative dipstick test is one criterion of severe preeclampsia)

3. **Liver function tests**
   a. AST: Elevated (normal, 8–20 mU/ml)
   b. ALT: Elevated (normal, 8–20 mU/ml)

4. **Hematology tests**
   a. Hematocrit: Elevated secondary to hemoconcentration
   b. Hemolysis may be noted on blood smear

5. **Coagulation studies**
   a. Platelet count: Decreased (normal, 140,000–440,000/mm^3)
   b. Serum fibrinogen: Decreased (normal, 300–600 mg/dl)
   c. PT: Increased (normal, 11–12 seconds)
   d. PTT: Increased (normal, 24–36 seconds)
   e. Fibrin D-dimer: Elevated (normal, <0.05 μg/ml)

■ MANAGEMENT OF PREGNANCY-INDUCED HYPERTENSION

The optimal management for the mother is always delivery, because preeclampsia is reversible and begins to resolve after delivery. The goal of management for the mother is the prevention of eclampsia. When the fetus is considered, however, the risk of fetal prematurity must be weighed against the maternal and the fetal risks of continuing a preeclamptic pregnancy.

1. Decision to deliver

The decision to deliver the infant or to manage the patient expectantly is based on the degree of severity of the patient's preeclampsia and the gestational age of the fetus. The route of delivery is determined by the usual obstetrical factors. If the fetus is stable, a vaginal delivery is preferable to a cesarean birth, because it does not impose surgical stress on a patient who is already ill.

a. Severe preeclampsia

(1) Gestational age >32 weeks—Delivery

Delivery should be considered when the gestational age is >32 weeks because severe preeclampsia is associated with a high risk of eclampsia, impaired renal function, and significant morbidity and mortality. Furthermore, infants born at >32 weeks usually do well and have normal long-term development.

(2) Gestational age <32 weeks—Delivery or expectant management

Some patients with severe preeclampsia improve somewhat on bedrest and with administration of antihypertensive agents and magnesium sulfate. Studies have shown that expectant management can be attempted in such patients. However, extreme care must be taken and delivery should be planned if the patient has persistent or recurrent signs and symptoms of severe preeclampsia. Renal failure, persistent blood pressures >160/110, CNS symptoms, and HELLP syndrome are all indications for delivery. Management of the patient at <28 weeks of gestation is especially difficult because expectant management is often associated with significant morbidity, including placental abruption, eclampsia, and impaired renal function.

b. Mild preeclampsia

(1) Term gestational age—Delivery

In term patients with mild preeclampsia, there is little to be gained by delaying delivery. If the gestational age of the fetus is 33 to 35 weeks, amniocentesis and phospholipid analysis for fetal lung maturity should be considered. If phospholipid analysis shows that lung maturity has been attained, the infant should be delivered. Expectant management is reasonable only to achieve ripening of the cervix in the patient with an unfavorable cervix (see Chapter 10).

(2) Premature gestational age—Expectant management

In the absence of fetal distress or severe intrauterine growth retardation, a preterm patient with mild preeclampsia can be managed expectantly. Because worsening of the disease is likely, both the mother and the infant should be monitored closely. Bedrest is commonly recommended but is only palliative and will only slow the progression of preeclampsia, rather than cure the disease. If both maternal and fetal conditions are stable, the patient should be seen at least once a week. If there is evidence that the preeclampsia is progressing, the patient should be seen more often, as frequently as every 2 or 3 days. Hospitalization of these patients should be considered for closer monitoring. The following maternal parameters should be monitored:

(a) BP
(b) Urine output
(c) Daily weights
(d) Repeat renal function tests: Urinalysis, serum creatinine, BUN, uric acid, 24-hour creatinine clearance, and 24-hour urine protein
(e) Repeat liver function tests: AST, ALT
(f) Repeat coagulation studies: Platelet count, PT, PTT, serum fibrinogen, fibrin split products
(g) Onset of epigastric pain
(h) Onset of neurological symptoms such as headaches or confusion; visual symptoms

The fetus should be monitored with the following tests:

(i) Nonstress testing or
(j) Contraction stress testing with either oxytocin-stimulated or breast-stimulation contractions
(k) Ultrasound examination

Ultrasound examination is used to monitor interval fetal growth and the amount of amniotic fluid present, because intrauterine growth restriction associated with preeclampsia is often accompanied by oligohydramnios. The amount of amniotic fluid can be followed quantitatively (amniotic fluid index [AFI]). AFI is determined by adding the lengths of the largest vertical fluid pockets not containing umbilical cord in each of the four quadrants of the uterus. Normal AFI measurements for different gestational ages are shown in Figure 8–1.

Because preeclampsia usually worsens gradually, the use of corticosteroids should be considered if the fetus is very premature. Antepartum corticosteroid therapy should be considered when the gestational age of the fetus is 24 to 34 weeks. Corticosteroid therapy reduces

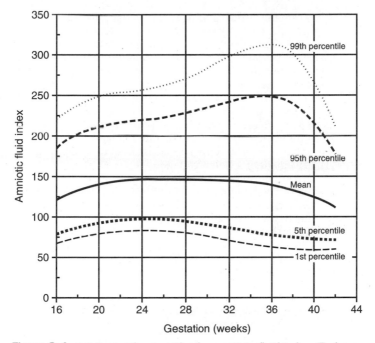

Figure 8–1 □ Mean and percentiles for amniotic fluid index. (Redrawn from Moore TR, Cayle JE: Amniotic fluid index in normal human pregnancy. Am J Obstet Gynecol 1990;162:1168.)

the incidence of respiratory distress syndrome and intraventricular hemorrhage in the neonate. Although the maximum benefits occur 24 hours after the start of treatment, some benefits can be gained sooner. Therefore, corticosteroid therapy should be begun unless delivery is imminent. **Administer 2 ml of betamethasone (Celestone Soluspan) solution intramuscularly (IM); then repeat the dose in 24 hours** (1 ml of Celestone Soluspan contains 3 mg of betamethasone sodium and 3 mg of betamethasone acetate). The effects of treatment last for 7 days, and therefore, a repeat dose should be administered if the infant is not delivered.

2. **Intrapartum management**
   The key issues that must be addressed are as follows: management of fluids and intravascular volume, prophylactic anticonvulsant therapy, and treatment of hypertension. In patients with severe preeclampsia, oliguria and coagulopathy must also be treated in a timely fashion.

a. **Management of fluids and intravascular volume**

In preeclamptic patients, vasospasm results in generalized vasoconstriction, contraction of the intravascular space, and increased vascular permeability. The end result is decreased intravascular fluid and increased extravascular fluid, making the preeclamptic patient extremely sensitive to fluid administration. Fluids must be given carefully to keep the contracted intravascular space expanded without causing excessive spillage into the extravascular space, which results in pulmonary edema. Intrapartum management of fluids and intravascular volume should include the following:

(1) Placement of a Foley catheter

(2) Recording of input and output

(3) Intensive cardiovascular monitoring with either a Swan-Ganz catheter or a central venous pressure (CVP) catheter in patients with eclampsia or severe preeclampsia. Normal central hemodynamic measurements for the pregnancy are shown in Table 8–2.

b. **Prophylactic anticonvulsant therapy**

Most eclamptic seizures occur in the intrapartum and

Table 8–2 □ NORMAL CENTRAL HEMODYNAMIC MEASUREMENTS IN NONPREGNANT AND PREGNANT PATIENTS

Parameter	Nonpregnant	Pregnant
Cardiac output (L/min)	4.3 ± 0.9	6.2 ± 1.0
Heart rate (beats/min)	71 ± 10.0	83 ± 10.0
Systemic vascular resistance ($dyne \times cm \times sec^{-5}$)	1530 ± 520	1210 ± 266
Pulmonary vascular resistance ($dyne \times cm \times sec^{-5}$)	119 ± 47.0	78 ± 22
Colloid oncotic pressure (mm Hg)	20.8 ± 1.0	18.0 ± 1.5
Colloid oncotic pressure–pulmonary capillary wedge pressure (mm Hg)	14.5 ± 2.5	10.5 ± 2.7
Mean arterial pressure (mm Hg)	86.4 ± 7.5	90.3 ± 5.8
Pulmonary capillary wedge pressure (mm Hg)	6.3 ± 2.1	7.5 ± 1.8
Central venous pressure (mm Hg)	3.7 ± 2.6	3.6 ± 2.5
Left ventricular stroke work index ($g \times m \times m^{-2}$)	41 ± 8	48 ± 6

From Clark SL, Cotton DB, Lee W, et al: Central hemodynamic assessment of normal term pregnancy. Am J Obstet Gynecol 1989;161:1439.

postpartum periods. Therefore, prophylactic anticonvulsant therapy should be initiated in the intrapartum period and continued into the postpartum period. Prophylaxis should be given to all preeclamptic patients, because there are no signs or symptoms that can be used with absolute reliability to predict the onset of seizures. Headaches are absent in 17% of patients who develop eclampsia, and hyperactive reflexes are absent in 20% (see Table 8–1). Magnesium sulfate is the most commonly used anticonvulsant agent. The effects of magnesium sulfate are threefold, as follows:

(1) Inhibition of neuromuscular transmission and the cardiac conducting system
(2) Reduction of smooth muscle contractility
(3) Depression of CNS irritability.

The following are the two regimens for the administration of magnesium sulfate:

(1) **Magnesium sulfate 2 to 4 g IV over 5 minutes, as a loading dose, followed by 1.0 g/hr IV, as the maintenance dose**, or
(2) **Magnesium sulfate 2 to 4 g IV over 2 to 4 minutes, concurrently with 10 g IM as the loading dose, followed by 5 g IM every 4 hours**.

Magnesium sulfate therapy should be continued after delivery for at least 24 hours. Undesired side effects of magnesium sulfate include flushing, nausea, and decreased uterine contractility. More serious complications resulting from magnesium toxicity include respiratory depression and cardiac arrest. Therefore, serum magnesium levels should be monitored. The desired serum level for anticonvulsant therapy is 4 to 7 mEq/L. Toxic effects of serum magnesium levels are listed in Table 8–3. If respiratory arrest or cardiac arrest develops, the magnesium sulfate infusion should be discontinued and calcium gluconate should be administered as follows: **Calcium gluconate (10% solution) 10 ml (1 g) IV over 3 minutes.**

Table 8–3 □ SERUM MAGNESIUM LEVELS AND CLINICAL EFFECTS

Clinical Effect	Serum Level (mEq/L)
Loss of patellar reflexes	10
Respiratory depression	10
Respiratory arrest	12
General anesthesia	15
Cardiac arrest	25

c. **Treatment of hypertension**

Antihypertensive therapy is recommended only for patients in whom diastolic blood pressure is persistently >105 mm Hg. Treatment is recommended in these patients to prevent hemorrhagic strokes. There is no evidence that antihypertensive therapy prevents eclampsia. The goal of treatment is not to attain normal blood pressures but to lower the blood pressure to a safer level. Because patients with preeclampsia have a decreased intravascular volume, overly aggressive treatment of hypertension decreases cardiac output and uterine blood flow further and may result in fetal compromise. Because they further reduce intravascular volume, diuretics are not appropriate antihypertensive agents for women with preeclampsia. Antihypertensive agents that can be used for acute hypertension in patients with preeclampsia are listed in Table 8–4. Hydralazine (Apresoline), an antihypertensive commonly used in preeclamptic patients, is a vasodilator. It increases cardiac output and uterine blood flow, and it should be administered as follows:

(1) **Hydralazine 1 mg IV over 1 minute, as a test dose to detect idiosyncratic hypotension; then 5 to 25 mg IV over 2 to 4 minutes.** After 20 minutes, if a diastolic blood pressure of between 90 and 100 mm Hg is not attained, a repeat dose or lower dose can be given.

In rare cases in which hydralazine is not effective, the following antihypertensive agents can be used:

(2) **Nifedipine 10 mg by mouth, and repeat in 4 to 8 hours**
(3) **Labetalol 20 mg IV bolus dose, followed by 10 to 50 mg IV every 10 minutes**

d. **Management of oliguria**

Oliguria in pregnancy is defined as a urine output of less than 20 to 30 ml/hr. Oliguria in preeclamptic patients may be of prerenal or renal origin. Furthermore, oliguria in pregnancy may be secondary to elevated antidiuretic hormone (ADH) resulting from stress or from high-dose oxytocin administration, which also has an antidiuretic effect. If pulmonary edema is not present and there is no history of congestive heart failure, management of oliguria in the preeclamptic patient is as follows:

(1) Intensive cardiovascular monitoring with either a Swan-Ganz catheter or a CVP catheter, and
(2) **IV infusion of 500 to 1000 ml of isotonic crystalloid solution over 1 hour**

e. **Management of DIC**

Management of DIC and blood loss in preeclamptic or eclamptic patients consists of the following:

(1) Red blood cells
Units of packed red blood cells (RBCs) and whole

Table 8–4 □ ANTIHYPERTENSIVE AGENTS USED IN PREECLAMPSIA

| Drug | Time Course of Action | | | Dosage | | Interval Between Doses | Mechanism of Action |
	Onset	Maximum	Duration	IM	Dosage IV		
Hydralazine	10–20 min	20–40 min	3–8 hr	10–50 mg	5–25 mg	3–6 hr	Direct dilatation of arterioles
Trimethaphan camsylate	1–2 min	2–5 min	10 min	—	IV solution, 2 g/L IV infusion rate, 1–5 mg/min		Ganglionic blockade
Sodium nitroprusside	$\frac{1}{2}$–2 min	1–2 min	3–5 min	—	IV solution, 0.01 g/L IV infusion rate, 0.2–0.8 mg/min		Direct dilatation of arterioles and veins
Labetalol	1–2 min	10 min	6–16 hr	—	20–50 mg	3–6 hr	Alpha- and beta-adrenergic blockade
Nifedipine	5–10 min	10–20 min	4–8 hr	—	10 mg orally	4–8 hr	Calcium channel blockade

From Creasy RK, Resnik R: Maternal-Fetal Medicine: Principles and Practice, 4th ed. Philadelphia, WB Saunders Co, 1999, p 860.

blood have volumes of 250 ml and 450 ml, respectively. Each unit of RBCs should increase the hematocrit by 3% and the hemoglobin concentration by 1 g/dl. Coagulation studies should be obtained after every 5 to 10 units of RBCs transfused.

(2) Platelets

Platelets should be transfused for a platelet count of <20,000/mm^3, or for a platelet count of <50,000/mm^3 in patients for whom a cesarean section is planned. Each unit of platelets should increase the platelet count by 5000 to 10,000/mm^3.

(3) Fresh frozen plasma

Fresh frozen plasma should be given to patients with coagulopathy due to deficiency of clotting factors, usually if PT or PTT is >1.5 times normal. Each unit given increases any clotting factor by 2 to 3%. The usual initial dose is 2 units, and each unit has a volume of 200 to 250 ml.

(4) Cryoprecipitate

Cryoprecipitate should be administered to patients with coagulopathy due to deficiency of factor VIII, von Willebrand's factor, factor XIII, fibrinogen, and/or fibronectin. Cryoprecipitate is concentrated from fresh frozen plasma, and each bag has a volume of 10 to 15 ml. Each bag contains at least 150 mg of fibrinogen.

As is the case with fluid administration, the transfusion of blood products must be performed carefully in preeclamptic and eclamptic women to prevent fluid overload and pulmonary edema.

3. **Treatment of eclampsia**

Eclamptic seizures usually resolve spontaneously in 1 to 2 minutes; therefore, protection of the patient from injury, prevention of aspiration, and establishment of an airway are the initial goals in addition to drug therapy. If seizures develop before the administration of prophylactic magnesium, the following should be given:

a. **Magnesium sulfate 4 g IV or IM**

A maintenance dose of either 1.0 g/hr IV or 5 g IM every 4 hours can then be given. If seizures develop while the patient is already receiving magnesium sulfate, treatment with one of the following anticonvulsant drugs should be initiated:

(1) **Diazepam (Valium) 5 g IV**, or

(2) **Pentobarbital (Nembutal) 125 mg IV**

9 | Incompetent Cervix

■ BACKGROUND AND DEFINITION

Incompetent cervix: Painless cervical dilatation and/or efface-ment that occurs in the second or early third trimester of preg-nancy in the absence of uterine contractions. The natural history includes the ballooning of the fetal membranes into the vagina with subsequent rupture of membranes and delivery of an imma-ture fetus. Incompetent cervix is a common cause of pregnancy loss in the second trimester (Table 9–1).

■ CLINICAL PRESENTATION

Painless cervical dilatation
Painless cervical effacement
Vaginal discharge
Vaginal bleeding or spotting
Premature rupture of membranes

■ PHONE CALL

Questions

1. What is the gestational age of the fetus?
2. Has the patient had rupture of membranes?
3. Does the patient appear to be having uterine contrac-tions?

Table 9–1 ◻ COMMON CAUSES OF PREGNANCY LOSS IN THE
SECOND TRIMESTER

Incompetent cervix
Fetal chromosomal abnormality
Uterine anomaly
Uterine leiomyomata
Premature rupture of membranes
Premature labor
Systemic infection (pyelonephritis, appendicitis)

Degree of Urgency

Incompetent cervix can progress quickly from cervical dilatation, to prolapse of the amniotic sac into the vagina, to rupture of membranes, and finally, to the delivery of an often nonviable fetus. The success of treatment of this condition depends on early diagnosis and intervention. Therefore, patients with suspected incompetent cervix should be seen immediately.

■ ELEVATOR THOUGHTS

What are the causes of incompetent cervix?
- Previous cervical trauma
    1. Cervical conization or amputation
    2. Extensive cervical dilatation as done in second-trimester pregnancy terminations
    3. Cervical laceration at the time of a prior vaginal delivery
- In utero exposure to diethylstilbestrol (DES)

    DES exposure in utero has been associated with an increased risk of cervical incompetence, spontaneous abortion, and preterm labor and delivery. The absence of structural abnormalities commonly seen in DES-exposed patients, such as cervical collars, hoods, and cock's combs, does not necessarily preclude cervical incompetence.

■ MAJOR THREAT TO FETAL LIFE

- Prematurity

    Cervical incompetence is not life threatening to the mother but can result in delivery of a previable or premature infant.

■ BEDSIDE

Quick Look Test

Does the patient appear to be having uterine contractions?

Is there evidence of gross rupture of membranes?

Both rupture of membranes and uterine contractions are poor prognostic signs that make surgical intervention with cervical cerclage placement contraindicated.

Vital Signs

Vital signs are usually normal. The presence of a fever may be a result of chorioamnionitis secondary to premature rupture of membranes.

Selective History and Chart Review

1. What is the gestational age of the fetus?
    The gestational age of the fetus affects the management of the patient.
2. Has the patient had a prior ultrasound examination?
    A prior ultrasound examination can be used to confirm gestational age; more importantly, it can also be used to rule out fetal anomalies before placement of a cervical cerclage.

Selective Physical Examination

Abdominal	Normal
Pelvic	
External genitalia and vagina	Normal or prolapsing of membranes into the vagina
Cervix	Dilated, effaced, and shortened
Uterus and adnexa	Normal unless patient is in labor or has chorioamnionitis, which results in uterine tenderness

Orders

1. Place the patient at bedrest in Trendelenburg position.
2. Start an intravenous access line.
3. Begin electronic fetal heart rate monitoring and uterine monitoring.

■ DIAGNOSTIC TESTING

There are no specific diagnostic tests for incompetent cervix; the diagnosis is based on clinical findings.

1. Ultrasound examination

Not only is an ultrasound examination useful for confirming gestational age of the fetus and for evaluating the fetus for fetal anomalies, but it can also be used to measure cervical length and dilatation. Serial ultrasound examinations can be used to detect change in cervical dilatation and change in cervical shortening. The length of the normal cervix remains constant at 5.2 ± 1.2 cm until 34 weeks of gestation, when gradual shortening of the cervix begins. Furthermore, ultrasound examination can detect ballooning or beaking of the membranes through the dilated cervix. This is the hallmark ultrasound finding in a patient with an incompetent cervix.

■ MANAGEMENT

1. Cervical cerclage

Cervical cerclage is best performed at a fetal gestational age of >14 weeks, so that the patient is beyond the first trimester, when spontaneous abortion of an abnormal fetus frequently occurs. The success of cervical cerclage is inversely related to the amount of cervical dilatation, and it is best performed before the cervix has dilated >2 cm. Cervical cultures for gonorrhea, for group B streptococcus, and for chlamydia should be performed, and patients with positive cultures should be treated before cerclage placement.

The two most common types of cervical cerclage are the McDonald cerclage and the Shirodkar cerclage. There is usually less cervical trauma and blood loss with the McDonald cerclage. The success rate for both procedures is 75 to 90%. After placement of the cerclage, tocolytics such as **terbutaline 2.5 mg by mouth (PO) every 4 hours** or **0.25 mg subcutaneously (SC) every 4 hours** or **indomethacin 25 mg PO every 6 hours** can be administered for 24 hours, although the benefits of tocolytics have not been clearly established. Sexual intercourse should be prohibited for at least 1 week after the procedure. The patient should have cervical examinations every 1 to 2 weeks to detect any cervical dilatation in the presence of the cerclage.

Cervical cerclage is contraindicated if the patient has ruptured membranes, uterine contractions, vaginal bleeding of unknown cause, intrauterine infection, cervical infection, or fetal anomalies. Complications of cervical cerclage include rupture of membranes, chorioamnionitis, vesicovaginal and urethrovaginal fistulas, and displacement of the suture. Rupture of membranes usually occurs in the perioperative period, but it can also occur intraoperatively, especially if advanced cervical dilatation has occurred.

The cerclage should be cut when the fetus has reached term, and preferably before onset of labor. If this is not performed before labor begins, the patient can incur uterine rupture or cervical laceration. Even after removal of the cerclage, the patient in labor can develop a cervical laceration because of the prior cerclage placement. Furthermore, the cervix might dilate abnormally because of scarring from the cerclage. Alternatively, if the patient intends another pregnancy and the cerclage placement was difficult to achieve, the cerclage can be left in place and a cesarean section can be planned. The optimal management has not been established for the patient with a cerclage who undergoes preterm premature rupture of membranes. Some advocate removal of the cerclage in order to avoid infection, while others have found no difference in infectious complications if the cerclage is left in place until the onset of labor. The incidence rates of complications resulting from cervical cerclage are listed in Table 9–2.

Table 9–2 □ **INCIDENCE RATES OF COMPLICATIONS OF CERVICAL CERCLAGE**

Complication	Incidence (%)
Rupture of membranes	1–9
Chorioamnionitis	1–8
Cervical laceration	1–13
Displacement of the suture	3–13
Vesicovaginal or urethrovaginal fistulas	Rare
Uterine rupture	Rare
Abnormal cervical dilatation	Rare

2. Bedrest without cervical cerclage

If there are contraindications to the placement of a cervical cerclage, the patient should be managed expectantly with bedrest. This management can also be used for patients with advanced cervical dilatation. The tocolytic drugs described previously can also be administered to these patients, or more aggressive drug therapy, as discussed in Chapter 21, can be used.

10 | Induction of Labor and Cervical Ripening

■ BACKGROUND AND DEFINITIONS

Approximately 18% of all deliveries in the United States are induced. This represents a twofold increase from 10 years ago.

Induction of labor: The artifical stimulation of uterine contractions before the onset of spontaneous labor

Augmentation of labor: The artificial stimulation of uterine contractions after labor has already begun spontaneously

Cervical ripening: The artificial means by which the cervix is made more favorable for induction of labor

■ CLINICAL PRESENTATION

Indications

Common indications for induction of labor include the following:
- Abruptio placentae
   When the hemodynamics and coagulation status of the mother are stable and the fetal heart rate pattern is reassuring, induction of labor may be considered in patients with abruptio placentae.
- Chorioamnionitis
- Fetal demise
- Hypertensive disorders
- Logistical reasons
   Logistical reasons are nonmedical reasons. These may include availability of the delivering health care provider, risk of rapid labor, distance from the hospital, availability of transportation to the hospital, and availability of the father of the baby and other support persons.
- Maternal medical conditions
   These include cardiac disease, diabetes mellitus, chronic pulmonary disease, and renal disease. Under many of these conditions, pregnancy causes exacerbation of the disease, which in turn may jeopardize fetal well-being.
- Nonreassuring fetal status
   These include severe intrauterine growth restriction, oligohydramnios, and isoimmunization.

- Postterm pregnancy

    A postterm pregnancy is one that persists beyond 42 weeks after the last menstrual period in a woman with regular 28-day menstrual cycles. Approximately 10% of all pregnancies are postterm, and postterm pregnancy is the most common indication for induction of labor. In some series, postterm pregnancy was the indication for 45% of all labor inductions.
- Premature rupture of membranes

Contraindications

Contraindications to induction of labor are generally the same as contraindications to labor and vaginal delivery. These include the following:
- Active genital herpes simplex infection
- Placenta previa
- Prior classical cesarean section
- Prolapsed umbilical cord
- Transverse fetal lie
- Vasa previa

Precautions Needed

There are clinical conditions under which induction of labor is not contraindicated but extra precaution should be taken. These include the following:
- Abnormal fetal heart rate pattern not requiring emergency delivery
- Breech presentation
- Grand multiparity
- History of one or more low transverse cesarean sections
- Maternal cardiac disease
- Multiple gestation
- Polyhydramnios
- Presenting fetal part above the pelvic inlet
- Severe pregnancy-induced hypertension

■ MAJOR THREAT TO FETAL LIFE

Uterine hyperstimulation and fetal heart rate deceleration are potential side effects of both labor induction and cervical ripening. These complications are dose-related and resolve with either a decrease in the dose or discontinuation of the induction or ripening agent.

■ MAJOR THREAT TO MATERNAL LIFE

- Uterine rupture
    Uterine rupture is rare, but caution should be used with patients who have had prior cesarean sections.
- Water intoxication
    Oxytocin has an antidiuretic effect, and water intoxication can occur after prolonged administrations at high doses (>40 mIU/min).

■ BEDSIDE

Quick Look Test

If induction of labor is planned for a maternal medical condition, a hypertensive disorder, or abruptio placentae, is the patient stable enough to undergo induction?

Does the fetal heart rate pattern show fetal well-being?

It is rare for vaginal delivery to be achieved in less than 6 hours after initiation of induction of labor. If cervical ripening is necessary, delivery may not be achieved for 24 hours or longer. Therefore, if either maternal or fetal status is deteriorating, cesarean section might be more appropriate.

Selective History and Chart Review

1. Do the benefits of labor induction outweigh the potential risks of the procedure?
2. If labor induction is elective, is there sufficient evidence of fetal maturity?
    The American College of Obstetricians and Gynecologists (ACOG) recommends that at least one of the criteria listed in Table 10–1 be met or that fetal lung maturity be confirmed by amniotic fluid testing if labor induction is elective and performed for logistical reasons.

Table 10–1 □ ACOG CONFIRMATION OF TERM GESTATION

Fetal heart tones have been documented for 20 weeks by nonelectronic fetoscope or for 30 weeks by Doppler ultrasound.

It has been 36 weeks since a positive serum or urine human chorionic gonadotropin pregnancy test was performed by a reliable laboratory.

An ultrasound measurement of the crown-rump length, obtained at 6–12 weeks, supports a gestational age of at least 39 weeks.

An ultrasound study obtained at 13–20 weeks confirms a gestational age of at least 39 weeks determined by clinical history and physical examination.

Table 10–2 □ BISHOP SCORE

Factor	Points Assigned			
	0	1	2	3
Cervical effacement (%)	0–30	40–50	60–70	>80
Cervical dilation (cm)	0	1–2	3–4	5–6
Cervical consistency	Firm	Average	Soft	—
Cervical position	Posterior	Midposition	Anterior	—
Station	−3	−2	−1 or 0	+1 or +2

Selective Physical Examination

Pelvic
   Cervix   Effacement, dilation, consistency, position, pre-
               senting part, and the station of the presenting
               part should be determined

   Induction of labor is more often successful if the patient has a
favorable cervix. The Bishop score (Table 10–2) can be used to
quantify the status of the cervix. To calculate the Bishop score,
points are given for effacement, dilation, consistency, and position
of the cervix as well as the station of the presenting part of the
fetus. The cervix is given a score between 0 and 13, and a score
of 9 or more is considered favorable. Induction with an unfavorable cervix is associated with increased maternal and fetal morbidity and a higher risk of prolonged labor, failed induction, and
cesarean section.

Orders

1. Initiate external electronic fetal heart rate monitoring to assess the fetal status.
2. Prepare the patient for a cervical examination to assess the
   Bishop score.

■ DIAGNOSTIC TESTING

1. **Ultrasound examination**
      An ultrasound examination can be ordered to confirm gesta-
   tional age and fetal presentation.
2. **Tests for fetal lung maturity**
      The benefits of labor induction must be weighed against
   potential risks to the fetus. In some cases, the benefits of
   induction outweigh the risks associated with prematurity. In
   other cases, fetal lung maturity is a factor in the decision to
   induce labor. Amniocentesis and phospholipid analysis can be

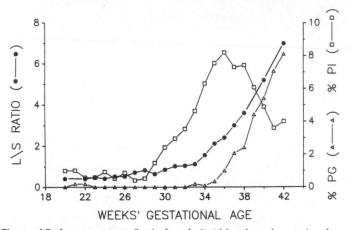

Figure 10–1 □ Amniotic fluid phospholipid levels and gestational age. L/S = lecithin-to-sphingomyelin; PG = phosphatidylglycerol; PI = phosphatidylinositol. (From Creasy RK, Resnik R: Maternal-Fetal Medicine: Principles and Practice, 4th ed. Philadelphia, WB Saunders Co, 1999, p 417. Data from Gluck L, et al: Am J Obstet Gynecol 1974;120:142, and Hallman M, et al: Am J Obstet Gynecol 1976;125:613, as shown in Jobe A: The developmental biology of the lung. In Fanaroff AA, Martin RJ [eds]: Neonatal-Perinatal Medicine. St Louis, Mosby–Year Book, 1992, p 792.)

performed to document fetal lung maturity. A **lecithin-to-sphingomyelin (L/S) ratio** >2 and the presence of **phosphatidylglycerol (PG)** are suggestive of fetal lung maturity (Fig. 10–1). Alternatively, a foam stability test or "shake test" can be performed, as described in Chapter 21.

■ MANAGEMENT

1. Cervical ripening

Mechanical cervical ripeners including intracervical balloon-tipped catheters, hygroscopic dilators, and *Laminaria* have been used in the past, but they have been replaced by prostaglandin agents. The two prostaglandins used are dinoprostone (prostaglandin E_2) and misoprostol, a prostaglandin E_1 analog. Currently, there are three prostaglandin agents available for cervical ripening: dinoprostone gel (Prepidil), dinoprostone vaginal insert (Cervidil), and misoprostol (Cytotec). Because of the low dose of prostaglandins in these agents, maternal side effects such as fever, vomiting, and diarrhea are rare. Furthermore, because prostaglandin E_2 is a bronchodilator, there have been no reports of bronchoconstriction.

a. **Dinoprostone gel (Prepidil) 0.5 mg intracervical every 6 hours**

Dinoprostone gel is available in a prefilled applicator containing 0.5 mg of dinoprostone in 2.5 ml of triacetin and colloidal silicon dioxide gel. The gel should be stored in the refrigerator and warmed to room temperature just before use. Administration requires the use of a speculum. Repeat doses may be administered every 6 hours. The maximum recommended dose is 3 gel applications or 1.5 mg of dinoprostone in 24 hours. Typically, oxytocin is started after ripening with the gel. It is recommended that oxytocin not be started until 6 to 12 hours after the last gel application. Dinoprostone gel is associated with a 1% rate of uterine hyperstimulation. In these patients, irrigation of the cervix and vagina is not beneficial.

b. **Dinoprostone vaginal insert (Cervidil) 10 mg every 12 hours**

Dinoprostone vaginal insert consists of 10 mg of dinoprostone contained in a thin, flat hydrogel chip that is encased within a knitted polyester pouch with a removal cord. Dinoprostone is released at a rate of 0.3 mg/hr over 12 hours. The insert should be placed transversely in the posterior fornix of the vagina, and the removal cord should be left in the vagina. A speculum is not needed for insertion. After insertion, the patient should remain supine for 2 hours but thereafter may ambulate. Oxytocin can be administered 30 minutes after removal of the insert. The use of dinoprostone inserts is associated with a 5% rate of uterine hyperstimulation. In these patients, removal of the insert usually results in resolution of the hyperstimulation within 2 to 13 minutes.

c. **Misoprostol (Cytotec) 25 to 50 μg intravaginally or orally every 3 to 6 hours**

Misoprostol is used for the prevention of peptic ulcers. It is not approved by the U.S. Food and Drug Administration for cervical ripening or induction of labor, although its use for these indications is common and is supported by the ACOG. Currently, misoprostol is available in 100-μg and 200-μg tablets. Typically a 100-μg tablet is broken into halves or quarters. Misoprostol is not recommended for cervical ripening in patients with prior uterine surgery, including cesarean section.

2. **Induction of labor**
   a. **Membrane stripping**

Membrane stripping is performed by using a finger through a partially dilated cervix to separate the amniotic membranes from the wall of the cervix and the lower uterine segment. Even though this procedure is often used for the induction of labor, its efficacy is not well established.

Membrane stripping is most successful in postterm pregnancies. The mechanism of action is increased prostaglandin $F_{2\alpha}$ and phospholipase A_2 activity.

b. **Amniotomy**

Amniotomy, or artificial rupture of amniotic membranes, can be performed with or without oxytocin administration to induce labor. In order to perform amniotomy safely, there must be adequate cervical dilation, and the presenting fetal part must be well applied to the cervix. Risks associated with this procedure include prolapse of the umbilical cord and maternal and fetal infection.

c. **Oxytocin (Pitocin)**

Oxytocin is typically administered in a **dilute solution of 10 IU oxytocin in 1000 ml of 5% dextrose and lactated Ringer's solution (D5 LR) or 5% dextrose and 0.5 normal saline (D5 1/2 NS).** This solution has a concentration of 10 mIU/ml and is administered intravenously by an infusion pump. Several dose regimens can be used.

(1) Low-dose regimens

Low-dose regimens use a starting dose of 0.5 to 2 mIU/min and increase in increments of 1 to 2 mIU/min every 15 to 40 minutes.

A commonly used regimen uses a starting dose of 1 mIU/min. The dose is then increased by 1 mIU/min every 20 to 30 minutes up to a dose of 8 mIU/min. Thereafter, the dose is increased by 2 mIU/min every 20 to 30 minutes up to a dose of 20 mIU/min.

(2) High-dose regimens

High-dose regimens use a starting dose of 6 mIU/min and increase in increments of 1 mIU/min, 3 mIU/min, or 6 mIU/min every 20 to 40 minutes up to a maximum dose of 42 mIU/min.

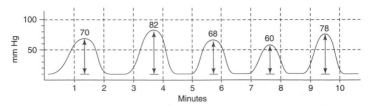

Figure 10–2 □ Calculation of Montevideo units. The term "Montevideo units" was coined by Caldeyro-Barcia and Alvarez in 1960. Montevideo units are calculated by summing the intensity (mm Hg) of all uterine contractions in a 10-minute period. In this example, the sum of all contractions yielded 358 Montevideo units.

In this regimen, increments of 6 mIU/min are used under normal circumstances. If hyperstimulation is encountered, then increments of 3 mIU/min are used. If the hyperstimulation is recurrent, then increments of 1 mIU/min are used.

Uterine response usually occurs 3 to 5 minutes after intravenous administration, and a steady state in the plasma is achieved after 40 minutes. Adequate uterine contractions usually generate between 95 and 395 Montevideo units. Montevideo units are calculated by adding the differences between the peak uterine pressure and the baseline uterine pressure (as measured by internal uterine pressure catheter) for each contraction in a 10-minute period (Fig. 10–2). Low-dose regimens are associated with a lower frequency of uterine hyperstimulation than high dose regimens whereas high-dose regimens are associated with shorter labor and a lower frequency of cesarean section. Because oxytocin has a plasma half-life of 1 to 6 minutes, hyperstimulation usually resolves minutes after oxytocin infusion is decreased or discontinued.

If high doses (>40 mIU/min) of oxytocin are administered for a prolonged period, water intoxication can occur. These patients should be placed on fluid restriction. Furthermore, more concentrated solutions of oxytocin should be used to further restrict fluid intake.

11 | Malpresentation

■ BACKGROUND AND DEFINITIONS

Malpresentation: Any fetal presentation other than vertex. The most common malpresentation is the breech presentation. Other abnormal presentations are brow presentation, face presentation, transverse lie, oblique lie, and compound presentations. The term malpresentation can also be used to refer to a vertex presentation that is not normal. Vertex presentations with severe extension of the fetal head or asynclitism are not normal and can result in dystocia.

Breech presentation: The presenting fetal part is the buttock, the sacrum, or the lower extremities (Fig. 11–1)

> **Frank breech:** Both lower extremities are flexed at the hips but extended at the knees, resulting in a U-shaped fetus with the feet close to the head
>
> **Complete breech:** Both lower extremities are flexed at the hips and one or both of the knees are also flexed
>
> **Incomplete breech:** One or both of the lower extremities are extended at the hips and one or both knees are extended so that the knees or the feet are presenting
>
> > **Single footling breech:** Incomplete breech presentation with one foot presenting

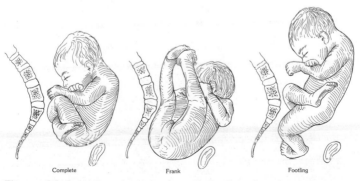

Complete   Frank   Footling

Figure 11–1 □ Complete, frank, and footling breech presentations. (From Hacker NF, Moore JG: Essentials of Obstetrics and Gynecology, 3rd ed. Philadelphia, WB Saunders Co, 1998, p 271.)

Double footling breech: Incomplete breech presentation with both feet presenting

Transverse lie: The axis of the fetus is perpendicular to that of the mother so that the shoulder is often the presenting part (Fig. 11–2). When a patient with a transverse lie is encountered before 39 weeks of gestational age, there is an 80 to 85% incidence of spontaneous conversion to a longitudinal lie, either vertex or breech.

Oblique lie: The axis of the fetus forms an acute angle with the axis of the mother. This malpresentation is usually transitory and converts to either a longitudinal lie (vertex or breech) or a transverse lie. Therefore, it is also referred to as an **unstable lie**.

Face presentation: The presenting part is the fetal chin or the mentum (Fig. 11–3). This malpresentation is the result of full extension of the fetal head so that the occiput comes into contact with the fetal back.

Brow presentation: The presenting part is the fetal brow, that portion of the head between the anterior fontanel and the orbital ridge (Fig. 11–4). Brow presentation is caused by partial extension of the head.

Compound presentations: A fetal extremity, usually an arm or a hand and less often a lower extremity, prolapses down and presents simultaneously with the presenting part.

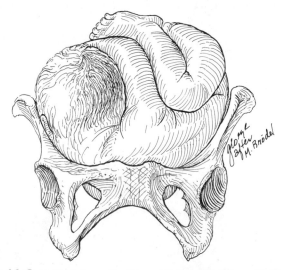

Figure 11–2 □ Transverse lie. (From Hacker NF, Moore JG: Essentials of Obstetrics and Gynecology, 3rd ed. Philadelphia, WB Saunders Co, 1998, p 279.)

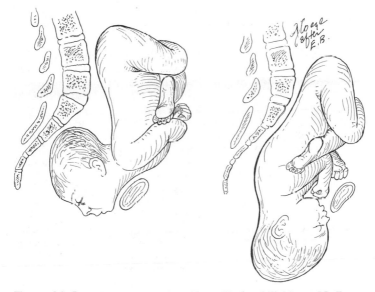

Figure 11–3 □ Face presentation. (From Hacker NF, Moore JG: Essentials of Obstetrics and Gynecology, 3rd ed. Philadelphia, WB Saunders Co, 1998, p 277.)

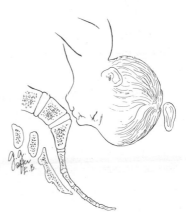

Figure 11–4 □ Brow presentation. (From Hacker NF, Moore JG: Essentials of Obstetrics and Gynecology, 3rd ed. Philadelphia, WB Saunders Co, 1998, p 278.)

Asynclitism: Deflection of the head so that the sagittal suture does not lie exactly midway between the promontory of the sacrum and the pubic symphysis. Asynclitism is anterior if the sagittal suture is deflected toward the sacral promontory and posterior if the sagittal suture is deflected toward the pubic symphysis (Fig. 11–5).

The most commonly encountered malpresentation is the breech presentation. Approximately 3 to 4% of singleton term pregnancies are complicated by this malpresentation. The incidence of breech presentation decreases with increasing gestational age. At 18 to 22 weeks of gestation, the incidence of breech presentation is almost 25%. At 28 to 34 weeks, the incidence is 7 to 8%, and at term, the incidence is 2.8%. Other malpresentations occur much less frequently than breech presentation. Transverse lie has a frequency of 0.24 to 0.3%. The incidence of face presentation is between 0.17 and 0.2%; and brow presentation is encountered in only 0.02%. Compound presentations are found in 0.05 to 0.14% of pregnancies. The incidence of all malpresentations is higher in pregnancies of earlier gestational ages.

At every gestational age, the fetal morbidity and mortality rates are higher for breech fetuses, compared with vertex fetuses. The overall mortality rate for breech fetuses is approximately 8.5%, even with cesarean delivery, compared with 2.2% for vertex fetuses. This increase is a result not only of complications encountered during labor and delivery but also of the increased incidence of preterm delivery, intrauterine growth restriction, and congenital anomalies in breech fetuses. Furthermore, it is possible that fetuses that do not spontaneously change their presentation to vertex may be abnormal and compromised in some way.

■ CLINICAL PRESENTATION

When the patient is not in labor or is in early labor, there may be no specific symptoms that are associated with malpresentation.
- Prolapsed umbilical cord
  Malpresentation is associated with a higher incidence of umbilical cord prolapse once membranes are ruptured.
- Abnormal labor
  Malpresentation is associated with a greater frequency of abnormal labor.

■ PHONE CALL

Questions

1. What is the fetus' gestational age?
If the fetus is not near term, breech presentation is a

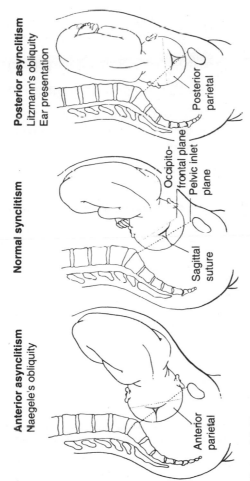

Anterior asynclitism
Naegele's obliquity

Anterior parietal

Normal synclitism

Occipito-frontal plane
Pelvic inlet plane

Sagittal suture

Posterior asynclitism
Litzmann's obliquity
Ear presentation

Posterior parietal

Figure 11-5 □ Synclitism and asynclitism. (From Cunningham FC, MacDonald PC, Gant NF, et al: Williams' Obstetrics, 19th ed. Norwalk, CT, Appleton & Lange, 1993, p 365. Reproduced with permission of The McGraw-Hill Companies.)

common and normal finding. If the patient is not in labor and membranes have not ruptured, the fetus may spontaneously turn to a vertex presentation. Therefore, these patients may be managed expectantly. As the gestational age approaches term, the likelihood of spontaneous version diminishes.

2. Is the patient in active labor?

In the patient in active labor with a malpresentation, the decision on the route of delivery must be made. Active labor is a contraindication to external cephalic version of the fetus in the breech presentation.

3. Is there evidence or a history of rupture of membranes?

Rupture of membranes makes external cephalic version technically more difficult. In patients with a breech presentation other than frank breech, rupture of membranes places the fetus at risk for prolapse of the umbilical cord.

4. Is there evidence of fetal compromise found on fetal heart rate monitoring?

The presence of nonreassuring fetal heart rate patterns is a contraindication to external cephalic version of a breech fetus. The management of patients with malpresentations and abnormal fetal heart rate patterns should be the same as the management of patients with vertex presentations. The only exception is that internal fetal monitoring is not recommended in the patient with a face presentation because of potential scarring of the fetus' face.

Degree of Urgency

If the patient is in labor or has ruptured membranes, she should be evaluated immediately so that a plan for management in labor and the route of delivery can be made.

■ ELEVATOR THOUGHTS

What factors increase the incidence of breech presentation?
- Early gestational age
- Multiple gestation
- Fetal anencephaly
- Fetal hydrocephalus
- Polyhydramnios
- Oligohydramnios
- Uterine anomaly
- Uterine or pelvic mass
- Multiparity resulting in uterine relaxation
- Placenta previa

- Fundal or cornual implantation of the placenta
- Previous pregnancy with breech presentation

What complications are associated with abnormal presentations?

- Increased perinatal morbidity and mortality from difficult delivery

    Vaginal delivery of the breech infant is complicated because the diameter of the fetal head is normally larger than that of the buttocks. This discrepancy is even greater when the fetus is premature. Furthermore, in the breech presentation, the fetal head does not undergo molding as it does in the vertex presentation. Therefore, the fetal buttocks and torso can be delivered through a cervix that is not dilated enough to allow delivery of the head. Once entrapment of the head occurs, if delivery is not accomplished soon, fetal hypoxia develops because of compression of the umbilical cord in the vagina. If an excessive amount of traction is applied to the fetus in an attempt to facilitate delivery, fetal trauma can occur. The most commonly injured organs are the brain, spinal cord, liver, spleen, adrenal glands, and brachial plexus. Although cesarean delivery of the breech fetus is often less traumatic than vaginal delivery, it does not preclude birth injury, because the fetus still must be delivered as a breech through the uterine incision.

- Preterm delivery
- Congenital anomalies

    The incidence of congenital anomalies in pregnancies complicated by breech presentation is 6 to 7%, compared with 2 to 2.5% for pregnancies with normal presentations.

- Abnormal labor

    Labor usually progresses normally with a fetus in the frank breech presentation. However, with certain malpresentations, such as transverse lie and face presentation with the fetal chin posterior, referred to as the mentum posterior position, labor progresses abnormally and vaginal delivery is impossible.

- Increased risk of cesarean section
- Intrauterine growth restriction
- Umbilical cord prolapse

    Transverse lie, complete breech, and incomplete breech presentations are all associated with an increased risk of umbilical cord prolapse after rupture of membranes, because in these presentations, there is no fetal part that is applied to the dilating cervix to act as a plug. The incidence of umbilical cord prolapse with a frank breech presentation is approximately 0.5%, which is comparable to the incidence of cord prolapse in vertex presentation (almost 0.4%). The incidence of cord prolapse is 5 to 6% with a complete breech presentation and 15 to 18% with a footling breech presentation.

■ MAJOR THREAT TO FETAL LIFE

- Birth trauma
- Prematurity
- Congenital anomalies

The major threat is to the life of the fetus. Maternal mortality is increased only very slightly because of the greater frequency of cesarean section.

■ BEDSIDE

Quick Look Test

Does the patient appear to be in labor?

If the patient is in active labor, external cephalic version is contraindicated, and therefore a management plan should be made for delivery of the breech fetus.

Are there abnormal fetal heart rate patterns suggestive of fetal compromise?

If abnormal fetal heart rate patterns suggestive of fetal compromise are present on electronic fetal monitoring, prolapse of the umbilical cord should be ruled out.

Does the patient appear to have a premature pregnancy?

If the patient is in labor with a breech fetus and the estimated fetal weight is less than 1500 g, vaginal delivery is not usually recommended, and cesarean section should be performed if progression of labor cannot be halted.

Vital Signs

Vital signs are usually normal.

Selective History and Chart Review

1. Has the patient had an ultrasound examination during her pregnancy to rule out congenital anomalies?

    Lethal fetal anomalies such as anencephaly must be ruled out by ultrasound examination so that an unnecessary cesarean section is not performed.

2. What is the best estimate of the gestational age of the fetus based on the date of the patient's last menstrual period and ultrasound examinations performed early in pregnancy?

    Knowledge of the gestational age of the fetus is essential

for developing a plan for delivery of the fetus with a malpresentation.

Selective Physical Examination

Abdominal

Breech presentation: Round, hard fetal head is palpable high in the fundal region of the uterus. Fetal heart sounds are heard loudest above the umbilicus.

Transverse lie: Abdomen is wide from one side to the other. Fundal height is low, often extending only slightly above the umbilicus. A hard band is palpable across the front of the abdomen if the fetal back is anterior. Irregular nodular fetal extremities or "small parts" are palpable across the front of the abdomen if the fetal back is posterior.

Oblique lie: Fetal head is palpable in the right or left lower quadrant.

Pelvic
External genitalia
and vagina

Footling breech: Fetal feet can be palpable in the vagina if the cervix is dilated.

Transverse lie: Prolapsed arm may be palpable if the cervix is dilated.

Cervix

Frank breech: Fetal buttock is palpable with the anus and both ischial tuberosities forming a straight line. This is in contrast to the triangle formed by the mouth and malar eminences in a face presentation.

Complete and incomplete breech: Fetal feet or buttock is palpable.

Transverse and oblique lie: Early in labor, when the fetus is high in the uterus, no fetal parts or presenting parts are palpable. Later in labor, when the cervix has dilated and the fetus is lower, an arm or shoulder may be palpable.

Face presentation: Fetal mouth, nose, orbital ridges, and malar eminences are palpable. The fetal mouth and malar eminences can feel similar to the anus and ischial tuberosities of a breech fetus. The difference is that the mouth and malar eminences form a triangle, whereas the anus and ischial tuberosities form a straight line.

Brow presentation: Fetal orbital ridges, root of the nose, and anterior fontanel are palpable. The absence of a palpable mouth or chin distinguishes the brow presentation from the face presentation.

Compound presentation: Fetal hand or arm and, less frequently, the fetal feet are palpable along with the vertex or buttock.

Uterus and adnexa   Same findings as abdominal examination.

Orders

1. Start an IV.
2. Obtain a complete blood count (CBC).
3. Begin continuous electronic fetal monitoring.
4. Type and crossmatch blood.
5. Notify the pediatrician and anesthesiologist of the possible need for an emergency cesarean section.

■ DIAGNOSTIC TESTING

The diagnosis of malpresentation can often be made by abdominal and vaginal examination. Radiographic studies are useful, however, in confirming the diagnosis and providing additional information that is crucial for the management of the patient.

1. **Ultrasound examination**

   Ultrasound examination should be performed to confirm the diagnosis of fetal malpresentation and to rule out congenital anomalies. A fetal anomaly of particular concern is anencephaly, which not only is associated with an increased incidence of breech presentation but also is a lethal anomaly. Fetal measurements can also be taken to estimate the birth weight. Furthermore, the degree of flexion or extension of the fetal head can also be determined by sonogram. These are all essential to planning the route of delivery of the breech fetus. Unfortunately, ultrasound examination cannot always distinguish among the different types of breech presentations.

2. **Pelvic radiography**

   Pelvic x-ray studies not only confirm the diagnosis of malpresentation but also, in the case of breech presentation, distinguish among the different types. Furthermore, if vaginal delivery of a breech fetus is being contemplated, pelvimetry can also be performed by pelvic x-ray.

3. **Computed tomography (CT)**

   CT can provide all the information provided by pelvic x-ray with less radiation exposure. Magnetic resonance imaging pelvimetry is usually more expensive and more time-consuming than CT pelvimetry.

■ MANAGEMENT

1. **Previable fetus—Attempt vaginal delivery**

   If the gestational age is <24 weeks or if the fetus is not viable for other reasons, vaginal delivery should be considered for all types of malpresentation.

2. **Breech presentation**
   a. **Nonfrank breech at any viable gestational age—Cesarean section**

   The increased incidence of prolapse of the umbilical cord and risk of birth trauma make vaginal delivery of a fetus in the complete or the incomplete breech presentation too risky. Unless imminent vaginal delivery precludes it, cesarean section should be performed.

   b. **Frank breech with fetal weight of <1500 g—Cesarean section**

   The mortality rate for breech fetuses weighing <1500 g is as high as 45% when delivered vaginally, compared with 18% when delivered by cesarean section. If premature labor cannot be treated successfully, cesarean section should be performed.

   c. **Frank breech with an estimated fetal weight of >1500 g**
      (1) Vaginal delivery

      Vaginal delivery of the frank breech fetus weighing >1500 g has been shown to be safe. However, the following criteria should be met before a vaginal delivery is attempted:
      (a) The physician must be experienced in performing a vaginal breech delivery.
      (b) Continuous electronic fetal monitoring should be used.
      (c) There must be the capability to perform an emergency cesarean section if complications are encountered.
      (d) An anesthesiologist or a nurse-anesthetist must be available.
      (e) The maternal pelvis should be adequate based on either x-ray or CT scan pelvimetry measurements (Table 11–1).
      (f) The estimated fetal weight should be <4000 g.
      (g) The fetal head must not be hyperextended and, optimally, should be flexed.
      (h) Labor must be progressing normally.

      Although studies have shown that the use of oxytocin is safe in patients with a frank breech fetus, this issue remains controversial.

Table 11–1 □ NORMAL PELVIMETRY MEASUREMENTS

	Anterior-Posterior Diameter (cm)	Transverse Diameter (cm)
Pelvic inlet	≥10.5	≥11.5
Midpelvis	≥11.5	≥10.0

(i) The patient must be counseled in detail concerning the risks of both vaginal delivery and cesarean birth of the breech fetus, and she must consent to the attempt at vaginal delivery.

(2) Cesarean section

If the criteria listed above cannot be met, then a cesarean section is usually recommended.

(3) External cephalic version

External cephalic version can be attempted if the patient is not in labor and if the gestational age is >36 weeks. Version is usually not recommended before 36 weeks, because of the possibility of spontaneous conversion to the vertex presentation when remote from term. Successful cephalic version requires the following:

(a) A physician who is familiar with the technique of external cephalic version.

(b) Continuous electronic fetal heart rate monitoring during the procedure.

(c) Ultrasound examination to follow the fetal head during the version.

(d) Uterine tocolytics to relax the uterus (e.g., **terbutaline 0.25 mg subcutaneously (SC) once or magnesium sulfate 4.0 to 6.0 g IV over 20 minutes once)**.

External cephalic version is successful in 60 to 70% of all cases. Factors that improve the success rate are frank breech presentation, multiparity, adequate amniotic fluid, and fetal back located anteriorly. The most common complication of cephalic version is abnormal fetal heart rate patterns, including variable decelerations, tachycardia, and bradycardia. These heart rate patterns are usually the result of cord compression and are in most cases transient. More serious complications are rare and include fetal trauma, such as brachial plexus injury and spinal cord transection, and fetal-maternal hemorrhage.

3. **Transverse lie**

a. **External cephalic version**

A fetus with a gestational age >25 weeks with a persistent transverse lie cannot usually be delivered vaginally. If the patient is not in active labor, external cephalic version to the vertex presentation can be attempted. Version of a fetus in the transverse lie does not usually need to be attempted until after 39 weeks of gestation because of the high likelihood of spontaneous conversion to a longitudinal lie, either vertex or breech, before 39 weeks. The criteria for cephalic version and the possible complications associated with version are the same as those listed for cephalic version of the breech fetus.

b. Cesarean section

If external cephalic version attempted after 39 weeks is unsuccessful or the patient is in active labor at any viable gestational age, then a cesarean section should be performed. Because the fetus is not in the lower uterus, a vertical uterine incision may be required, instead of the more common low transverse incision.

4. Face presentation

a. Mentum posterior position—Cesarean section

Vaginal delivery is usually not possible if the fetus is in a persistent mentum posterior position in which the fetal chin is posterior in the maternal pelvis. Cesarean section is usually required in these patients.

b. Positions other than mentum posterior—Attempt vaginal delivery

Vaginal delivery should be attempted if the position is other than mentum posterior. Vaginal delivery is usually successful if the pelvis is not contracted. External continuous electronic fetal heart rate monitoring should be performed. Internal fetal heart rate monitoring with a scalp electrode is not recommended because of the risk of scarring of the face. Face presentation is sometimes caused by a contracted pelvis. Therefore, the need for a cesarean section for arrest of cervical dilatation or arrest of descent of the fetal head is increased in these patients, compared with those with a vertex presentation.

5. Brow presentation—Attempt vaginal delivery

The brow presentation is usually transient. In patients with this presentation, approximately two-thirds spontaneously convert to either the vertex presentation by flexion of the head or the face presentation by extension of the head. If the brow presentation persists, there is an increased incidence of arrest of cervical dilatation or arrest of descent of the fetal head and, therefore, a greater likelihood that a cesarean section will be needed.

6. Compound presentation

a. Attempt vaginal delivery

The prolapsed fetal extremity, usually the arm, usually does not interfere with labor and therefore should not be manipulated. In many cases, the extremity will spontaneously be pulled back and away from the presenting part.

b. Reduce the extremity

If the prolapsing extremity prevents descent of the fetus during labor, a gentle attempt should be made to reduce it by pushing it upward. If this attempt fails and labor remains obstructed, then a cesarean section is usually required.

■ BACKGROUND AND DEFINITIONS

Mastitis: Infection of the connective tissue of the breast. Mastitis occurs most often in lactating women but can also be encountered in nonpuerperal women.

Endemic mastitis: Mastitis that occurs 2 weeks to several months after delivery due to bacteria in the infant's oropharynx and nose

Epidemic mastitis: Mastitis that occurs in hospitalized women because their infants are infected from contact with infected nursery personnel

■ CLINICAL PRESENTATION

Tender and erythematous breast, usually unilateral
Breast indurated and engorged
Fever
Chills and rigor
Malaise
Breast abscess in approximately 10% of patients with mastitis

■ PHONE CALL

Questions

1. How ill does the patient appear?
Breast abscess and, less commonly, septic shock and toxic shock syndrome (TSS) should be considered in the severely ill patient.

Degree of Urgency

Unless the rare complications of septic shock or TSS are encountered, mastitis is not life threatening and the patient does not need to be seen immediately.

■ ELEVATOR THOUGHTS

What causes the most common type of mastitis?
Mastitis is usually caused by transmission of bacteria in the

infant's oropharynx and nose into the breast through breast abrasions and fissures that develop from breast feeding.

What bacteria usually cause mastitis?
Staphylococcus aureus
Streptococcus viridans
Group A and B streptococci
Haemophilus influenzae
Haemophilus parainfluenzae

■ MAJOR THREAT TO MATERNAL LIFE

- Septic shock
- Toxic shock syndrome

Both of these life-threatening complications are rare.

■ BEDSIDE

Quick Look Test

Does the patient appear to be severely ill?
   Breast abscess, septic shock, and TSS should be considered in severely ill patients.

Vital Signs

Fever is almost always present. Other vital signs are normal unless the patient has developed septic shock or TSS.

Selective History and Chart Review

1. Does the patient have a prior history of breast conditions?
      Other breast diseases, such as cancer, can mimic mastitis.
2. Is the patient already taking antibiotics for other reasons, and is she allergic to any antibiotics?

Selective Physical Examination

Dermatological	"Sunburn-like" skin rash with desquamation is suggestive of TSS
Breasts	Tender, hard, engorged, and erythematous breast, usually unilateral; a fluctuant mass would be suggestive of a breast abscess
Abdominal	Normal
Pelvic	Normal

Orders

1. Collect breast milk for culture if the diagnosis is unclear.

In the severely ill patient, the following orders should also be given:

2. Start IV.
3. Insert Foley catheter.
4. Record input and output.
5. Obtain a complete blood count (CBC) with differential.
6. Obtain chemistry panel.
7. Obtain blood cultures.
8. Obtain urinalysis.

■ DIAGNOSTIC TESTING

The diagnosis of mastitis can usually be made from the patient's history and physical examination. Further testing is usually not necessary unless the diagnosis is unclear or a breast abscess is suspected.

1. **Culture of the breast milk**
   Culturing of the milk may aid in selection of the appropriate antibiotic to administer, but it is not necessary for making the diagnosis of mastitis if the clinical picture is clear.
2. **Leukocyte and bacterial colony count of the breast milk**
   In patients with mastitis, the breast milk leukocyte count is usually >1 million/ml, and the bacterial colony count is usually >1000/ml.
3. **Ultrasound examination**
   Ultrasound examination of the breast can be used to diagnose breast abscesses that appear as discrete fluid collections within the breast tissue.

■ MANAGEMENT

1. **Pain relief**
   a. **Ice packs** should be applied to the breast.
   b. **Breast support** of some form should be used.
   c. **Analgesics and antipyretics** can be used.
2. **Breast feeding should be continued** to prevent further breast engorgement.
   Patients should continue breast feeding from the unaffected breast and pump from the affected breast.

3. **Antibiotic therapy**

Although penicillin and sulfonamides have been used successfully, the following are the antibiotics of choice in the treatment of mastitis:

a. **Dicloxacillin 125 to 250 mg by mouth (PO) four times per day for 10 days** for penicillin-resistant staphylococci.

b. **Erythromycin 250 mg PO four times per day for 10 days** if the patient is allergic to penicillin.

c. **Vancomycin 250 to 500 mg PO four times per day for 10 days** if a methicillin-resistant staphylococcus is suspected.

d. **Cephalosporins PO for 10 days.**

4. **Surgical incision and drainage** is performed if a breast abscess is present. The abscess fluid should be cultured for both aerobic and anaerobic bacteria.

■ BACKGROUND AND DEFINITIONS

Meconium: Meconium is first found in the fetal intestine between 10 and 12 weeks of gestation. Water makes up 70 to 80% of the composition of meconium. Other components include bile acids and salt, squamous cells, vernix, mucopolysaccharides, protein, lipid, and enzymes.

Meconium passage: The passage of meconium from the fetal rectum into the amniotic fluid. Meconium passage usually does not occur before 34 weeks of gestation.

Meconium aspiration: The finding of meconium below the vocal cords and in the lungs of the neonate.

Meconium aspiration syndrome: A syndrome caused by either antepartum or intrapartum aspiration of meconium by the fetus. This syndrome is characterized by varying degrees of respiratory distress, caused by both mechanical obstruction of the airways and chemical pneumonitis. The hallmark findings of meconium aspiration syndrome are hypoxia, persistent fetal circulation, and pulmonary hypertension. Fetal breathing and gasping is thought to be the mechanism for meconium aspiration.

Meconium passage can occur in either the antepartum or the intrapartum period. The incidence of intrapartum meconium passage at term is between 7 and 22%. In postterm pregnancies, the incidence of meconium passage can be as high as 40%. Intrapartum meconium passage has been associated with a higher incidence of fetal acidosis and low Apgar scores. This finding is not consistent, however, and some studies have not found this association. In the presence of normal reassuring fetal heart rate patterns, meconium passage is not a sign of fetal compromise.

Meconium aspiration can be found in as many as 33% of neonates who have passed meconium. However, meconium aspiration syndrome is encountered in only 2 to 8% of neonates delivered in the presence of meconium passage. Mild cases of meconium aspiration syndrome consist of mild tachypnea that resolves in a few days. More severe cases can lead to severe hypoxia, respiratory failure, and even death.

■ CLINICAL PRESENTATION

The amniotic fluid is green or brown; it can be thin and watery or thick and particulate, like pea soup.

■ PHONE CALL

Questions

1. Is the meconium thin or thick?

Meconium aspiration syndrome is caused only by thick meconium, and thin meconium is usually not significant.

2. Are there abnormal fetal heart rate patterns?

Degree of Urgency

Because meconium passage can be associated with fetal compromise, the fetal heart rate tracing should be evaluated immediately.

■ ELEVATOR THOUGHTS

What are factors that can be associated with meconium passage?
- Fetal acidosis
- Postterm pregnancy
- Idiopathic

■ MAJOR THREAT TO FETAL LIFE

- Fetal meconium aspiration syndrome
- Fetal asphyxia

Meconium passage is not life threatening to the mother, but it can be associated with abnormal fetal heart rate patterns and fetal acidosis that can result in fetal morbidity and mortality.

■ BEDSIDE

Quick Look Test

Is the patient in labor?

Are there abnormal fetal heart rate patterns?

Vital Signs

Vital signs are usually normal.

Selective History and Chart Review

1. What is the gestational age of the fetus based on the patient's last menstrual period and ultrasound examination?

   Meconium is found in up to 40% of postterm pregnancies.

2. Does the patient have any predisposing factors for fetal compromise such as intrauterine growth restriction, post-term status, or placental abruption?

Selective Physical Examination

Abdominal	Usually normal
Pelvic	
External genitalia and vagina	Stained green or brown with meconium
Cervix	Normal
Uterus and adnexa	Usually normal

Orders

1. Place the patient on external electronic fetal heart rate monitoring if not already being monitored.
2. Start IV.
3. Have available a fetal scalp electrode for internal fetal heart rate monitoring.
4. Have available at the delivery a DeLee suction catheter, a neonatal laryngoscope, and an endotracheal tube to allow for endotracheal suctioning of meconium below the vocal cord.
5. Notify the pediatric team so that they can be present at the delivery.

■ DIAGNOSTIC TESTING

The diagnosis of meconium passage is based on physical examination after rupture of the amniotic sac.

■ MANAGEMENT

Management of a patient with meconium passage is twofold.

1. Monitor the fetus closely for evidence of fetal compromise
   a. Electronic fetal heart rate monitoring

When meconium passage is detected, the fetal heart rate should be monitored electronically. Internal monitoring with a fetal scalp electrode should be considered. If nonreassuring fetal heart rate patterns are present, the following steps, as discussed in Chapter 4, should be taken to improve fetal oxygenation:

   (1) Place the patient in the lateral position to relieve uterine compression of the vena cava and to improve venous return and cardiac output.

(2) Administer supplemental oxygen at a rate of 8 to 10 L/min via face mask.

(3) Decrease uterine contractions by either discontinuing oxytocin or administering a tocolytic drug.

(4) Correct maternal hypotension, if present.

If the above steps do not result in resolution of the abnormal fetal heart rate patterns, fetal scalp blood sampling or fetal scalp stimulation testing should be performed to identify the asphyxic fetus.

2. Prevent meconium aspiration syndrome

a. Suctioning of the fetal oropharynx

After delivery of the fetal head but before delivery of the thorax, the fetal oropharynx should be suctioned. The DeLee suctioning device is commonly used, but no one suctioning device has been shown to be clearly superior to others. The goal of this procedure is to suction the oropharynx clear of meconium before the infant can take its first breath and aspirate meconium. If the meconium is thick or if the neonate appears to be depressed, endotracheal suctioning under laryngoscopic visualization should be performed, preferably by the pediatric team immediately after the delivery of the infant. Unfortunately, suctioning of the oropharynx, as described above, does not entirely eliminate the risk of meconium aspiration syndrome because suctioning does not remove meconium that has already been aspirated into the lungs.

b. Amnioinfusion

Intrauterine infusion of saline or amnioinfusion has been used to dilute the meconium. Amnioinfusion may also benefit the fetus by decreasing the severity and frequency of variable decelerations through decreasing umbilical cord compression. This procedure has been shown to decrease the finding of meconium below the vocal cords of the neonate. However, it has not been shown that amnioinfusion decreases the incidence of meconium aspiration syndrome. Amnioinfusion can be performed as a bolus or as a continuous infusion.

(1) **Bolus infusion:** 500 to 800 ml of room-temperature normal saline infused via intrauterine catheter at a rate of 10 to 15 ml/min and repeated as needed.

(2) **Continuous infusion:** 10 ml/min of room-temperature normal saline for 1 hour followed by maintenance infusion of 3 ml/min via intrauterine catheter.

■ BACKGROUND AND DEFINITION

Multiple gestation or multiple pregnancy: The incidence of multiple gestation is approximately 3%, and most are twin gestations. The incidence has been increasing because of the availability of ovulation-inducing drugs and assisted reproductive technologies. Up to 25% of pregnancies resulting from assisted reproductive technologies are twins, and up to 5% are triplets. In both spontaneous pregnancies and pregnancies resulting from assisted reproductive technologies, the true incidence of twin gestations is probably higher, because early demise of one of the twins is common. One-third of all multiple gestations are monozygotic, resulting from cleavage of a single fertilized ovum. The incidence of monozygotic twins is independent of maternal race, age, parity, and heredity. Two-thirds of all multiple gestations are dizygotic and are due to the fertilization of two ova. The incidence of dizygotic twins is influenced by maternal race, heredity, age, parity, and the use of ovulation-inducing drugs.

The perinatal mortality rate of twin gestations is 50 to 120 per 1000 births, approximately fivefold higher than that of singleton pregnancies. Monozygotic twins have an even higher perinatal mortality rate, because they have a 1% risk of having a monoamniotic sac. This results in a fetal mortality rate of 50% because of umbilical cord entanglement. In triplets, the perinatal mortality rate is 95 to 200 per 1000 births. Even with the widespread use of ultrasonography, approximately 20% of twin gestations are not diagnosed until the patient is admitted to the hospital in labor.

■ CLINICAL PRESENTATION

Size greater than dates
> Beginning with the second trimester, a patient with a multiple gestation frequently presents with a uterus larger than expected for the gestational age. This size–date discrepancy is often unreliable and not helpful in patients who begin labor having had no prenatal care or with unclear pregnancy dating. In a similar manner, the palpation of multiple fetuses and the auscultation of multiple fetal heartbeats do not diagnose a multiple gestation reliably.

Persistent labor and enlarged uterus after delivery
> A multiple gestation should be suspected in a patient who

continues to labor and also has an enlarged uterus after delivery of one fetus.

■ PHONE CALL

Questions

1. **Is the patient in active labor?**
2. **What is the gestational age of the fetus?**

The gestational age and the presentation of the fetuses are the two most important factors in the management of the patient who is in labor with multiple gestation.

Degree of Urgency

Because of the potential for complications to occur during delivery, a patient who presents in labor with a multiple gestation must be seen immediately.

■ ELEVATOR THOUGHTS

What are the fetal complications encountered in a multiple gestation?

- Spontaneous abortion

  The incidence of spontaneous abortion is twofold higher in multiple gestations than in singleton pregnancies. Fewer than 50% of patients diagnosed with twin gestations in the first trimester actually deliver twins. Some twins are absorbed without maternal symptoms, whereas other demises cause vaginal bleeding, uterine contractions, and spontaneous abortion. Occasionally, the dead fetus and placenta remain as a fetus papyraceus and are found at the subsequent delivery of the surviving twin.

- Preterm delivery

  Preterm birth is the most common cause of perinatal morbidity and mortality in multiple gestations. The average duration of gestation decreases proportionately as the number of fetuses increases. Almost 50% of twin gestations deliver prematurely, before 37 weeks of gestation. Furthermore, if one of the fetuses is anomalous, there is an even higher incidence of preterm delivery. Measures taken to prevent preterm birth, including bedrest, serial cervical examinations, home uterine monitoring, and the use of prophylactic tocolytic drugs, have not been universally successful.

- Preterm rupture of membranes

  Preterm rupture of membranes occurs more frequently in

multiple gestations than singleton gestations. The sac of the presenting twin is the one that most often is ruptured. The nonpresenting twin develops respiratory distress syndrome more frequently than the presenting twin does.

- Intrauterine growth restriction

  Intrauterine growth restriction is defined as an estimated fetal weight below the 10th percentile for a singleton gestation. Growth restriction accounts for increased neonatal morbidity and mortality. The incidence of intrauterine growth restriction in a multiple gestation is approximately 70%. Furthermore, the degree of growth restriction increases as the pregnancy approaches term.

- Growth discordancy

  The accepted definition of growth discordancy is a difference of >20% in the estimated fetal weights of the two twins based on a percentage of the weight of the larger twin. The incidence of growth discordancy is 4 to 23%. The most severe cases of growth discordancy result from twin-to-twin transfusion, in which there are vascular anastomoses between the two twins in a monochorionic, monoamniotic placenta. The incidence of twin-to-twin transfusion in monochorionic twins is approximately 15%. The perinatal mortality rate increases proportionately with the degree of discordancy. When the degree of discordancy is >25%, the fetal death rate is increased 6.5-fold and the neonatal death rate is increased 2.5-fold.

- Umbilical cord accidents

  The incidence of cord accidents (e.g., cord entanglement) is highest with monochorionic, monoamniotic multiple gestation.

- Congenital anomalies

  The frequency of major congenital malformations is approximately 2% in twins, compared with 1% in singletons. The incidence of anomalies in monozygotic twins is twice that in dizygotic twins.

- Complications at delivery

  Multiple gestation is associated with a higher incidence of fetal malpresentation. Furthermore, after delivery of the first fetus, premature placental separation may occur before the delivery of the remaining fetus, due to contraction of the uterus. For these reasons, in patients with more than two fetuses, delivery is usually by cesarean section.

- Neurological abnormalities

  Cerebral palsy, microcephaly, and encephalomalacia are encountered more frequently in multiple gestation. The incidence of cerebral necrosis is as high as 14% in fetuses of multiple gestation delivered prematurely.

- Conjoined twins

    This is an extremely rare complication of monochorionic gestation.

What are the maternal complications associated with a multiple gestation?

- Hyperemesis gravidarum

    Hyperemesis is probably due to the increased levels of human gonadotropins found in multiple gestation.
- Placental abruption
- Placenta previa
- Preeclampsia

    The incidence of preeclampsia is increased threefold in patients with multiple gestation, compared with singleton pregnancies. Furthermore, there is also an increase in the severity of the disease in patients with multiple gestation.
- Polyhydramnios

    Polyhydramnios is found in 5 to 8% of patients with multiple gestation and represents one of the causes of preterm labor in these patients.
- Anemia

    Both iron deficiency anemia and folic acid deficiency anemia are more commonly encountered in patients with multiple gestation because of increased fetal demands.
- Postpartum hemorrhage

    The risk of postpartum hemorrhage is increased in patients with multiple gestation because of uterine atony caused by overdistention of the uterus.
- Cholestasis of pregnancy
- Increased risk of cesarean section

    The higher incidences of prematurity and malpresentation contribute to the higher frequency of cesarean sections.

■ MAJOR THREAT TO FETAL LIFE

- Prematurity

    The major threat to life for the fetuses is that of prematurity. This risk of prematurity increases with the number of fetuses.

■ MAJOR THREAT TO MATERNAL LIFE

- Hemorrhage and hypovolemic shock

    Several of the maternal complications in a multiple gestation, such as placental abruption, postpartum hemorrhage, and the increased rate of cesarean section, all increase the risk of hemorrhage and hypovolemic shock.

■ BEDSIDE

Quick Look Test

Are abnormal fetal heart rate patterns present?

Because of the increased incidence of prematurity, intrauterine growth restriction, and growth discordancy, patients with multiple gestation are at higher risk for developing fetal distress when in labor.

If the first infant has already been delivered, what is its approximate size and gestational age?

In patients with no prenatal care and/or unclear dates, assessing the size and estimating the gestational age of the delivered infant can be useful in the management of the undelivered fetus.

If the first infant has already been delivered, is there significant vaginal bleeding?

Heavy vaginal bleeding that occurs between the deliveries of the twins may be indicative of premature separation of the placenta. This usually necessitates immediate delivery, either by operative vaginal delivery or cesarean section.

Vital Signs

Vital signs are usually normal.

Selective History and Chart Review

1. What is the best estimate of gestational age based on early examinations and ultrasound measurements?
2. Has there been appropriate and concordant fetal growth during the pregnancy?
3. If the patient has had prior ultrasound examinations, has a membrane been detected between the twins, thereby ruling out monoamniotic twins (Fig. 14–1)?
4. Has the patient had any complications during her pregnancy such as preeclampsia or polyhydramnios?

Selective Physical Examination

Abdominal	Patient's uterus appears large for the gestational age
	Uterus still enlarged after delivery of the first twin
Pelvic	
External genitalia and vagina	Normal

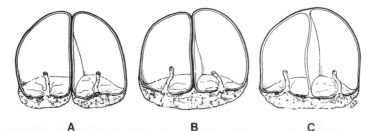

Figure 14–1 □ Placenta and membranes in twin gestations. *A*, Two placentas, two amnions, and two chorions. *B*, Single placenta, two amnions, and two chorions. *C*, One placenta, one chorion, and two amnions. (From Cunningham FC, MacDonald PC, Gant NF, et al: Williams Obstetrics, 19th ed. Norwalk, Connecticut, Appleton & Lange, 1993, p 892. Reproduced with permission of The McGraw-Hill Companies.)

Cervix	After delivery of the first twin, fetal parts of the second twin may be palpable through the dilated cervix
Uterus and adnexa	Large for dates
	Uterus still enlarged and contracting after delivery of the first twin

Orders

In the patient who is in labor with a multiple gestation, the following orders should be given:
1. Initiate continuous electronic monitoring of the fetuses.
2. Begin IV.
3. Type and crossmatch 2 units of blood.
4. Notify the anesthesiologist of the possible need for an emergency cesarean section.
5. Notify the pediatrician of the imminent delivery of the multiple gestation.

■ DIAGNOSTIC TESTING

1. Ultrasound examination

Ultrasound examination is the quickest test available to determine not only the presence of a multiple gestation but also the presentation of the fetuses and their approximate gestational age. If an ultrasound examination is not possible, a portable abdominal x-ray study should be performed. Ultrasound examination can also be used to diagnose intrauterine growth restriction, growth discordancy, and most cases of significant congenital anomalies. Furthermore, polyhydramnios and placenta previa can be diagnosed by ultrasound examination.

■ MANAGEMENT

1. **Antepartum surveillance**

   Serial ultrasound examinations should be used to diagnose intrauterine growth restriction and growth discordancy. If those conditions are found, weekly nonstress testing and/or biophysical profile assessment should be performed.

2. **Detection of preterm labor**

   Efforts should be made to detect and treat preterm labor even though neither the detection nor the treatment of preterm labor has been completely successful.

3. **Management in labor**

   a. **Continuous electronic fetal heart rate monitoring**

   b. **Decision on the route of delivery**

   The route of delivery depends on the presentation, size, and gestational age of the fetuses, the condition of the mother and the fetuses, the experience of the deliverer, and the availability of an anesthesiologist and pediatrician. A flowchart of intrapartum management of the patient with multiple gestation is presented in Figure 14–2. The most common presentation in twin gestations is vertex–vertex, followed in frequency by vertex–breech. The frequency of presentations in twin gestations is presented in Table 14–1.

   (1) Twin A vertex with twin B vertex

   Vaginal delivery should be attempted in the patient with a vertex–vertex presentation. It is estimated that 70 to 80% of vertex–vertex twins can be delivered safely vaginally. Immediately after delivery of the first twin,

Table 14–1 □ **INCIDENCE OF PRESENTATIONS IN TWIN DELIVERIES**

Presentation	Incidence (%)
Vertex–vertex	40
Vertex–breech	26
Breech–vertex	10
Breech–breech	10
Vertex–transverse	8
Miscellaneous	6

From Creasy RK, Resnik R: Maternal-Fetal Medicine: Principles and Practice, 3rd ed. Philadelphia, WB Saunders Co, 1994, p 597.

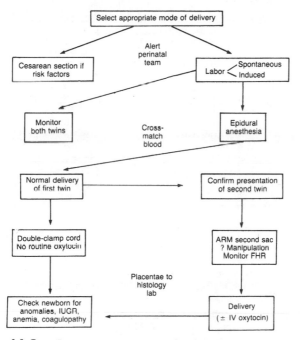

Figure 14–2 □ Intrapartum management of multiple gestation. ARM, artificial rupture of membranes; FHR, fetal heart rate; IUGR, intrauterine growth retardation. (From Creasy RK, Resnik R: Maternal-Fetal Medicine: Principles and Practice, 3rd ed. Philadelphia, WB Saunders Co, 1994, p 594.)

the presentation and heart rate tracing of the undelivered twin should be evaluated. Potential complications encountered in vaginal delivery of the second twin include premature placental separation, prolapse of the umbilical cord, and abnormal presentation.

In the absence of these complications, the time interval between the deliveries of the first and second twins is not critical to the well-being of the second twin.

(2) Twin A vertex with twin B nonvertex

Although cesarean section is often performed for this presentation, an attempt at vaginal delivery is a reasonable alternative if the estimated fetal weight is >1500 g. Vaginal delivery of the breech fetus with an estimated weight of <1500 g is controversial, and many advocate cesarean section for these patients because of increased

Table 14–1 □ INCIDENCE OF PRESENTATIONS
IN TWIN DELIVERIES

Presentation	Incidence (%)
Vertex–vertex	40
Vertex–breech	26
Breech–vertex	10
Breech–breech	10
Vertex–transverse	8
Miscellaneous	6

From Creasy RK, Resnik R: Maternal-Fetal Medicine: Principles and Practice, 3rd ed. Philadelphia, WB Saunders Co, 1994, p 597.

perinatal morbidity and mortality. As an alternative, external cephalic version can be attempted on twin B after delivery of twin A.

(3) Twin A nonvertex

When twin A has a nonvertex presentation, a cesarean section is usually advisable regardless of the presentation of twin B. External cephalic version of twin A is not technically possible because of the presence of twin B.

4. Management of the surviving twin after the death of one twin

Fetal demise of one fetus can occur at any gestational age in a multiple gestation, although most deaths occur in the first trimester; the incidence is higher in monochorionic, monoamniotic twins. The incidence of fetal demise is as high as 25% in the first trimester and is between 0.5 and 6.8% after the first trimester. Early in pregnancy, the twin that has died is usually resorbed and the prognosis for survival of the viable twin is very good. Later in pregnancy, the prognosis for the surviving twin depends on the cause of the death, the gestational age, and the existence of vascular anastomoses between the two twins. The greatest risk to the surviving twin is preterm labor. Disseminated intravascular coagulation (DIC) can occur in rare cases. Before 34 to 35 weeks, management should be expectant. Fetal surveillance should be performed with weekly nonstress tests and/or biophysical profile assessment. Furthermore, weekly maternal coagulation studies should be obtained. Delivery should be performed if there is evidence of fetal compromise or once fetal lung maturity has been attained. After 34 to 35 weeks, labor should be induced and cesarean section should be performed only for the usual obstetrical indications.

5. Multifetal reduction

The risks of preterm delivery and poor perinatal outcome increase with the number of fetuses. Multifetal reduction can be performed to decrease the number of fetuses and decrease the risk of preterm delivery and associated morbidity and mortality. This procedure is especially beneficial in quadruplet pregnancies and higher-order multiple gestations. The decision on the part of the patient considering multifetal reduction is an extremely difficult one, and there are ethical issues to consider. A common method for selective fetal reduction is ultrasound-guided intracardiac injection of potassium chloride. Loss of the entire pregnancy is the most common risk; it occurs in 10 to 25% of patients. Furthermore, a risk of preterm delivery still remains after successful reduction.

■ BACKGROUND AND DEFINITIONS

Placenta previa: Abnormal implantation of the placenta either over or near the internal os of the cervix. The incidence of placenta previa is approximately 1 in 200 to 250 births. It is found more commonly in multiparous patients than in nulliparous patients. The incidence in nulliparous patients is approximately 1 in 1500 births, whereas the incidence in grand multiparous patients, patients who have had ≥5 deliveries, is approximately 1 in 20 births. The incidence of placenta previa has also been found to be increased by as much as 15 times in patients who have had previous cesarean sections. The risk of recurrent placenta previa in subsequent pregnancies is 4 to 8%. These findings support the theory that placenta previa is caused by defective decidual vascularization or endometrial damage that might occur with each pregnancy, especially when delivered by cesarean section. Placenta previa results in a maternal mortality rate of less than 1% and a perinatal mortality rate of less than 10%. There are four degrees of placenta previa, defined as follows (Fig. 15–1):

Total or complete placenta previa: Placenta covers the entire internal cervical os

Partial placenta previa: Placenta partially covers the cervical os

Marginal placenta previa: Edge of the placenta is at the margin of the internal os

Low-lying placenta: Placenta is implanted in the lower uterine segment, so that the placental edge is near the cervical os but does not actually reach the os

■ CLINICAL PRESENTATION

Painless vaginal bleeding, usually in the second or third trimester
Bleeding often increases with labor

The peak incidence of bleeding is in the early third trimester. Bleeding may begin without a precipitating cause such as labor, intercourse, or digital or speculum examination. Placenta previa is not ruled out by the absence of bleeding before labor, because approximately 10% of patients with this condition have their initial bleeding episode at the onset of labor.

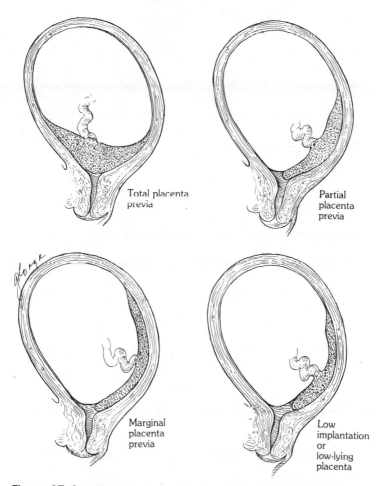

Figure 15-1 □ Degrees of placenta previa. (From Hacker NF, Moore JG: Essentials of Obstetrics and Gynecology, 3rd ed. Philadelphia, WB Saunders Co, 1998, p 189.)

■ PHONE CALL

Questions

1. How much is the patient bleeding?
2. What are the patient's vital signs?

Degree of Urgency

Bleeding from a placenta previa can be severe enough to be life threatening. Patients with bleeding from a suspected placenta previa should be seen immediately.

■ ELEVATOR THOUGHTS

What are risk factors and corresponding relative risks for placenta previa?
- Previous cesarean section, relative risk up to $15\times$
- Previous placenta previa, relative risk $8\times$
- Previous uterine curettage, relative risk $1.3\times$
- Maternal age >35 years, relative risk $5\times$
- Maternal age >40 years, relative risk $9\times$
- Smoking, relative risk 1.5 to $3\times$

What are other causes of painless vaginal bleeding?
- Mild placental abruption, also referred to as "marginal separation"
- Normal "bloody show" from cervical effacement and dilatation
- Cervical or vaginal lesion
- Vasa previa

■ MAJOR THREAT TO FETAL LIFE

- Prematurity
  Preterm delivery performed for severe bleeding is the most common cause of perinatal morbidity and mortality.
- Fetal compromise
  Severe hemorrhage can result in maternal hypovolemic shock and fetal compromise.

■ MAJOR THREAT TO MATERNAL LIFE

- Hypovolemic shock
  Bleeding from placenta previa can be severe enough to result in hypovolemic shock.

■ BEDSIDE

Quick Look Test

Does the patient appear to be in shock?

Is there ongoing bleeding, and if so, how severe is the bleeding?

Is the fetal heart rate pattern nonreassuring?
A nonreassuring fetal heart rate pattern may result from severe bleeding and decreased transplacental blood flow or from placental abruption which can manifest with signs and symptoms similar to those of placenta previa.

Is the patient having pain?
Uterine contractions and cervical dilatation exacerbate bleeding from a placenta previa because they cause further separation of the placenta. Laboring patients can be given tocolytic medications to stop the progression of labor. Pain can also be a result of placental abruption.

Vital Signs

A patient in hypovolemic shock from placenta previa will be hypotensive and tachycardic. The patient might have postural hypotension. Changes in blood pressure (BP) and pulse should be measured when the patient is assisted in sitting or standing from a supine position. A fall in systolic or diastolic BP >15 mm Hg or a rise in pulse >15 beats/min is indicative of hypovolemia.

Selective History and Chart Review

1. What is the gestational age of the fetus?
   The gestational age is one of the key factors that influences the management of a patient bleeding from a placenta previa, especially if the bleeding is not severe.
2. Has the patient had an ultrasound examination during the pregnancy?
   A prior ultrasound examination might help to confirm the diagnosis of placenta previa. However, of all patients who are identified as having placenta previa on ultrasound examination performed before 30 weeks of gestation, no more than 5% have placenta previa at delivery. This is because the placenta in effect moves away from the cervical os as the lower uterine segment develops late in pregnancy. A previous ultrasound examination also provides information concerning the gestational age.

Selective Physical Examination

Abdominal   Nontender and benign

Pelvic

External genitalia and vagina	Blood-stained
Cervix	Digital or speculum examination either should not be performed or, if absolutely necessary, should be performed with extreme care in an operating room in case the examination results in severe bleeding. A double setup is described in the section on Diagnostic Testing
Uterus and adnexa	Nontender and benign

Orders

1. Start a large-bore IV.
2. Do not allow anyone to perform a digital or speculum vaginal examination on the patient.
3. Obtain a complete blood count (CBC).
4. Type and crossmatch 2 or more units of blood.
5. Initiate external electronic fetal monitoring.
6. Insert a Foley catheter if the patient appears to be in shock.
7. Notify the anesthesiologist and pediatric team of the possible need for an emergency cesarean delivery.

■ DIAGNOSTIC TESTING

1. Ultrasound examination

Ultrasound examination is the simplest and safest diagnostic test for localization of the placenta. It has an accuracy rate of >95% in the diagnosis of placenta previa. Distention of the bladder can result in false-positive readings, and therefore patients who are diagnosed as having placenta previa should have a repeat ultrasound examination after emptying the bladder.

2. Double-setup digital examination

With the availability and resolution of current sonography techniques, there are very few indications for a double-setup examination. However, when ultrasound examination is either equivocal or unavailable, the diagnosis of placenta previa can be established by digitally palpating the placenta through the cervical os. This type of examination should be performed only if delivery is planned, because heavy bleeding can be caused even by very gentle digital examination. Furthermore, this type of examination should be performed only in an operating room with the patient prepared for both vaginal delivery and cesarean section, so that an immediate cesarean section can be performed if a placenta previa is found. At least 2 to 4 units of blood should be available. A double-setup examination is not indicated if the patient is having bleeding severe enough to require immediate delivery by cesarean section.

■ MANAGEMENT

The management of the patient with placenta previa depends on the following factors: presence and severity of the bleeding, gestational age of the fetus, and presence of labor.

1. Minimal or no bleeding, premature gestational age
a. Expectant management

Expectant management consists of the severe restriction of physical activity, either in the hospital or at home. The goals of expectant management are attainment of fetal maturity and resolution of the placenta previa. Depending on the gestational age when placenta previa is diagnosed, there is a possibility of resolution as the lower uterine segment develops. Patients who present to the hospital with bleeding from a placenta previa should be observed.

If the bleeding has not been severe and it is thought that the patient is stable, discharge home and expectant management can be considered. If the patient's bleeding makes premature delivery likely, the administration of corticosteroids should be considered to decrease the risk of respiratory distress syndrome and intraventricular hemorrhage. **Celestone Soluspan solution, 2 ml IM, should be given with a repeat dose in 24 hours.** The maximal beneficial effects of steroids are seen after 24 hours, although some benefits may be attained sooner. Delivery should not be delayed if it is indicated by the maternal and/or fetal condition. Effects of steroids last for approximately 7 days, so the dose should be repeated at that time.

A patient who is managed expectantly at home must be compliant with the restriction of physical activity, including sexual intercourse. Furthermore, she must be able to be transported to the hospital immediately if bleeding occurs. Autologous blood donation may be appropriate for the patient who is stable and not anemic. A hemoglobin concentration ≥ 11 g/dl and a hematocrit $\geq 34\%$ are usually required for autologous blood donation.

2. Minimal or no bleeding, mature gestational age
a. Amniocentesis for fetal lung maturity
b. Cesarean section if mature

Once the fetus has reached a gestational age of 35 to 36 weeks, little is gained by expectant management, and there remains the risk of sudden unexpected bleeding. Therefore, amniocentesis should be performed and a phospholipid fetal lung profile should be obtained. The fetus should be delivered if the fetal lung profile is mature. The route of delivery should in almost all cases be cesarean section. An exception would be for the patient with a low-lying placenta, who could be allowed to labor if she is monitored closely for the onset of bleeding. In a patient undergoing cesarean section, blood should be available even if the patient is not actively bleeding, because intraoperative blood loss can be heavy. This is because the placental implantation site is in the lower uterine segment, where there is not the thick uterine musculature found in the uterine fundus that provides for hemostasis through uterine contractions. Furthermore, placenta accreta is commonly associated with placenta previa, occurring in approximately 15% of cases. This is a condition in which the placenta is abnormally attached to the uterine myometrium, resulting in difficult removal and postpartum hemorrhage (see Chapter 19).

3. **Minimal bleeding associated with premature labor**
   a. **Administration of tocolytic drugs**
   b. **Expectant management if labor is successfully stopped**
   c. **Cesarean section if labor is not stopped and bleeding continues**
   d. **Consideration of steroid administration**
   Labor can often precipitate bleeding because progressive cervical dilatation results in further separation of the placenta. The administration of tocolytic drugs such as magnesium sulfate or terbutaline can result in cessation of bleeding in the patient with premature labor and can also be used to temporize with patients who are being prepared for cesarean section.

4. **Severe bleeding, any gestational age**
   a. **Cesarean section**
      Patients who have severe, life-threatening vaginal bleeding should be delivered by cesarean section regardless of the gestational age of the fetus.

■ BACKGROUND AND DEFINITION

Placental abruption: Separation of a normally implanted placenta before delivery of the fetus; also referred to as abruptio placentae

Placental abruption is one of the common causes of third-trimester bleeding, but it can also occur any time after 20 weeks of gestation. The severity of placental abruption is based on how much of the placenta has undergone separation. Depending on the location of the placenta, bleeding from placental abruption may be concealed, resulting in hypotension out of proportion to the amount of visible bleeding (Fig. 16–1). The incidence of placental abruption is approximately 1 in 150 deliveries, and the perinatal mortality rate associated with this condition is 15 to 20%. Severe abruption may result in Couvelaire uterus or uterine apoplexy, in which there is extravasation of blood into the myometrium, underneath the uterine serosa, and sometimes even into the broad ligament and fallopian tube serosa. This is usually

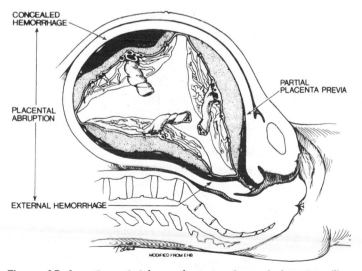

Figure 16–1 □ Concealed hemorrhage in placental abruption. (From Cunningham FC, MacDonald PC, Gant NF, et al: Williams Obstetrics, 19th ed. Norwalk, Connecticut, Appleton & Lange, 1993, p 826. Reproduced with permission of The McGraw-Hill Companies.)

observed at the time of cesarean delivery. Furthermore, blood may dissect beyond the edge of the placenta and between the uterine decidua and fetal membranes. Blood may then pass through the fetal membranes into the amniotic fluid, resulting in the classic port-wine discoloration of amniotic fluid.

■ CLINICAL PRESENTATION

Vaginal bleeding
Hypovolemic shock, often out of proportion to the amount of visible bleeding
Port-wine discoloration of amniotic fluid
Coagulopathy
Uterine pain and tenderness
Uterine irritability
Hypertonic uterine contractions
Back pain
Nonreassuring fetal heart rate pattern
Fetal demise

A grading system, originally published by Page and colleagues (Page EW, King EB, Merrill JA: Abruptio placentae: dangers of delay in delivery. Obstet Gynecol 1954;3:385) can be used to classify cases of placental abruption depending on maternal and fetal signs and symptoms (Table 16–1).

■ PHONE CALL

Questions

1. **What are the patient's vital signs?**
2. **Does the patient appear to be in pain?**
   Placental abruption commonly results in uterine contractions and/or hypertonus of the uterus, which causes abdominal and back pain.

Degree of Urgency

Placental abruption is an obstetrical emergency that can be associated with serious morbidity and even mortality for both the patient and the fetus. The patient should be seen immediately.

■ ELEVATOR THOUGHTS

What factors are associated with placental abruption?
■ Hypertensive disorders

Table 16-1 □ GRADING OF PLACENTAL ABRUPTION

Grade	Concealed Hemorrhage	Uterine Tenderness	Maternal Shock	Coagulopathy	Fetal Distress	Comments
0	−	−	−	−	−	Asymptomatic, based on retrospective examination of placenta
1	−	−	−	−	−	Includes "marginal sinus rupture," bleeding variable
2	+	+	−	Rare	+	Progresses to grade 3 unless delivery is achieved
3	+ +	+ +	+	Common	Fetal death	Major maternal morbidity

− = absent; + = present; + + = severe.
Adapted from Creasy RK, Resnik R: Maternal-Fetal Medicine: Principles and Practice, 3rd ed. Philadelphia, WB Saunders Co, 1994, p 610.

Both pregnancy-induced hypertension and chronic hypertension are associated with a higher risk of abruption. Up to 50% of patients with severe abruption have a hypertensive disorder.

- Cocaine abuse

    The mechanism is unclear but may involve cocaine-induced vasoconstriction. Abruption can be found in as many as 10% of mothers who use cocaine late in pregnancy.

- Cigarette smoking

    Smoking is associated with the pathological finding of decidual necrosis in the placenta.

- Trauma

    Trauma is rarely the cause of abruption because only severe cases of trauma have been associated with abruption. Most patients present within 24 hours of the trauma.

- High parity
- Sudden decompression of the uterus

    This can occur after delivery of the first twin in a multiple gestation or after rupture of membranes in any pregnancy but especially a pregnancy complicated by polyhydramnios.

- Short umbilical cord
- Preterm premature rupture of membranes
- Uterine anomaly
- Uterine leiomyomata
- History of placental abruption

    The risk of recurrence of abruption with subsequent pregnancies is between 6 and 17%. This represents an almost 30-fold increase over the rate in the normal population.

■ MAJOR THREAT TO FETAL LIFE

- Fetal demise

    Severe placental abruption can result in fetal compromise and fetal death.

- Prematurity

    Preterm delivery performed for severe abruption is a common cause of perinatal morbidity and mortality. Perinatal mortality rates associated with abruption range from 1 to 4 per 1000 births.

■ MAJOR THREAT TO MATERNAL LIFE

- Hypovolemic shock
- Disseminated intravascular coagulation (DIC)

■ BEDSIDE

Quick Look Test

Does the patient appear to be in shock?

Patients with placental abruption may appear to be in shock even in the absence of significant external bleeding because of concealed retroplacental bleeding, which is encountered in approximately 10% of all patients with abruption.

Is the fetal heart rate tracing nonreassuring?

Significant placental abruption can cause fetal compromise and even fetal death from placental separation, maternal hemorrhage, fetal hemorrhage, uterine hypertonus, or a combination of these factors. The incidence of fetal compromise in the presence of placental abruption is approximately 60%.

Vital Signs

A patient in hypovolemic shock from placental abruption will be hypotensive and tachycardic. The patient might have postural hypotension. Changes in blood pressure (BP) and pulse should be measured when the patient is assisted in sitting or standing from a supine position. A fall in systolic or diastolic BP >15 mm Hg or a rise in pulse >15 beats/min is evidence of hypovolemia.

Selective History and Chart Review

1. What is the gestational age of the fetus?

    The gestational age affects the management of the patient.

2. Has the patient had a prior obstetrical ultrasound examination?

    A prior ultrasound examination provides an estimate of the gestational age. Furthermore, it can rule out placenta previa, which manifests with bleeding similar to that seen with placental abruption.

3. Does the patient have pregnancy-induced or chronic hypertension?

    Both of these conditions are most commonly associated with placental abruption.

4. Has the patient had a previous pregnancy complicated by abruption?

Selective Physical Examination

Abdominal	Uterine fundus hard and tender
Pelvic	
External genitalia and vagina	Blood-stained or negative
	Port-wine–colored amniotic fluid if there has been rupture of membranes

Cervix	Blood-stained or negative
Uterus	Fundus hard and tender
	Irritable on palpation

Orders

1. Start a large-bore IV.
2. Initiate electronic fetal heart rate monitoring.
3. Obtain a complete blood count (CBC).
4. Obtain coagulation studies: prothrombin time (PT), partial thromboplastin time (PTT), platelet count, fibrinogen, fibrin split products.
5. Type and crossmatch blood if bleeding is severe or if the patient is in hypovolemic shock.
6. Insert a Foley catheter.
7. Record input and output.
8. Notify the anesthesiologist and pediatric team of the possible need for an emergency cesarean section.

■ DIAGNOSTIC TESTING

The diagnosis of placental abruption is usually made clinically and should be suspected in any patient with bleeding, abdominal pain, uterine tenderness, or uterine irritability.

1. Ultrasound examination

Ultrasound examination cannot absolutely exclude or diagnose placental abruption. Acute hemorrhage is usually hyperechoic and therefore can sometimes be detected between the placenta and the uterine wall. However, only large retroplacental clots can be reliably detected by current ultrasound technology. A normal ultrasound examination does not exclude placental abruption because acute hemorrhage can appear isoechoic and therefore be misinterpreted as part of a thick placenta. Ultrasound examination is more useful in diagnosing placenta previa, which can manifest with signs and symptoms similar to those of placental abruption.

■ MANAGEMENT

The options in the management of placental abruption are **(1) expectant management** with close monitoring of both the maternal and the fetal status, **(2) induction of labor and vaginal delivery**, and **(3) immediate cesarean section**. The management of placental abruption is dependent on maternal status, fetal status, and gestational age of the fetus. Transfusion of blood, platelets, fresh frozen plasma, or cryoprecipitate may be necessary regardless of the management option chosen. Postpartum hysterectomy may be necessary in rare cases.

1. **Expectant management**
   Expectant management is especially preferable in premature pregnancies. Expectant management is usually appropriate if all of the following criteria are met:
   a. Degree of placental abruption is mild with minimal bleeding
   b. Maternal status is stable and there is no evidence of hypovolemic shock or severe coagulopathy
   c. There is no evidence of fetal compromise
   Expectant management consists of close continuous monitoring of maternal hemodynamic and coagulation status with serial CBCs and coagulation studies. The fetus should also be monitored with electronic fetal heart rate monitoring.
   If it is anticipated that preterm delivery will eventually occur, the administration of steroids should be considered. Celestone Soluspan solution 2 ml intramuscularly (IM) is administered with a repeat dose in 24 hours. Each milliliter of Celestone contains 3 mg of betamethasone sodium and 3 mg of betamethasone acetate. Maximal beneficial effects—decrease in respiratory distress syndrome and intraventricular hemorrhage—are seen after 24 hours, although some benefit is attained sooner. Delivery should not be delayed in an attempt to attain maximal beneficial effects if the maternal and/or fetal status makes delivery advisable. The beneficial effects from one dose of steroids last for 1 week, and therefore a repeat dose should be given at that time if the fetus is still premature.
2. **Induction of labor and vaginal delivery**
   Induction of labor can be considered in the term pregnancy with mild abruption and stable maternal and fetal status. Induction of labor is also appropriate under the following circumstances:
   a. Degree of placental abruption is moderate with ongoing bleeding, but the mother is not in immediate jeopardy and there is no evidence of hypovolemic shock or coagulopathy
   b. There is no evidence of fetal compromise
   Even when the degree of placental abruption is mild, uterine contractions may be hypertonic and labor may be rapid and tumultuous. During labor, the degree of placental separation may increase and result in deterioration of maternal or fetal status, making cesarean delivery necessary. Induction of labor and vaginal delivery is also the management of choice for fetal demise when the mother is stable. It is also the best management for the pregnancy with a previable fetus when the degree of placental abruption is severe enough to make delivery nec-

essary. Induction of labor should be attempted with an oxytocin infusion, and amniotomy should be performed as soon as it is safe. As an alternative, in early pregnancies, **20-mg prostaglandin E₂ (dinoprostone) vaginal suppositories administered every 4 hours** or **misoprostol (Cytotec) 200- to 800-μg tablets intravaginally every 12 hours,** can be used to induce labor.

3. **Cesarean section**

   Immediate cesarean section should be performed for any one of the following:

   a. Degree of placental abruption is severe with brisk ongoing bleeding
   b. Maternal status is unstable with signs of hypovolemic shock or coagulopathy
   c. There is evidence of fetal compromise

   In a patient who is already unstable, cesarean section almost always results in further deterioration of maternal status. Furthermore, patients with a coagulopathy caused by placental abruption may bleed excessively intraoperatively and postoperatively. Therefore, aggressive efforts to correct anemia, hypovolemic shock, and coagulopathy must be taken before surgery. Red blood cells (RBCs), platelets, fresh frozen plasma (FFP), or cryoprecipitate should be transfused accordingly.

4. **Transfusion of blood products**

   a. **Red blood cells**

      RBCs can be transfused to increase oxygen-carrying capacity in anemic patients. One unit of packed RBCs has a volume of 250 ml, and 1 unit of whole blood has a volume of 450 ml. Each unit of RBCs should increase the hematocrit by 3% and the hemoglobin concentration by 1 g/dl. Coagulation studies should be obtained after transfusion of every 5 to 10 units of RBCs.

   b. **Platelets**

      Platelets should be transfused for a platelet count of <20,000/mm³ or, in patients in whom a cesarean delivery is planned, for a platelet count of <50,000/mm³. Each unit of platelets should increase the platelet count by 5000 to 10,000/mm³.

   c. **Fresh frozen plasma**

      FFP is transfused for coagulopathy due to deficiency of clotting factors, usually if PT or PTT is >1.5 times normal. Each unit of FFP will increase any clotting factor by 2 to 3%. The usual initial dose is 2 units, and each unit has a volume of 200 to 250 ml.

   d. **Cryoprecipitate**

      Cryoprecipitate is transfused for coagulopathy due to deficiency of factor VIII, von Willebrand's factor, factor XIII, fibrinogen, or fibronectin. Cryoprecipitate is concentrated from FFP, and each bag has a volume of 10 to 15 ml. Each bag contains at least 150 mg of fibrinogen.

5. **Postpartum hysterectomy**

   Postpartum hysterectomy is performed only if there is severe and persistent uterine bleeding that is not responsive to correction of the coagulopathy or the administration of oxytocin, methergine, or prostaglandin. Before hysterectomy, selective angiographic arterial embolization should be considered. Consideration should also be given to bilateral ligation of the hypogastric arteries, which will decrease pulse pressure enough to allow the patient's coagulation system to decrease blood loss. Bilateral hypogastric artery ligation, however, precludes the use of angiographic arterial embolization. If the patient has already lost a significant amount of blood or is unstable, supracervical or subtotal hysterectomy should be performed. The presence of Couvelaire uterus is not, by itself, an indication for hysterectomy.

17 | Postpartum Depression

■ BACKGROUND AND DEFINITIONS

Postpartum blues: Also referred to as **maternity blues**, it affects 50 to 70% of postpartum women. This condition develops early in the postpartum period, usually in the first few days. It is transient and rarely persists beyond 2 weeks.

Postpartum depression: Also known as **postpartum neurotic depression**, it occurs in approximately 10% of postpartum patients. It can develop anytime in the first 6 months of the postpartum period and often lasts for more than 2 weeks.

Postpartum psychosis: It occurs in 1 to 2 of 1000 puerperal women. It most often begins in the first 3 weeks postpartum and rarely begins after 6 weeks postpartum.

■ CLINICAL PRESENTATION

Postpartum blues
  Insomnia
  Weepiness
  Depression
  Fatigue
  Anxiety
  Headaches
  Poor concentration
  Confusion
Postpartum depression—symptoms of postpartum blues plus
    the following:
  Despondency
  Emotional lability
  Apathy
  Listlessness
  Irritability
  Guilt
  Ambivalent feelings toward the infant
  Feelings of inadequacy as a mother
  Anorexia
  Self-derogatory feelings
  Indecisiveness
  Somatic complaints, especially involving the gastrointestinal
    tract

Postpartum psychosis—symptoms of postpartum blues and postpartum depression plus the following:
Suicidal thoughts or actual attempts
Threats of violence or actual violence toward the infant
Delusional and paranoid thoughts
Cognitive disorders
Psychomotor retardation or catatonic features
Motor agitation
Inappropriate affect
Hallucinations, especially ones that command her to harm her infant
Excessive concern over the infant's health
Delusions that the baby is either dead or defective
Schizophrenic features
Manic features

■ PHONE CALL

Questions

1. Does the patient pose a danger to herself or to her infant?

Patients with postpartum psychosis can have suicidal ideations and may attempt suicide. Furthermore, they can exhibit violent behavior toward their infants.

2. When did the patient deliver?

A patient is more likely to have postpartum depression or psychosis, as opposed to the very common postpartum blues, if her symptoms have been present for more than several weeks after her delivery.

Degree of Urgency

Patients who appear to have postpartum psychosis should be seen immediately.

■ ELEVATOR THOUGHTS

What factors contribute to postpartum blues?
- Emotional letdown after the long-anticipated labor and delivery
- Fatigue from labor and delivery and from caring for the infant
- Postpartum pain from the delivery process, especially if a cesarean section was performed

- Recovery from complications of the pregnancy and delivery such as infection and blood loss
- Changes in body image after pregnancy

What are predictive factors for postpartum depression?
- Marital difficulties
- Undesired or unplanned pregnancy
- Single or separated marital status
- Family history of depression
- Prior history of postpartum depression
- History of physical violence in the patient's family
- High level of anxiety during pregnancy

What are predictive factors for postpartum psychosis?
- History of bipolar affective disorder
- History of postpartum psychosis
- First-degree relatives with bipolar affective disorders
- First pregnancy
- Cesarean delivery

What medical conditions may contribute to postpartum depression?
Between 4 and 7% of postpartum women have abnormalities in thyroid function. Postpartum thyroiditis can cause delayed postpartum depression. Postpartum thyroiditis usually manifests with a thyrotoxic phase 2 to 3 months after delivery. In this phase, patients experience nonspecific symptoms including fatigue, weight loss, and palpitations. This phase is followed by a hypothyroid phase that usually occurs 4 to 8 months postpartum. Most patients eventually return to a euthyroid state, although between 10 and 30% develop permanent hypothyroidism.

■ MAJOR THREAT TO INFANT'S LIFE

- Physical violence to infant
  Threat to the life of the infant is a concern only with postpartum psychosis.

■ MAJOR THREAT TO MATERNAL LIFE

- Suicide
  Suicide is a concern only with postpartum psychosis.

■ BEDSIDE

Quick Look Test

Does the patient exhibit motor agitation or catatonic features?
These are symptoms suggestive of psychosis.

Vital Signs

Vital signs are usually normal.

Selective History and Chart Review

1. Does the patient have a past history of postpartum depression or psychosis?
2. Does the patient have any of the predictive factors listed for postpartum depression or psychosis?

Selective Physical Examination

Physical examination is usually normal.

Orders

If the patient appears to be potentially harmful to either herself or her infant, she should have an attendant with her and not be left alone. Furthermore, she should not be allowed to leave before being evaluated by a physician.

■ DIAGNOSTIC TESTING

For the majority of patients, there is no evidence for a direct causative effect of the postpartum physiological and hormonal changes on the incidence of postpartum blues, depression, or psychosis. Therefore, there are no diagnostic laboratory tests available to confirm the diagnosis of these conditions in most patients. If postpartum thyroiditis is suspected, thyroid function tests including free thyroxine (T_4) and thyroid-stimulating hormone (TSH) should be ordered.

■ MANAGEMENT

1. **Postpartum blues**

   No specific treatment is indicated for postpartum blues. The patient should be reassured that her symptoms are very common and transient, rarely persisting for more than 2 weeks. Emotional support, encouragement, and aid and education in the care of the infant can be helpful.

2. **Postpartum depression**

   a. **Psychotherapy**

   Although psychiatric consultation is recommended for severe cases of postpartum depression, more mild cases can be managed by the primary physician if he or she is comfortable dealing with the patient's psychological problems and has the time to provide psychotherapy.

b. **Antidepressant medication**
   (1) **Imipramine (Tofranil) 75 to 300 mg/day PO**
   (2) **Amitriptyline (Elavil) 75 to 300 mg/day PO**
   (3) **Fluoxetine (Prozac) 20 to 60 mg/day PO**
   (4) **Alprazolam (Xanax) 0.75 to 4 mg/day PO**

   All of these antidepressant medications can be detected in the breast milk of nursing mothers, usually at a level 10% of that found in maternal serum. Alprazolam has been shown to cause lethargy, weight loss, and impaired temperature regulation in breast-feeding infants. No adverse effects have been found in breast-feeding infants whose mothers use fluoxetine or the two tricyclics imipramine and amitriptyline. Nevertheless, caution is advised in the use of these antidepressant medications in breast-feeding mothers. When in doubt, if the medication is believed to be absolutely necessary, breast feeding should be discontinued.

c. **Thyroid hormone replacement**

   Thyroid hormone replacement should be initiated in patients with persistent hypothyroidism: **Levothyroxine sodium (Levo-thyroxine, Synthroid, Levothyroid) 0.025 to 0.50 mg/day PO** as a starting dose with incremental increases of 0.025 mg/day every 4 weeks until euthyroid state is reached.

3. **Postpartum psychosis**
   a. **Psychiatric consultation**

      Patients with postpartum psychosis should be admitted to the hospital and should be seen by a psychiatrist.

   b. **Antipsychotic medication**
      (1) **Chlorpromazine (Thorazine) 400 to 600 mg/day PO or 25 mg IM initially for acute psychosis**
      (2) **Haloperidol (Haldol) 0.5 to 5.0 mg PO two or three times per day or 2 to 5 mg IM initially for acute psychosis**

      Both chlorpromazine and haloperidol are excreted in the breast milk of breast-feeding mothers; therefore, consideration should be given to cessation of breast feeding.

■ BACKGROUND AND DEFINITIONS

Standard puerperal morbidity: Temperature of 100.4°F or 38.0°C, which occurs in any 2 of the first 10 days postpartum, exclusive of the first 24 hours taken orally at least four times daily.

Endometritis, endomyometritis, endoparametritis, and metritis with pelvic cellulitis: All are synonymous and defined as uterine infection, the most common cause of a postpartum fever. The incidence of endometritis after vaginal delivery is between 1.3 and 6%. However, the incidence is significantly higher after cesarean section, increasing to 12 to 51%. Endometritis is caused by aerobic and anaerobic organisms that ascend into the uterine cavity from the lower genital tract. Anaerobic organisms can be isolated in approximately half of endometrial cultures. Commonly encountered organisms are listed in Table 18–1.

Table 18–1 □ ORGANISMS RESPONSIBLE FOR ENDOMETRITIS

Aerobic organisms

Groups A, B, and D streptococci and *streptococcus viridans*
Staphylococcus aureus
Enterococcus
Escherichia coli
Proteus mirabilis
Klebsiella
Enterobacter
Gardnerella vaginalis

Anaerobic organisms

Bacteroides fragilis, B. bivius, and *B. disiens*
Clostridium
Peptococcus
Peptostreptococcus
Mobiluncus
Prevotella
Porphyromonas asaccharolyticus
Fusobacterium
Neisseria gonorrhoeae

Miscellaneous

Chlamydia trachomatis
Mycoplasma hominis

■ CLINICAL PRESENTATION

Fever
Chills and rigor
Malaise
Uterine pain and tenderness
Abdominal pain and tenderness
Foul-smelling lochia

■ PHONE CALL

Questions

1. What are the patient's vital signs?
2. How ill does the patient appear?

Degree of Urgency

Endometritis and other causes of postpartum fever are rarely life threatening, and the patient does not need to be seen immediately.

■ ELEVATOR THOUGHTS

What is the differential diagnosis of postpartum fever?
- Endometritis
- Pyelonephritis
- Mastitis
- Breast engorgement
- Respiratory complications
- Wound infection
    Infection of cesarean section incision
    Infection of episiotomy repair
    Infection of spontaneous obstetrical lacerations
- Thrombophlebitis
    Septic pelvic thrombophlebitis
    Thrombophlebitis of the lower extremities
- Bacterial endocarditis

What are factors that increase the risk for postpartum endometritis?
- Cesarean section
- Prolonged labor
- Prolonged rupture of membranes
- Multiple vaginal examinations

- Use of internal fetal monitoring
- Use of internal uterine monitoring by pressure catheter
- Low socioeconomic status
- Chorioamnionitis
- Bacterial vaginosis
- Anemia
- Major obstetrical trauma of the cervix or vagina
- Intrauterine instrumentation (e.g., uterine curettage)

■ MAJOR THREAT TO MATERNAL LIFE

- Sepsis

    Sepsis is a rare complication of endometritis. It is most often caused by *Escherichia coli*, *Clostridium*, or *Bacteroides*.

■ BEDSIDE

Quick Look Test

Does the patient appear to be severely ill?

In patients who appear severely ill, sepsis, septic pelvic thrombophlebitis, and pelvic abscess should be considered.

Vital Signs

Patients are febrile, but otherwise the vital signs are usually normal. The findings of hypotension and tachycardia are suggestive of sepsis or ruptured pelvic abscess.

Selective History and Chart Review

1. Does the patient have symptoms of a nonpelvic cause of postpartum fever such as pyelonephritis, mastitis, or pneumonia?
2. What was the route of delivery?

    Patients who undergo cesarean section are at a much higher risk for endometritis and wound infection.
3. When did the patient give birth?

    Late-onset endometritis, occurring more than 5 to 7 days after delivery, is commonly caused by *Chlamydia trachomatis*.
4. If the patient gave birth vaginally, did she have any risk factors for endometritis, such as prolonged labor, prolonged rupture of membranes, internal monitoring, or chorioamnionitis?
5. Did the patient have bacterial vaginosis or anemia?

Selective Physical Examination

Breast	Tender, hard, and erythematous in mastitis
Back	Costovertebral angle (CVA) tenderness in pyelonephritis
Abdominal	Tender in uncomplicated endometritis
	Surgical incision erythematous, indurated, and draining purulent fluid in wound infection
	Rigid with rebound tenderness and involuntary guarding in ruptured pelvic abscess
Pelvic	
External genitalia and vagina	Episiotomy or laceration sites tender, erythematous, indurated, and draining purulent fluid in infection
Cervix	Usually normal, although a foul-smelling purulent discharge may be present with endometritis
Uterus and adnexa	Tender to palpation in endometritis

Orders

1. Obtain a complete blood count (CBC) with differential.
2. Obtain a urinalysis.
3. Obtain blood and urine cultures if the patient appears to be severely ill.

■ DIAGNOSTIC TESTING

The diagnosis of endometritis is based on the clinical findings of uterine tenderness, fever, foul-smelling discharge, and malaise. Laboratory tests may be helpful in confirming the diagnosis and in ruling out other causes of fever.

1. **CBC with differential**
   The white blood cell count is elevated in endometritis, as also occurs in other infections.
2. **Gram stain and culture of foul-smelling lochia**
   Cultures are often contaminated with vaginal flora, but they can still be helpful in identifying clostridia, anaerobes, and chlamydia.
3. **Ultrasound examination**
   Ultrasound examination is helpful in detecting a pelvic abscess.

4. Urinalysis

The finding of white blood cell casts is diagnostic of pyelonephritis.

5. Blood cultures

Positive blood cultures can result from many types of infection; cultures are positive in 25% of cases of septic pelvic thrombophlebitis.

6. Computed tomography scan

A CT scan may be helpful in patients who do not respond to antibiotic therapy and who have negative ultrasound examinations, because this test can detect occult abscesses and can also detect the thrombus in septic pelvic thrombophlebitis.

■ MANAGEMENT

1. Intraoperative prophylactic antibiotics

Intraoperative administration of prophylactic antibiotics decreases the risk of endometritis and wound infection after cesarean section. Several regimens have been shown to be effective:

a. Ampicillin 1 to 2 g IV or

b. Cefazolin 1 g IV or

c. Clindamycin 900 mg and gentamicin 1.5 mg/kg IV

Ampicillin provides better coverage of enterococcus, but cefazolin has a longer half-life. Clindamycin and gentamicin can be used in patients who are allergic to penicillin. Typically, the antibiotic chosen is administered intraoperatively after clamping of the umbilical cord.

2. Endometritis

Antibiotic regimens for the treatment of endometritis are numerous and depend on the organisms suspected.

a. Clindamycin 300 to 600 mg IV every 6 hours or 900 mg IV every 8 hours plus gentamicin 1.0 to 1.5 mg/kg IV every 8 hours

This regimen has a cure rate of 95%, and most failures result from poor coverage of enterococcus. A possible adverse effect of clindamycin is diarrhea from pseudomembranous colitis caused by an overgrowth of enterotoxin-producing *Clostridium difficile*. This can be caused by other antibiotics as well. Pseudomembranous colitis usually responds to vancomycin or metronidazole and discontinuation of clindamycin.

b. Ampicillin 0.5 to 2.0 g IV every 6 hours plus gentamicin 1.0 to 1.5 mg/kg IV every 8 hours

This regimen has a cure rate of 70 to 85%, although it does not provide optimal coverage for anaerobes.

c. Clindamycin 300 to 600 mg IV every 6 hours or 900 mg IV every 8 hours plus aztreonam 1.0 to 2.0 g IV every 8 hours

Aztreonam is a monobactam antibiotic that provides excellent coverage for aerobic gram-negative organisms. It can be used instead of gentamicin in those patients who are at risk for aminoglycoside toxicity. Aztreonam is more expensive than gentamicin.

d. **Beta-lactamase inhibitor combined with penicillin**
   (1) **Ampicillin and sulbactam (Unasyn) 1.5 g (1.0 g ampicillin and 0.5 g sulbactam) to 3.0 g (2.0 g ampicillin and 1.0 g sulbactam) IV every 6 hours**
   (2) **Ticarcillin and clavulanic acid (Timentin) 50 to 75 mg/kg IV every 6 hours**

e. **Cephalosporins**
   (1) **Cefoxitin (Mefoxin) 1.0 to 2.0 g IV every 6 hours**
   (2) **Cefotetan (Cefotan) 1.0 to 2.0 g IV every 12 hours**
   (3) **Cefoperazone (Cefobid) 0.5 to 1.0 g IV every 6 hours**

With the administration of the appropriate antibiotics, 90% of patients respond within a few days. Antibiotics should be continued until the patient has been afebrile for 24 to 48 hours. There is no need for a course of oral antibiotics to follow the parenteral antibiotics.

Of those patients who do not respond initially to antibiotic therapy, approximately 20% fail because of resistant organisms. When the regimen of gentamicin and clindamycin fails, the addition of ampicillin or penicillin should be considered to cover enterococcus. Peak serum levels of gentamicin can also be obtained to ensure adequate dosing. Normally, it is not necessary to obtain serum levels of gentamicin in patients with normal renal function. Neurotoxicity and nephrotoxicity are uncommon when the antibiotic is administered for less than 1 week. Furthermore, metronidazole can be substituted for clindamycin to better cover resistant gram-negative anaerobes. If a patient continues to be nonresponsive to antibiotic therapy and nonpelvic sources for fever have been ruled out, septic pelvic thrombophlebitis and pelvic abscess should be considered.

2. **Septic pelvic thrombophlebitis**

Septic pelvic thrombophlebitis has also been referred to as "enigmatic" or "obscure" fever, because fever usually persists after prolonged therapy with multiple antibiotics. It is caused by the extension of endometritis along venous routes, especially the ovarian veins. Patients typically do not appear ill but have multiple fever spikes, giving the temperature curve a "sawtooth" appearance. There is usually either no pain or mild and vague abdominal pain. Findings on pelvic and abdominal examination are vague and unremarkable.

a. **Heparin**
   (1) **Loading dose:** 5000 units IV

(2) **Maintenance dose:** 1000 to 1500 U/hr IV to achieve PTT of ≥1.5-fold control

Anticoagulation therapy with IV heparin is both diagnostic and therapeutic. Patients with septic pelvic thrombophlebitis respond with rapid defervescence within 2 to 3 days. If there is no such improvement, the diagnosis should be questioned. After successful heparinization, the patient should be placed on oral warfarin therapy. The total duration of anticoagulation therapy should be 10 to 14 days.

3. **Pelvic abscess**

Antibiotic therapy for patients with pelvic abscess must include agents such as clindamycin that cover anaerobic bacteria. Pelvic abscesses that do not respond to antibiotics must be drained. This can be performed percutaneously with radiographic guidance if the abscess is accessible. If the abscess is inaccessible or if rupture of the abscess is suspected, exploratory laparotomy is indicated.

■ BACKGROUND AND DEFINITIONS

Postpartum hemorrhage: Blood loss of more than 500 ml after vaginal delivery, 1000 ml after cesarean delivery, or 1500 ml after repeat cesarean delivery

Early postpartum hemorrhage: Postpartum hemorrhage occurring in the first 24 hours after delivery

Late postpartum hemorrhage: Postpartum hemorrhage occurring 24 hours to 6 weeks after delivery

Postpartum hemorrhage is difficult to diagnose because the diagnosis is based on a subjective estimate of blood loss. Blood loss is often underestimated by as much as 50%. It has been advocated that a 10% decrease in hematocrit between admission and the postpartum period or the need for blood transfusion should be used instead of clinical estimation of blood loss to diagnose postpartum hemorrhage. Using these criteria, the incidence of postpartum hemorrhage is approximately 4% after vaginal delivery and 6% after cesarean delivery.

Early postpartum hemorrhage is more acute and is associated with greater blood loss and morbidity than late postpartum hemorrhage, which tends to be more chronic. Fortunately, blood volume expands in pregnancy, and this expansion can compensate for most cases of normal blood loss. However, postpartum hemorrhage remains a common cause of maternal mortality, ranking third behind thromboembolism and hypertensive disorders. It has been estimated that postpartum hemorrhage accounts for approximately 30% of all maternal mortality.

■ CLINICAL PRESENTATION

Vaginal bleeding
Hypovolemic shock in severe cases

■ PHONE CALL

Questions

1. What are the vital signs?
2. How severe is the bleeding?

3. How long has the patient been bleeding?
4. Is the patient currently receiving intravenous oxytocin?

Degree of Urgency

Postpartum hemorrhage is a potentially life-threatening complication that accounts for 4 to 5% of all maternal mortality. Patients should be seen immediately.

■ ELEVATOR THOUGHTS

What are the causes of early postpartum hemorrhage?
- Uterine atony
    Risk factors for uterine atony include uterine distention from multiple gestation, polyhydramnios, or fetal macrosomia; prolonged administration of oxytocin; grand multiparity; prolonged labor; chorioamnionitis; administration of tocolytic agents; and use of halogenated anesthetics.
- Lacerations of the vulva, vagina, or cervix
    Lacerations of the genital tract are often associated with forceps or vacuum-assisted delivery, fetal macrosomia, rapid labor and delivery, and uncontrolled delivery. Lacerations may result in hematoma formation of the vulva and/or vaginal vault. High hematomas are often not found unless digital vaginal and bimanual examinations are performed.
- Retained fragments of placenta
- Retained placenta due to abnormal placental implantation (Fig. 19–1)
    1. Placenta accreta
        Placenta accreta is the most common of the abnormal implantations, occurring at a frequency of 1 in 2500 deliveries. Risk factors include placenta previa, previous cesar-

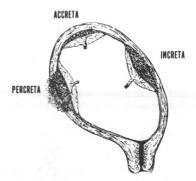

Figure 19–1 □ Placenta accreta, increta, and percreta. (From Breen JL, Neubecker R, Gregori CA, et al: Placenta accreta, increta, and percreta. A survey of 40 cases. Obstet Gynecol 1977; 49:43. Reprinted with permission from The American College of Obstetricians and Gynecologists.)

ean delivery, high parity, previous myomectomy, and previous uterine curettage. Placenta previa in a patient with a prior cesarean delivery is associated with an incidence of placenta accreta of approximately 25%.
2. Placenta increta
3. Placenta percreta

- Coagulopathy
  Disseminated intravascular coagulopathy (DIC) may result from placental abruption, severe chorioamnionitis with sepsis, amniotic fluid embolism, and fetal demise. Furthermore, thrombocytopenia may result from severe preeclampsia and HELLP syndrome. Inherited coagulopathy may also be present.

- Uterine rupture
  The incidence of uterine rupture is approximately 1 in 2000 deliveries overall, but it is 0.5 to 1.0% in patients with a prior low transverse cesarean section and as high as 10% in patients with a prior vertical uterine incision.

- Inversion of the uterus (Fig. 19–2)

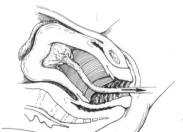
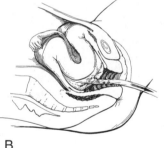

A   B

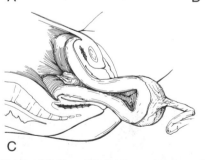

C

Figure 19–2 □ Uterine inversion secondary to cord traction. *A*, Partial uterine inversion. *B*, Complete uterine inversion. *C*, Complete uterine inversion with prolapse. (From Plauche WC, Morrison JC, O'Sullivan M: Surgical Obstetrics. Philadelphia, WB Saunders Co, 1992, p 219.)

Uterine inversion occurs in approximately 1 in 2500 deliveries. Risk factors include abnormal placental implantation, fundal implantation, administration of oxytocin, uterine anomalies, and excessive traction on the cord after delivery of the newborn.

What are the causes of late postpartum hemorrhage?
- Endometritis
- Subinvolution of the uterus
    Subinvolution is the delay in involution, the shrinking of the enlarged postpartum uterus back to its normal nonpregnant size. It is the most common cause of late postpartum hemorrhage.
- Retained placental fragments
- Coagulopathy

■ MAJOR THREAT TO MATERNAL LIFE

- Hypovolemic shock

■ BEDSIDE

Quick Look Test

Does the patient appear to be in shock?
    A patient in hypovolemic shock will usually appear distressed, ill, and apprehensive. She will appear pale and will have cold and clammy skin.

Vital Signs

A patient in hypovolemic shock will be hypotensive and tachycardic. Furthermore, the patient might have postural hypotension. Changes in BP and pulse should be measured when the patient is assisted in sitting or standing from a supine position. A fall in systolic or diastolic BP >15 mm Hg or a rise in pulse >15 beats/min is evidence of hypovolemia.

Selective History and Chart Review

1. Did the patient have any of the risk factors for uterine atony?
2. What was the route of delivery?
    Vulvar, vaginal, or cervical lacerations are possible causes of postpartum hemorrhage if the patient had a difficult forceps- or vacuum-assisted delivery. Uterine rupture should be considered if the patient had a vaginal delivery after a prior cesarean section. Retained placental fragments are

possible after a vaginal delivery but unlikely after a cesarean section, because the placenta is removed manually under direct visualization.

3. Was the delivery of the placenta difficult?

    Retained placental fragments or abnormal placental implantation should be suspected if the delivery of the placenta was difficult. Furthermore, if excessive traction was applied to the umbilical cord in an attempt to deliver the placenta, uterine inversion can result.

4. Did the patient have preeclampsia or placental abruption?

    Severe preeclampsia and placental abruption are common causes of coagulopathy in pregnancy.

5. Did the patient complain of excessive pain in the postpartum period?

    Excessive pain that is unrelieved by usual analgesics could indicate hematoma formation and/or extensive genital tract lacerations.

Selective Physical Examination

Abdominal	Uterine atony: uterine fundus is soft and sometimes difficult to palpate
Pelvic	
External genitalia and vagina	Lacerations or hematomas of the vulva or vagina are easily seen, although the detection of high hematomas might require speculum examination or bimanual examination
Cervix	Lacerations are possible after vaginal delivery
Uterus and adnexa	Uterine atony: uterine fundus is soft and sometimes difficult to palpate
	Uterine rupture: hematoma in the broad ligament sometimes detected lateral to the uterus
	Uterine inversion: bleeding mass present in the vagina just inside the introitus
	Subinvolution: uterus large and boggy

Orders

1. Start a large-bore IV if the patient does not already have one.
2. Obtain a complete blood count (CBC).
3. Obtain coagulation studies: platelet count, prothrombin time (PT), partial thromboplastin time (PTT), fibrinogen, and fibrin split products.
4. Type and crossmatch blood if the patient has had significant bleeding.
5. Insert a urethral catheter to monitor urinary output.
6. Administer supplemental oxygen.

■ DIAGNOSTIC TESTING

1. Complete blood count (CBC)
2. Coagulation studies: platelet count, PT, PTT, fibrinogen, fibrin split products
3. Examination of the placenta

    If examination of the placenta reveals that segments of placenta are absent, retained placental fragments or abnormal placental implantation should be suspected.
4. Pelvic ultrasound examination

    If a pelvic mass is palpated lateral to the uterus, ultrasound examination might reveal a broad-ligament hematoma caused by uterine rupture.

■ MANAGEMENT

1. Uterine atony
    a. Massage the uterine fundus with one hand on the abdomen over the uterine fundus and the other hand in the vagina.
    b. Administer uterotonic drugs
        (1) Oxytocin 10 to 40 IU (1 to 4 ampules) IM or intramyometrial or IV in 500 to 1000 ml IV fluid by continuous infusion
        (2) Methylergonovine (Methergine) 0.2 mg IM or intramyometrial or IV every 2 to 4 hours
        (3) 15-Methyl prostaglandin $F_2\alpha$ (carboprost tromethamine) 0.25 mg IM or intramyometrial every 15 to 90 minutes up to a maximum of 8 doses
        (4) Prostaglandin E_2 (dinoprostone) 20-mg suppository per vagina or per rectum every 2 hours
    c. Surgical management: uterine artery ligation, hypogastric artery ligation, or hysterectomy

        Uterine packing is usually not helpful in treating postpartum hemorrhage from atony, because the uterus is merely distended by the packing. Packing also prevents the postpartum uterus from contracting and can conceal ongoing bleeding.

        If the medical measures listed above are unsuccessful, several surgical procedures should be considered. Ligation of the anterior branch of the uterine artery is technically the easiest of the surgical procedures to perform (Fig. 19–3). Uterine artery ligation is especially helpful for bleeding from the lower uterine segment. Ligation of the infundibulopelvic and utero-ovarian vessels can reduce uterine perfusion further. Hypogastric artery ligation decreases the pulse pressure to allow time for the normal clotting mechanisms

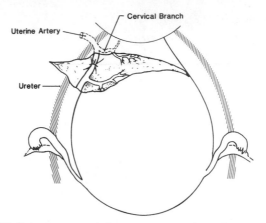

Figure 19-3 □ Ligation of the anterior branch of the uterine artery. (From Creasy RK, Resnik R: Maternal-Fetal Medicine: Principles and Practice, 4th ed. Philadelphia, WB Saunders Co, 1999, p 912.)

to function (Fig. 19-4). Hypogastric artery ligation is performed by ligating but not dividing the hypogastric artery distal to the posterior division. Unfortunately, hypogastric artery ligation precludes one other measure used to treat postpartum hemorrhage, namely selective arterial angio-

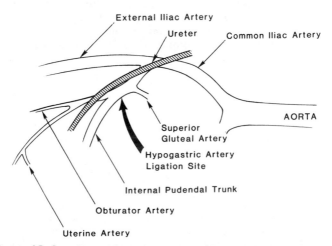

Figure 19-4 □ Site of hypogastric artery ligation. (From Creasy RK, Resnik R: Maternal-Fetal Medicine: Principles and Practice, 4th ed. Philadelphia, WB Saunders Co, 1999, p 912.)

graphic embolization, which is performed by interventional radiologists. Angiography is first performed to identify extravasation of contrast from bleeding pelvic vessels, and embolization is performed with Gelfoam pellets or wire coils.

Hysterectomy should be considered if bleeding is persistent despite all efforts. If the patient is unstable from severe bleeding, subtotal hysterectomy is recommended over total hysterectomy, because it can be accomplished in a shorter amount of time and is associated with less blood loss.

2. Lacerations of the vulva, vagina, or cervix
   a. Repair of lacerations
   b. Evacuation of expanding hematomas
   c. Vaginal packing
   d. Arterial angiographic embolization
   e. Hypogastric artery ligation

Stable hematomas do not require surgical intervention. Expanding hematomas, however, should be evacuated, and bleeding vessels should be ligated. Vaginal packing is often helpful and can be used in addition to the repair of vaginal lacerations. If bleeding persists despite these measures, selective arterial angiographic embolization is often successful. Hypogastric artery ligation can also be performed.

3. Retained placental fragments

Retained placental fragments can result from abnormal adherence of the placenta. Placental villi are attached to the myometrium in placenta accreta, invade into the myometrium in placenta increta, and penetrate through the entire layer of myometrium in placenta percreta (see Fig. 19–1).

   a. Manual removal of retained fragments
   b. Uterine curettage

Uterine curettage should be performed carefully with a large curette to prevent perforation of the postpartum uterus.

4. Treatment of coagulopathy and replacement of blood products
   a. Correct underlying cause of coagulopathy
   b. Transfusion with blood products
   c. Transfusion of platelets, initially 6 to 10 units, *or*
   d. Transfusion of fresh frozen plasma, initially 2 bags

In patients with severe blood loss, replacement of depleted intravascular volume can be achieved with crystalloid solutions if blood products are not immediately available. A 3:1 ratio should be used, with 3 units of crystalloid administered IV for every 1 unit of blood loss. In addition, blood and blood components should be administered. The use of blood components is superior to the use of whole blood because the patient can be given only those blood products that are needed.

Coagulation studies should be obtained after the transfusion of every 5 to 10 units of blood. Platelets should be transfused in patients with a platelet count of <20,000/mm³. If surgery such as hysterectomy is planned, platelets should be transfused if the platelet count is <50,000/mm³. Each unit of platelets will increase the platelet count by 5000 to 10,000/mm³. Fresh frozen plasma should be administered if the PT or PTT is >1.5 times normal.

5. **Uterine rupture**
   a. **Immediate laparotomy with either repair of the rupture site or hysterectomy**
   Although uterine rupture can occur in an unscarred uterus, most cases occur in women attempting vaginal delivery after a previous cesarean section. Uterine rupture usually occurs during labor but can also appear before labor.

6. **Inversion of the uterus**
   a. **Manual replacement of the uterine fundus with fingers or palm of the hand**

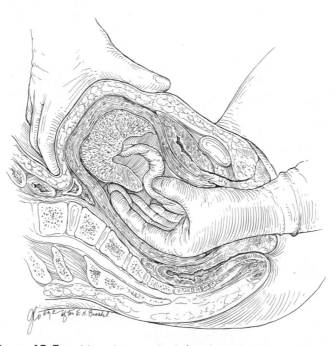

Figure 19-5 □ Manual removal of the placenta. (From Hacker NF, Moore JG: Essentials of Obstetrics and Gynecology, 3rd ed. Philadelphia, WB Saunders Co, 1998, p 338.)

 b. **If manual replacement is unsuccessful, emergency laparotomy with the use of traction sutures to replace the uterine fundus**

Tocolytic drugs such as terbutaline or magnesium sulfate are administered to relax the uterus and facilitate the repositioning. Oxytocin should not be administered until the uterine fundus has been replaced into its normal position. To prevent uterine inversion, manual removal of the placenta and gentle traction on the umbilical cord should be performed if the placenta does not spontaneously separate within 20 to 30 minutes after the delivery of the newborn (Fig. 19–5).

7. **Subinvolution of the uterus**
 a. **Methylergonovine (Methergine) 0.2 mg PO every 3 to 4 hours for 1 to 2 days**
 b. **Broad-spectrum antibiotics if endometritis is suspected: doxycycline 100 mg PO two times per day or erythromycin 500 mg PO four times per day for 7 days**

Endometritis can be the cause of subinvolution. Approximately one-third of cases of late endometritis are caused by *Chlamydia trachomatis*.

Premature Rupture of Membranes

■ BACKGROUND AND DEFINITIONS

Premature rupture of membranes (PROM): Rupture of membranes before the onset of labor

Preterm premature rupture of membranes: Rupture of membranes before the onset of labor at a gestational age of less than 37 weeks

Prolonged rupture of membranes: Rupture of membranes for more than 24 hours before delivery

Midtrimester premature rupture of membranes: Rupture of membranes prior to fetal viability or 24 to 26 weeks of gestation

Latency period: Period of time between PROM and the onset of labor

The incidence of premature rupture of membranes (PROM) in pregnancies of all gestational ages is between 3% and 18.5%. The incidence of PROM in full-term pregnancies is 8 to 10%. At term, approximately 95% of women with PROM deliver within 28 hours after rupture. When preterm premature rupture of membranes occurs, approximately 75% of women deliver within 1 week. Preterm premature rupture of membranes occurs in 25 to 33% of all preterm births.

Amniotic fluid is necessary for normal development of the fetal lungs. Amniotic fluid also protects the fetus from trauma and the umbilical cord from compression. Rupture of membranes and the subsequent loss of amniotic fluid result in the loss of these beneficial effects. Furthermore, prolonged rupture of membranes increases the risk of chorioamnionitis, which is associated with increased maternal and neonatal morbidity. The risk of infection increases with duration of rupture.

■ CLINICAL PRESENTATION

Gush of fluid from the vagina followed by persistent leakage of fluid
Chorioamnionitis
Active labor

A patient's complaint of a gush of fluid from the vagina followed by ongoing leakage is indicative of rupture of membranes in 90% of cases. In many cases, the patient has no symptoms until she develops labor or chorioamnionitis. Furthermore, a patient with intact membranes can present with leakage of urine, excessive normal vaginal discharge or mucus, or bloody show associated with labor, all of which may mimic the rupture of membranes.

■ PHONE CALL

Questions

1. **What is the gestational age of the fetus?**
   The gestational age of the fetus is the most critical factor in determining the management of PROM.
2. **Is the patient in labor?**

Degree of Urgency

The patient should be seen immediately if she has preterm labor, if she has chorioamnionitis, or if there is a suggestion of fetal distress. Otherwise she should be seen as soon as possible.

■ ELEVATOR THOUGHTS

What conditions are associated with a higher risk of PROM and preterm PROM?
■ Local infection
   Patients who are carriers of *Neisseria gonorrhoeae, Chlamydia trachomatis,* group B streptococci, *Trichomonas vaginalis,* or *Gardnerella vaginalis* are at an increased risk for PROM, probably because the local infection results in weakening of the membranes. These patients are also at a greater risk for chorioamnionitis and postpartum endometritis.
■ Multiple gestation
■ Polyhydramnios
■ Incompetent cervix
■ Cervical cerclage
■ Previous cervical laceration or operation
■ Smoking

What are potential complications that can result from PROM?
■ Preterm labor
   Preterm PROM is responsible for 25 to 33% of all preterm births. This percentage is higher for patients of lower socioeconomic class and patients with sexually transmitted diseases. In women with preterm PROM at 28 to 34 weeks of gestation, approximately 50% will be in labor within 24 hours

and 75% will be in labor within 1 week. In women with preterm PROM before 26 weeks, 50% will be in labor within 1 week.

- Maternal chorioamnionitis

  The incidence of chorioamnionitis in all cases of PROM is 0.5 to 1%. In patients with prolonged rupture of membranes, the incidence of chorioamnionitis is 3 to 15%. The incidence of chorioamnionitis is greatest in patients with preterm PROM, ranging from 13 to 60%. In these patients, there is also a 2 to 13% incidence of postpartum endometritis.

- Fetal infection

  Fetal pneumonia, sepsis, urinary tract infection, or conjunctivitis can occur. Serious neonatal infection is found in 5% of all cases of preterm PROM and in 15 to 20% of cases of maternal chorioamnionitis.

- Fetal compromise

  In patients with preterm PROM, the incidence of fetal compromise is 8.5%. This represents an almost sixfold higher incidence than the incidence of fetal compromise in patients with preterm labor with intact membranes. The cause is probably the increased frequency of umbilical cord compression when there is no longer adequate fluid to protect the cord. A higher incidence of umbilical cord prolapse, approximately 1.5%, also contributes to the increased risk of fetal compromise.

- Fetal deformations

  Preterm PROM at early gestational ages can result in impaired development of the fetal lungs, referred to as pulmonary hypoplasia, which is lethal. Furthermore, early preterm PROM can cause intrauterine growth restriction and compression malformations of the face and limbs. The incidence of these fetal deformations is 3.5% when preterm PROM occurs before 26 weeks of gestational age.

■ MAJOR THREAT TO FETAL LIFE

- Prematurity
- Sepsis
- Fetal compromise
- Fetal deformations

■ MAJOR THREAT TO MATERNAL LIFE

- Sepsis secondary to chorioamnionitis
- Sepsis secondary to endometritis

■ BEDSIDE

Quick Look Test

Is the patient in labor?

In the patient with a term pregnancy and PROM, labor is desirable. In the absence of chorioamnionitis and any other pre-existing complications, labor should be managed in the usual manner. However, in the patient with preterm PROM, labor is not necessarily desired despite the potential for chorioamnionitis because of the complications associated with prematurity. If premature birth is anticipated, the appropriate personnel, including the anesthesiologist and pediatrician or neonatologist, should be made aware of the patient's condition. Maternal transport to another medical facility better equipped to care for the premature infant should be considered.

Is there evidence of fetal compromise?

Abnormal fetal heart rate patterns suggestive of fetal compromise may be caused by umbilical cord compression or prolapse.

Vital Signs

A maternal fever is suggestive of chorioamnionitis. Otherwise, vital signs are usually normal.

Selective History and Chart Review

1. What is the gestational age of the fetus?

    The gestational age should be established by the patient's last menstrual period, early prenatal examinations, and previous ultrasound examinations.

2. When did rupture of membranes occur?

    The patient should be asked when rupture of membranes occurred. The time of rupture of membranes affects the likelihood of chorioamnionitis, fetal infection, and fetal deformation.

Selective Physical Examination

Abdominal	Uterine contractions may be palpable.
Pelvic	
External genitalia and vagina	Watery discharge is noted externally or in a vaginal pool.
Cervix	Watery discharge may be observed flowing from the cervical os when fundal pressure is applied or the patient performs Valsalva's maneuver.
	Cervical dilatation and effacement may be noted visually by sterile speculum examination.
	Digital cervical examination should not be performed in the patient with preterm PROM who is not in labor.

Uterus and adnexa   Uterine contractions may be palpable. Uterine
                     tenderness is suggestive of chorioamnionitis.

Orders

1. Prepare the patient for a sterile speculum examination and
   have available Nitrazine paper and microscope slides.
2. Begin external uterine monitoring.
3. Initiate external electronic fetal heart rate monitoring.
4. Obtain a complete blood count (CBC) with differential.
5. Do not perform digital cervical examination on the patient
   with preterm PROM who is not in labor.

■ DIAGNOSTIC TESTING

1. Tests to document rupture of membranes
   The diagnosis of rupture of membranes can be confirmed by
the presence of amniotic fluid pooling in the vagina or passing
through the cervical os. If the diagnosis is uncertain, the following tests should be performed to confirm or rule out rupture of membranes.
   a. Nitrazine test for pH of vagina
      Nitrazine paper should be used to test the pH of vaginal
   fluid. This test is performed by swabbing the vagina with
   a sterile cotton-tipped applicator and then touching the
   applicator to a strip of Nitrazine paper. As an alternative, a
   strip of Nitrazine paper can be applied to the vaginal introitus. The normal vaginal pH is 4.5 to 6.0. Amniotic fluid is
   more basic and has a pH of 7.1 to 7.3. The color of Nitrazine
   paper changes from yellow to blue at a pH >6.0. A false-
   positive Nitrazine test can be caused by contamination of
   the vagina by semen, blood, vaginal infection, and alkaline
   antiseptics.
   b. Microscope slide test for ferning of vaginal fluid
      This test is performed by swabbing the posterior fornix
   of the vagina with a cotton-tipped applicator and preparing
   a smear on a microscope slide. The smear is allowed to dry
   and is examined with a microscope under low power. A
   ferning pattern is seen in the presence of ruptured membranes.
   c. Intrauterine instillation of dye
      Under ultrasound guidance, a diluted solution of indigo
   carmine dye, 1 ml in 5 to 10 ml of sterile saline, is instilled
   with a spinal needle transabdominally into the uterus. Passage of blue fluid from the vagina is evidence of ruptured
   membranes.

2. Ultrasound examination

The gestational age of the fetus should be established by an ultrasound examination if the gestational age is unclear when reviewing menstrual dating, prenatal examinations, and prior ultrasound examinations. Ultrasound examination also establishes the presentation of the fetus. This is especially important in patients with preterm PROM who are not in labor, because digital examination should not be performed to determine fetal presentation in these patients. Ultrasound examination in some cases helps in confirming the diagnosis of PROM by demonstrating a low amniotic fluid index (AFI) (Figs. 20–1 and 20–2).

3. Tests to rule out chorioamnionitis

a. CBC with differential

An elevated white blood cell count with the presence of bands is suggestive of chorioamnionitis. Unfortunately, the white blood cell count is nonspecific and can be elevated in a patient during normal labor.

b. Amniocentesis and culture of amniotic fluid

In patients with preterm PROM who have adequate amounts of fluid, amniocentesis can be performed to confirm or rule out chorioamnionitis. A specimen should be submitted for Gram stain as well as amniotic fluid culture and sensitivity. The frequency of organisms found in the culture of amniotic fluid obtained by amniocentesis is listed in Table 20–1. Because results of amniotic fluid culture take 24 to 48 hours, amniotic fluid glucose can be measured. An

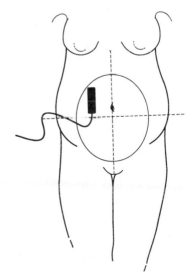

Figure 20–1 □ Technique for assessing the amniotic fluid index (AFI). (From Creasy RK, Resnik R: Maternal-Fetal Medicine: Principles and Practice, 3rd ed. Philadelphia, WB Saunders Co, 1994, p 621.)

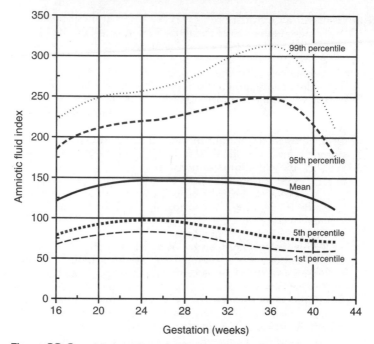

Figure 20-2 □ Mean and percentiles for amniotic fluid index. (Redrawn from Moore TR, Cayle JE: Amniotic fluid index in normal human pregnancy. Am J Obstet Gynecol 1990;162:1168.)

Table 20-1 □ **COMBINED FREQUENCY OF ORGANISMS CULTURED FROM AMNIOTIC FLUID OBTAINED BY AMNIOCENTESIS IN PATIENTS WITH PRETERM PROM (7 STUDIES)**

Group B streptococci	20%
Gardnerella vaginalis	17%
Peptostreptococcus/Peptococcus	11%
Fusobacteria	10%
Bacteroides fragilis	9%
Other streptococci	9%
Bacteroides species	5%

From Creasy RK, Resnik R: Maternal-Fetal Medicine: Principles and Practice, 4th ed. Philadelphia, WB Saunders Co, 1999, p 650.

amniotic fluid glucose concentration <20 mg/dl is suggestive of chorioamnionitis. The presence of white blood cells
without any other amnionitic fluid findings is not indicative
of chorioamnionitis.

c. **Nonstress test and biophysical profile**

Nonreactive nonstress tests are associated with perinatal
infection. Fetal biophysical profile testing can also be used
to detect fetal infection (Table 20–2). The loss of fetal movement, fetal tone, and breathing activity are suggestive of
fetal infection, although these signs are nonspecific. A biophysical profile score of ≤6 is associated with perinatal
infection and is furthermore suspicious for chronic asphyxia
(Table 20–3).

d. **Serum C-reactive protein**

An elevated serum C-reactive protein with a level >0.8
mg/dl is suggestive of chorioamnionitis, but this test is
nonspecific.

4. **Cervical cultures**

Cultures for *Chlamydia trachomatis, Neisseria gonorrhoeae,* and
group B streptococci should be obtained in patients at risk
for these sexually transmitted diseases. Patients with positive
cultures should be treated with the appropriate antibiotic to
decrease the risk of perinatal transmission.

5. **Tests for fetal lung maturity**

Fetal lung maturity is one of the most important factors that
is considered in the management of the patient with preterm
PROM. Phospholipid analysis of amniotic fluid is used to
document fetal lung maturity. A **lecithin-to-sphingomyelin
(L/S) ratio** of >2.0 and the presence of **phosphatidylglycerol
(PG)** are very assuring, although they do not provide absolute
guarantee of fetal lung maturity. Phospholipid levels as a function of gestational age are illustrated in Figure 20–3.

Unlike lecithin and sphingomyelin, PG is not present in
blood, vaginal secretions, or meconium, and therefore the presence of these contaminants in amniotic fluid does not affect
the interpretation of PG levels. The incidence of respiratory
distress syndrome is approximately 34% at 33 weeks of gestation, 14% at 34 weeks, 6% at 35 weeks, and 3 to 4% after 35
weeks. In the patient with PROM at 33 to 35 weeks of gestation, amniotic fluid can be collected for phospholipid measurements. If there is an adequate vaginal pool, fluid can be collected from the vagina with a sterile syringe and catheter. The
presence of PG is indicative of lung maturity at least a week
later than the L/S ratio. Therefore, PG determination in vaginal
pool fluid is considered a screening test; if it is absent, amniocentesis should be performed and the L/S ratio should be
determined. Insulin has been shown to interfere with surfactant synthesis. Therefore, the interpretation of the L/S ratio

Table 20-2 □ BIOPHYSICAL PROFILE SCORING: TECHNIQUE AND INTERPRETATION

Biophysical Variable	Normal Score	Abnormal (Score = 0)
Fetal breathing movements	At least one episode of FBM of at least 30-sec duration in 30-min observation	Absent FBM or no episode of ≥30 sec in 30 min
Gross body movement	At least three discrete body/limb movements in 30 min (episodes of active continuous movement considered as single movement)	Two or fewer episodes of body/limb movements in 30 min
Fetal tone	At least one episode of active extension with return to flexion of fetal limb(s) or trunk; opening and closing of hand considered normal tone	Either slow extension with return to partial flexion or movement of limb in full extension or absent fetal movement with fetal hand held in complete or partial deflection
Reactive FHR	At least two episodes of FHR acceleration of ≥15 beats/min and of at least 15-sec duration associated with fetal movement in 30 min	Fewer than two episodes of acceleration of FHR or acceleration of <15 beats/min in 30 min
Qualitative AFV*	At least one pocket of AF that measures at least 2 cm in two perpendicular planes	Either no AF pockets or a pocket <2 cm in two perpendicular planes

From Creasy RK, Resnik R: Maternal-Fetal Medicine: Principles and Practice, 4th ed. Philadelphia, WB Saunders Co, 1999, p 322.

FBM = fetal breathing movement; FHR = fetal heart rate; AFV = amniotic fluid volume; AF = amniotic fluid.

*Modification of the criteria for reduced amniotic fluid from <1 to <2 cm would seem reasonable.

and phospholipid levels is modified in patients with diabetes. An L/S ratio of ≥3.5 and a PG level of ≥3% are usually required as indicators of fetal lung maturity in the fetus of a patient with diabetes.

An alternative to laboratory measurement of phospholipids is the **foam stability test,** also referred to as the **"shake test."** This test evaluates amniotic fluid for sufficient surfactant to

Table 20–3 □ MANAGEMENT OF BIOPHYSICAL PROFILE SCORES

Score	Interpretation	Recommended Management
10	Normal infant, low risk for chronic asphyxia	Repeat testing at weekly intervals; repeat twice weekly in diabetic patients and patients ≥42 wk gestation
8	Normal infant, low risk for chronic asphyxia	Repeat testing at weekly intervals; repeat twice weekly in diabetic patients and patients ≥42 wk; oligohydramnios indication for delivery
6	Suspected chronic asphyxia	Repeat testing in 4–6 hr; deliver if oligohydramnios present
4	Suspected chronic asphyxia	If ≥36 wk and favorable, then deliver; if ≤36 wk and L/S <2.0, repeat test in 24 hr; if repeat score <4, deliver
0–2	Strong suspicion of chronic asphyxia	Extend testing time to 120 min; if persistent score <4 deliver, provided gestational age is sufficiently advanced to permit possible neonatal survival

L/S = amniotic fluid lecithin:sphingomyelin ratio.
From Creasy RK, Resnik R: Maternal-Fetal Medicine: Principles and Practice, 4th ed. Philadelphia, WB Saunders Co, 1999, p 322.

form a stable foam at the air-surface interface. The steps to perform the shake test are listed in Table 20–4. The presence of a ring of bubbles that persists at the air-fluid interface for 15 minutes is a positive test and is usually indicative of fetal lung maturity. A problem with the shake test is the frequency of false-negative tests, because a positive test requires an L/S ratio of 4.0 to 6.0.

■ MANAGEMENT

1. **Patients who present with PROM, along with advanced active labor, chorioamnionitis, or fetal compromise, should undergo delivery regardless of gestational age**
   Vaginal delivery should be attempted and cesarean section should be performed only for the usual obstetrical indications. In patients with chorioamnionitis, IV antibiotics should be given during labor. The choice of antibiotic agents depends on the organisms suspected. Ampicillin, gentamicin, and cephalosporins have been used successfully. There is much more controversy about the optimal management of patients with

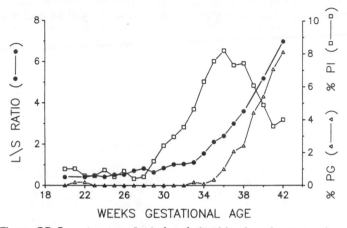

Figure 20-3 □ Amniotic fluid phospholipid levels and gestational age. (From Creasy RK, Resnik R: Maternal-Fetal Medicine: Principles and Practice, 4th ed. Philadelphia, WB Saunders Co, 1999, p 417. Data from Gluck L, et al: Am J Obstet Gynecol 1974;120:142, and Hallman M, et al: Am J Obstet Gynecol 1976;125:613, as shown in Jobe A: The developmental biology of the lung. In Fanaroff AA, Martin RJ, eds: Neonatal-Perinatal Medicine. St Louis, Mosby–Year Book, 1992, p 792.)

Table 20-4 □ **STEPS FOR PERFORMING AMNIOTIC FLUID "SHAKE TEST"**

Materials needed	Amniotic fluid recently collected
	95% ethanol (19 parts of absolute alcohol mixed with 1 part of distilled water)
	0.9% saline
	Two 13 × 100-mm glass tubes with Teflon-lined plastic screw cap
Steps of test	1. Mix 1 ml of amniotic fluid and 1 ml of ethanol in one tube.
	2. Mix 0.5 ml of amniotic fluid, 0.5 ml of saline, and 1 ml of ethanol in the second tube.
	3. Shake both tubes for 15 seconds and place tubes upright.
	4. Wait for 15 minutes and look for a ring of bubbles or foam at the air–liquid interface.
Results	Positive test: ring of bubbles is observed in both tubes
	Equivocal test: ring of bubbles is observed only in first tube
	Negative test: ring of bubbles is not observed in either tube

PROM without chorioamnionitis, advanced labor, or fetal compromise, especially if the patient has preterm PROM.

2. PROM at term

The goal of management of the term patient with PROM is delivery before the development of chorioamnionitis. Fortunately, 95% of patients at term enter into spontaneous labor within 28 hours after rupture of membranes. Therefore, one of two management plans can be used: expectant management for up to 72 hours, or immediate induction of labor. Fetal status, the status of the cervix, and the patient's wishes should be considered in deciding between these two management plans.

a. Expectant management for up to 72 hours

(1) Await spontaneous labor.

(2) Avoid digital cervical examinations until the patient is in labor.

(3) Initiate intermittent electronic fetal heart rate monitoring and antepartum testing with nonstress tests and / or biophysical profile assessment. Nonreactive nonstress tests and a biophysical profile score ≤6 are associated with chorioamnionitis.

(4) Perform serial temperature recordings and uterine palpation for clinical signs of chorioamnionitis.

(5) Obtain serial CBCs with differential. Serum C-reactive protein may also be monitored.

(6) Deliver if chorioamnionitis or fetal distress develops.

b. Induction of labor immediately

(1) Induce labor with IV oxytocin infusion.

(2) Administer prostaglandin agents for preinduction cervical ripening if the cervix is unfavorable for induction

   (a) **Dinoprostone gel (Prepidil) 0.5 mg intracervical every 6 hours**

   (b) **Dinoprostone vaginal insert (Cervidil) 10 mg every 12 hours**

   (c) **Misoprostol (Cytotec) 20 to 50 μg intravaginally or PO every 3 to 6 hours**

3. Preterm PROM

The major fetal risks of preterm PROM are prematurity and infection. Therefore, the goal of the management of preterm PROM without chorioamnionitis, labor, or fetal compromise is prolongation of the pregnancy until the risk of infection outweighs the risk of premature delivery. If there is pulmonary maturity, delivery after 32 to 36 weeks is rarely associated with significant neonatal morbidity.

a. Expectant management

Expectant management can be used in any patient with preterm PROM but is especially recommended before 30 to 32 weeks of gestation.

(1) Administer prophylactic antibiotics.

The use of prophylactic antibiotics increases the latency period and decreases the risks of chorioamnionitis, endometritis, neonatal sepsis, neonatal pneumonia, and intraventricular hemorrhage. Ampicillin, erythromycin, and the combination of ampicillin, gentamicin, and clindamycin have been used successfully. The use of prophylactic antibiotics is especially important if the patient is a known carrier of group B streptococci.

(2) Administer corticosteroids: **Celestone Soluspan solution 2 ml IM, repeat dose in 24 hours** (1 ml of Celestone contains 3 mg of betamethasone sodium and 3 ml of betamethasone acetate).

Steroid administration has been shown to decrease the incidence of respiratory distress syndrome, periventricular hemorrhage, and necrotizing enterocolitis. The benefits of steroids outweigh the possible risk of compromised maternal immune status between 24 and 32 weeks of gestation.

(3) Administer tocolytics.

Tocolytics such as beta-adrenergic drugs or magnesium sulfate can be given in an attempt to prolong the latency period.

(4) Order modified bedrest.

(5) Avoid digital cervical examinations until the patient is in labor.

(6) Initiate intermittent electronic fetal heart rate monitoring and antepartum testing with nonstress tests and/or biophysical profile assessment. Nonreactive nonstress tests and a biophysical profile score ≤6 are associated with chorioamnionitis.

(7) Perform serial temperature recordings and uterine palpation for clinical signs of chorioamnionitis.

(8) Obtain serial CBCs with differential. C-reactive protein could also be monitored.

(9) Obtain amniocentesis for Gram stain, glucose, and culture if needed to diagnose chorioamnionitis.

(10) Deliver if chorioamnionitis or nonreassuring fetal heart rate patterns develop.

b. Active management

Active management may be used in patients with preterm PROM between 32 and 36 weeks of gestation.

(1) Obtain amniotic fluid from the vagina or by amniocentesis for phospholipid analysis.

(2) If fetal lung maturity is confirmed, induction of labor can be considered, especially if the cervix is favorable. Cervical ripening can be considered if the cervix is not favorable for induction of labor.

c. Maternal transport

Extremely preterm infants who are delivered in a facility with specialized intensive perinatal and neonatal services have both a higher survival rate and lower rates of short-term and long-term morbidity than those who are transported to such a facility after birth. Therefore, if the patient with midtrimester preterm PROM is initially admitted to a medical facility where the necessary level of care for the infant cannot be provided, maternal transport to a proper facility should be considered unless delivery is imminent.

d. **Management of preterm labor after preterm PROM**

When the patient with preterm PROM begins labor, it should be remembered that preterm labor and delivery are associated with a higher incidence of complications, including fetal compromise, malpresentation, and birth trauma. The following steps should be taken:

(1) **Initiate continuous electronic fetal heart rate monitoring.**

(2) **Notify the anesthesiologist and pediatric team of the patient's status.**

(3) **Provide adequate anesthesia to ensure a controlled delivery.**

(4) **Consider amnioinfusion.**

Amnioinfusion has been used to decrease the incidence of fetal compromise by replacing, at least in part, the amniotic fluid that is lost with PROM and by reducing the risk of umbilical cord compression. The procedure is performed by infusing room-temperature normal saline into the uterine cavity through an intrauterine catheter. Amnioinfusion can be performed as a bolus infusion or continuous infusion. Bolus infusion is administered by infusing 500 to 800 ml of saline at a rate of 10 to 15 ml/min. A repeat infusion can be administered as needed if there is further loss of fluid.

Continuous infusion is administered by infusing saline at a rate of 10 ml/min for 1 hour, followed by a maintenance infusion of 3 ml/min. Overdistention should be avoided because it can cause abnormal fetal heart rate patterns.

(5) **Have available the proper personnel and equipment for an emergency cesarean section.**

(6) **Consider the use of low forceps and an episiotomy to reduce resistance and trauma to the fetal head, especially with a prolonged second stage of labor.**

(7) **Decide on the route of delivery for the preterm fetus by using the same guidelines that would normally apply to the term fetus.**

Cesarean section should be considered for the frank breech infant with an estimated weight of <1500 g because of the increased morbidity associated with vaginal delivery of these infants.

4. Midtrimester PROM

Approximately 1% of pregnancies are complicated by PROM between 16 and 26 weeks of gestation. The fetal survival rate after midtrimester PROM is approximately 30%. This survival rate is highly dependent on the gestational age at rupture, the presence of infection, fetal deformities, and pulmonary hypoplasia. Pulmonary hypoplasia rarely occurs in patients with PROM after 26 weeks, but it occurs in 1 to 27% of patients with midtrimester PROM.

Advances in neonatology have resulted in survival rates of up to 75% for infants born between 24 and 26 weeks. Furthermore, midtrimester PROM can be associated with a prolonged latency period in a small percentage of patients. In some studies, almost 20% of patients have latency periods of approximately 1 month. However, the risk of chorioamnionitis is almost 40%, and there is a risk of maternal sepsis and even death. Even if neonatal survival is achieved, delayed motor development, developmental delays, cerebral palsy, hydrocephalus, mental retardation, chronic lung disease, and blindness can occur. Therefore it is often difficult to decide on a management plan. Both parents must be counseled extensively concerning the options and the poor prognosis, so that they are then able to participate fully in deciding on an appropriate management plan. For patients with preterm PROM at a previable gestational age, there are generally two options:

a. Expectant management
  (1) Administer prophylactic antibiotics.
  (2) Avoid digital cervical examinations until the patient is in labor.
  (3) Expectant management can be carried out at home without fetal heart rate monitoring if the gestational age is remote from the age of fetal viability.
  (4) Order modified bedrest.
  (5) Advise against intercourse.
  (6) Perform serial temperature recordings and examinations for clinical signs of chorioamnionitis
  (7) Obtain serial CBCs with differential. Serum C-reactive protein may also be followed.
  (8) Deliver if chorioamnionitis develops.

b. Termination of the pregnancy
  If the patient elects termination, this can be performed with an intravenous oxytocin infusion, **prostaglandin E_2 20 mg by vaginal suppository every 4 hours or misoprostol (Cytotec) 200 µg intravaginally every 12 hours.**

chapter 21

Preterm Labor

■ BACKGROUND AND DEFINITION

Preterm labor: Onset of labor after 20 weeks of gestation but before the completion of 37 weeks, or 259 days, of gestation. Labor is defined as the presence of documented uterine contractions occurring at a frequency of at least four contractions in 20 minutes or eight contractions in 60 minutes with documented cervical change in dilatation, cervical dilatation of ≥2 cm, cervical effacement of ≥80%, or ruptured membranes. Delivery of a fetus before 20 weeks of gestational age is referred to as an **abortion** instead of preterm delivery.

The incidence of preterm labor is approximately 10%. Preterm birth accounts for nearly 85% of all neonatal mortality not caused by congenital anomalies. The predicted neonatal survival rates and weekly improvement in survival rates at various premature gestational ages are listed in Table 21–1. The largest weekly improvements in neonatal survival occur at 26 to 28 weeks of gestation. After 30 weeks, survival rates are greater than 90% and improve only slightly weekly. Even if the premature infant

Table 21–1 □ PREDICTED SURVIVAL BY GESTATIONAL AGE
AND WEEKLY IMPROVEMENT IN NEONATAL SURVIVAL

Gestational Age (weeks)	Survival by Gestational Age (%)	Weekly Improvement in Survival (%)
22	0.0	0.0
23	1.8	1.8
24	9.9	8.1
25	15.5	5.6
26	54.7	39.2
27	67.0	12.3
28	77.4	10.4
29	85.2	7.8
30	90.6	5.4
31	94.2	3.6
32	96.5	2.3
33	97.9	1.4

Adapted from Cooper RL, Goldenberg RL, Creasy RK, et al: A multicenter study of preterm birth weight and gestational age specific mortality. Am J Obstet Gynecol 1993;168:78.

survives, there is significant morbidity associated with prematurity, especially from intraventricular hemorrhage and respiratory distress syndrome secondary to immature lungs. Prematurity also results in significant long-term problems including chronic respiratory disease, neurological impairment, seizure disorders, developmental delays, visual impairment, hearing impairment, and cerebral palsy.

Although significant advances have been made in neonatology, resulting in improved survival rates of the preterm neonate, no concomitant advances have been made in the prevention of preterm births. Despite extensive research efforts in the prevention, early recognition, and treatment of preterm labor, the incidence of preterm labor has increased by 17% in the past 15 years. Even routine cervical examinations performed in the late second and early third trimesters and home uterine monitoring have not affected the incidence of preterm births.

■ CLINICAL PRESENTATION

Uterine contractions
Uterine tightening
Menstrual-like cramps
Pelvic pressure
Back pain
Rupture of membranes
Watery vaginal discharge
Vaginal spotting

The symptoms of preterm labor can be so vague and subtle that by the time the diagnosis of preterm labor is made, advanced cervical dilatation or rupture of membranes has already taken place. Uterine contractions are frequently painless, and fewer than 50% of patients in preterm labor are aware of their contractions. An increase in vaginal discharge, which is often watery and stained pink, is noticed by 30 to 50% of patients. To make the interpretation of these symptoms even more difficult, many of these symptoms are nonspecific and occur in 5 to 20% of normal patients.

■ PHONE CALL

Questions

1. **What is the gestational age of the fetus?**
2. **Does the patient complain of ruptured membranes?**
    Rupture of membranes can be an indication of advanced preterm labor. Furthermore, the treatment of preterm labor

with tocolytic drugs is controversial when there has been rupture of membranes.

3. **Is the patient febrile?**

A fever may be caused by chorioamnionitis resulting from premature rupture of membranes.

Degree of Urgency

The successful treatment of a patient with preterm labor is more likely if treatment is instituted early, before advanced cervical dilatation or rupture of membranes. Therefore, patients with suspected preterm labor should be seen and evaluated as soon as possible.

■ ELEVATOR THOUGHTS

What socioeconomic factors are associated with preterm labor?
- Nonwhite race

Black patients have an incidence of preterm labor of 18.9%, which is almost twice the incidence seen in white patients.
- Low socioeconomic status
- Low maternal age (younger than 20 years of age)
- Advanced maternal age (35 years of age or older)

The risk is greatest for women who are 35 years old or older at the time of their first delivery.
- Strenuous and physically demanding occupation

Occupations that require constant standing also appear to increase the incidence of preterm labor.
- Low prepregnancy maternal weight

Women with weights below their optimal weights at the beginning of pregnancy have a threefold increase in the incidence of preterm labor.

What medical conditions are associated with preterm labor?
- History of preterm delivery

After one preterm birth, the recurrence rate of preterm labor with subsequent pregnancies is 17 to 47%.
- Preterm premature rupture of membranes
- Multiple gestation

Prematurity is the most common cause of perinatal morbidity and mortality in patients with multiple gestation. Almost 50% of twin gestations deliver prematurely. Furthermore, the degree of prematurity increases with the number of fetuses.
- Chorioamnionitis
- Uterine anomaly

Overall, 5 to 15% of all preterm labor is associated with a

uterine anomaly. The risk of preterm labor varies with the specific type of uterine anomaly. A septate uterus is associated with a 4 to 17% incidence of preterm labor. A bicornuate uterus is associated with a 18 to 80% risk.

- Uterine leiomyomata
- Sepsis
  Sepsis from conditions such as acute pyelonephritis or acute appendicitis increases the risk of preterm labor. Endotoxins cause uterine contractions through stimulation of the myometrium.
- Genital infection
  Group B streptococci, *Chlamydia trachomatis, Ureaplasma urealyticum,* and *Trichomonas vaginalis* infections of the lower genital tract have all been associated with an increased risk of preterm labor. Bacterial vaginosis caused by *Gardnerella vaginalis* and multiple anaerobes has also been implicated as a cause of preterm labor.
- Incompetent cervix
- History of second-trimester abortion
  Some studies have also shown an increased risk of preterm labor after multiple first-trimester abortions.
- Placental abruption
- Placenta previa
- Fetal anomalies
- Abdominal surgery during pregnancy
  Abdominal surgery such as for acute appendicitis, cholecystitis, or ovarian neoplasms has been associated with preterm labor.
- Smoking
  The risk of preterm labor appears to be proportionate to the number of cigarettes smoked per day.
- Pregnancy complications
  Certain complications of pregnancy such as severe preeclampsia and intrauterine growth restriction are best treated by early delivery.

What are the causes of neonatal morbidity and mortality associated with prematurity?

- Respiratory distress syndrome (RDS)
  RDS, also referred to as hyaline membrane disease, is the most common neonatal problem associated with prematurity. Its incidence is as high as 93% for infants born at 26 weeks and decreases to 3 to 4% at 36 to 38 weeks of gestation.
- Patent ductus arteriosus (PDA)
  The incidence of PDA is as high as 61% in neonates delivered at 25 weeks and drops to less than 0.5% after 36 weeks of gestation.
- Intraventricular hemorrhage (IVH)

The incidence of IVH is as high as 30% in infants delivered at 26 weeks and is rarely encountered after 32 weeks of gestation.

- Sepsis
- Necrotizing enterocolitis
- Hyperbilirubinemia
- Hypoglycemia

■ MAJOR THREAT TO FETAL LIFE

- Prematurity

  Preterm delivery is the cause of approximately 85% of all perinatal mortalities, excluding fetuses with congenital anomalies.

■ BEDSIDE

Quick Look Test

A patient who appears to be having painful contractions is likely to be in advanced labor. If there has been advanced cervical dilatation, treatment of preterm labor in this patient may be futile.

Preterm labor can be associated with vaginal bleeding from placental abruption or placenta previa. In many cases, delivery even at a preterm gestational age is the treatment of choice if there is severe bleeding from either of these conditions.

Vital Signs

Vital signs are usually normal. If the patient is febrile, chorioamnionitis should be suspected.

Selective History and Chart Review

1. What is the estimated gestational age of the fetus, and has the patient had prior ultrasound examinations to confirm the gestational age?
2. Does the patient have any of the socioeconomic factors associated with preterm labor?
3. Had the patient experienced preterm labor in a previous pregnancy?
4. Does the patient have a history of premature rupture of membranes?
5. Does the patient have any medical conditions such as sepsis, chorioamnionitis, uterine anomalies, or multiple gestation that predispose to preterm labor?

6. Has the patient undergone any testing in an attempt to predict preterm labor, such as cervical length measurement by ultrasonography, fetal fibronectin measurements, or salivary estriol measurements?

Selective Physical Examination

Abdominal	Uterine tenderness with chorioamnionitis
	Uterine irritability with placental abruption
Pelvic	
External genitalia and vagina	Watery discharge or pooling of fluid in the vagina suggestive of rupture of membranes
	Vaginal bleeding is caused by placental abruption or placenta previa or may represent bloody show from cervical dilatation and effacement.
Cervix	Cervical dilatation, effacement, presenting part, and station of the presenting part should be determined.
Uterus and adnexa	Uterine contractions may be palpable.
	Tender with chorioamnionitis
	Tender and irritable with placental abruption

Orders

1. Place the patient at bedrest in the lateral decubitus position.
2. Begin external uterine monitoring.
3. Begin continuous electronic fetal heart rate monitoring.
4. Start IV with either 5% dextrose in water or 0.25% normal saline, and hydrate the patient with 500 ml of intravenous (IV) fluid.
5. Obtain a clean-catch urine specimen for urinalysis and urine culture and sensitivity testing.

■ DIAGNOSTIC TESTING

Tests have been proposed to predict preterm labor in patients with risk factors:

1. Cervical length measurements with transvaginal ultrasound
   The risk of preterm labor is greater at shorter cervical lengths (Fig. 21–1). A cervical length of 25 mm or less measured by transvaginal ultrasound is associated with a relative risk for preterm labor of 6.5 to 7.7.

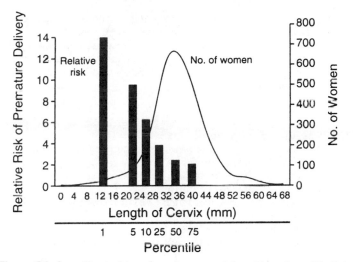

Figure 21–1 □ Cervical length and preterm labor. (From Iams JD, Goldenberg RL, Meis PJ, et al: The length of the cervix and the risk of spontaneous delivery. N Engl J Med 1996;334:567.)

2. Fetal fibronectin enzyme immunoassay

Fetal fibronectin is an extracellular matrix protein that is present between fetal membranes and the uterine decidua. It usually is not found in cervical secretions after 22 weeks of gestation. Its presence is thought to be an indication of disruption of the fetal membrane–decidual interface, especially as a result of infection associated with bacterial vaginosis. Fibronectin immunoassay should be performed only if the following criteria are met:

a. **Membranes are intact**

b. **Cervical dilatation is <3 cm**

c. **Gestational age is between 24 and 35 weeks**

A negative test has a high negative predictive value for delivery within 14 days.

3. Salivary estriol

Estriol is produced by the placenta from precursors that are derived from the fetal adrenal glands. Estriol can be detected as early as 9 weeks of gestation. Levels of estriol increase with gestational age and surge at approximately 3 to 5 weeks before labor. Estriol can be measured in saliva through commercially available kits using enzyme-linked immunosorbent assay (ELISA) technology. Saliva can be collected weekly or biweekly between 22 and 36 weeks of gestation. Normal levels increase from 0.74 ng/ml at 22 to 24 weeks of gestation to 1.77 ng/ml at 36 to 37 weeks of gestation. A level of 2.1 ng/ml or greater is considered abnormal. If a patient has one abnormal result, she should be examined and her risk factors for preterm labor should be assessed. A repeat estriol measurement should be obtained 1 week later. If the second result is also abnormally high, the patient is at high risk for preterm delivery and should be monitored closely.

All patients with suspected preterm labor should have the following diagnostic tests performed.

1. **Ultrasound examination**
   An ultrasound examination should be performed to
   a. **Confirm the gestational age**
   b. **Rule out multiple gestation**
   c. **Determine fetal presentation**
      There is a higher incidence of malpresentations at premature gestational ages.
2. **Serial cervical examinations**
   If membranes have not ruptured, serial cervical examinations should be performed, preferably by the same examiner, to document changes in cervical dilatation and effacement and to confirm the diagnosis of preterm labor. Although treatment of preterm labor is more likely to be successful if initiated early, waiting until there has been cervical change does not jeopardize the efficacy of treatment. The frequency of cervical examinations can be individualized for each patient, based on the strength and frequency of the uterine contractions and the level of patient discomfort.
3. **Tests to document rupture of membranes**
   If obvious pooling of amniotic fluid in the vagina is not seen on pelvic examination, either or both of the following tests should be performed to determine whether the membranes have ruptured. Testing for rupture of membranes should be performed even if the patient denies symptoms of ruptured membranes, because symptoms can be subtle or even absent.
   a. **Nitrazine test for pH of vagina**
      Nitrazine paper should be used to test the pH of vaginal fluid. This is performed by swabbing the vagina with a sterile cotton-tipped applicator and then touching a strip of Nitrazine paper. As an alternative, a strip of Nitrazine paper can be applied to the vaginal introitus. The normal vaginal pH is 4.5 to 6.0. Amniotic fluid is more basic and has a pH of 7.1 to 7.3. The color of Nitrazine paper changes from yellow to blue at a pH of >6.0. A false-positive Nitrazine test can be caused by contamination of the vagina by semen, blood, vaginal infection, and alkaline antiseptics.
   b. **Microscope slide test for ferning of vaginal fluid**
      This test is performed by swabbing the posterior fornix of the vagina with a cotton-tipped applicator and preparing a smear on a microscope slide. The smear is allowed to dry

and is examined under low power with a microscope. A ferning pattern is seen in the presence of ruptured membranes.

4. **External uterine monitoring**

External uterine monitoring is performed to aid in determining both the presence and the frequency of uterine contractions. Monitoring should be performed even if the patient does not report the presence of uterine contractions. Symptoms of preterm labor can be very subtle, and only approximately 45% of patients with preterm labor report the presence of uterine contractions.

5. **Microscopic urinalysis and culture**

Because of the high association between urinary tract infections and preterm labor, a urine specimen should be sent for microscopic urinalysis and for culture and sensitivity testing. Antibiotic and antipyretic therapy should be initiated if there is evidence of a urinary tract infection.

Certain patients with suspected preterm labor should have the following additional diagnostic tests performed.

6. **Cervical cultures**

In patients who are at high risk for a lower genital tract infection, cervical cultures for *C. trachomatis*, herpes simplex, and bacteria such as group B streptococci, *G. vaginalis*, and various anaerobes may be indicated. Although the treatment of cervical infections has not been shown to significantly influence the success of treatment of preterm labor, a positive culture could affect management during labor and the route chosen for delivery.

7. **Amniocentesis**

Amniocentesis can be performed for the following indications:

a. **Determination of fetal lung maturity**

The incidence of RDS is approximately 13.5% at 34 weeks of gestation, 6.4% at 35 weeks, and 3 to 4% after 35 weeks. Therefore, amniocentesis is an option at 33 to 35 weeks to determine whether the fetal lungs are mature based on phospholipid measurements. A **lecithin-to-sphingomyelin (L/S) ratio** >2.0 and the presence of **phosphatidylglycerol (PG)** are reassuring findings, although they do not provide absolute guarantees of fetal lung maturity.

Unlike lecithin and sphingomyelin, PG is not present in blood, vaginal secretions, or meconium; therefore, the presence of these contaminants in amniotic fluid does not affect the interpretation of PG levels. The levels of amniotic fluid phospholipids at various gestational ages are shown in Figure 21–2. Insulin has been shown to interfere with surfactant synthesis. Therefore, the interpretation of the L/S ratio and phospholipid levels is modified in patients with

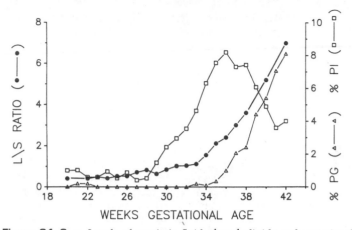

WEEKS GESTATIONAL AGE

Figure 21-2 □ Levels of amniotic fluid phospholipids and gestational age. (From Creasy RK, Resnik R: Maternal-Fetal Medicine: Principles and Practice, 4th ed. Philadelphia, WB Saunders Co, 1999, p 417. Data from Gluck L, et al: Am J Obstet Gynecol 1974;120:142, and Hallman M, et al: Am J Obstet Gynecol 1976;152:613, as shown in Jobe A: The developmental biology of the lung. In Fanaroff AA, Martin RJ, eds: Neonatal-Perinatal Medicine. St Louis, Mosby–Year Book, 1992, p 792.)

diabetes. An L/S ratio ≥3.5 and a PG level ≥3% are required to be assured of fetal lung maturity in the fetus of a patient with diabetes.

An alternative to laboratory measurement of phospholipids is the **foam stability test**, also referred to as the **"shake test,"** which tests amniotic fluid for sufficient surfactant to form a stable foam at the air-surface interface. Although it is inferior to laboratory measurement of phospholipids, the foam stability test can be performed more quickly and inexpensively. The steps taken to perform the shake test are listed in Table 21–2. The presence of a ring of bubbles that persists at the air-fluid interface for 15 minutes is a positive test, verifying fetal lung maturity. A problem with the shake test is the frequency of false-negative tests, because a positive test requires an L/S ratio of 4.0 to 6.0.

b. Tests to confirm chorioamnionitis

Not only is chorioamnionitis a cause of preterm labor, but it is also a contraindication for the use of tocolytic medications to treat preterm labor. It is therefore important to confirm the diagnosis of chorioamnionitis, especially because patients with this infection may be asymptomatic. Although the routine use of amniocentesis has not been established as efficacious in the management of all patients with preterm labor, it can be helpful in patients with sus-

Table 21–2 □ STEPS FOR PERFORMING AMNIOTIC FLUID "SHAKE TEST"

Materials needed	Amniotic fluid recently collected
	95% ethanol (19 parts of absolute alcohol mixed with 1 part of distilled water)
	0.9% saline
	Two 13 × 100-mm glass tubes with Teflon-lined plastic screw cap
Steps of test	1. Mix 1 ml of amniotic fluid and 1 ml of ethanol in one tube.
	2. Mix 0.5 ml of amniotic fluid, 0.5 ml of saline, and 1 ml of ethanol in the second tube.
	3. Shake both tubes for 15 seconds and place tubes upright.
	4. Wait for 15 minutes and look for a ring of bubbles or foam at the air–liquid interface.
Results	Positive test: ring of bubbles is observed in both tubes
	Equivocal test: ring of bubbles is observed only in first tube
	Negative test: ring of bubbles is not observed in either tube

pected chorioamnionitis, to confirm or rule out the diagnosis. A specimen should be submitted for Gram stain as well as amniotic fluid culture and sensitivity tests. Because results of amniotic fluid culture can take 24 to 48 hours, amniotic fluid glucose can be measured to help with the detection of chorioamnionitis. An amniotic fluid glucose concentration <14 mg/dl is suggestive of chorioamnionitis. Patients who have chorioamnionitis should be treated with parenteral antibiotics, and the pediatrician should be notified so that treatment of the infant can be initiated immediately after delivery.

■ MANAGEMENT

1. Bedrest in the lateral decubitus position

The patient should initially be placed at bedrest in the lateral decubitus position while the cervix is evaluated and uterine contraction and fetal heart rate monitoring is performed.

2. Intravenous fluid hydration

Intravenous hydration should be administered with 500 ml of 5% dextrose in water or 0.25% normal saline. Hydration may successfully treat preterm labor in dehydrated patients but has not been shown to be of benefit in hydrated patients. Because of the possible use of a tocolytic drug and the association between these drugs and pulmonary edema, fluid hydration should not be excessive.

3. **Tocolytic medications**

Administration of tocolytic drugs has been shown to be more successful in delaying delivery for a few days than in delaying until term. Although these drugs are commonly used, there is no convincing evidence that they significantly affect either neonatal survival or long-term morbidity. Tocolytic medications are used most often to treat preterm labor in patients with a gestational age <34 weeks. Because of the risk of complications associated with the use of tocolytic medication and the cost of not only the drug but also hospitalization, the use of tocolytics is individualized in patients with a gestational age >34 weeks. After the cervix has dilated beyond 4 to 5 cm, successful treatment of preterm labor with tocolytic medications is unlikely. The relative and absolute contraindications to the administration of tocolytic medications are listed in Table 21–3. Comparison studies have shown that tocolytic drugs are comparable with each other in efficacy and that their differences have more to do with side effects and complications associated with their use. Beta-adrenergic agonists and magnesium sulfate are the most commonly used tocolytic drugs. Prostaglandin inhibitors and calcium antagonists are considered third-line drugs, to be used if beta-adrenergic drugs and magnesium sulfate fail to achieve tocolysis.

a. **Beta-adrenergic agonists**

Beta-adrenergic agonists used to treat preterm labor pri-

Table 21–3 □ CONTRAINDICATIONS TO THE USE OF TOCOLYTIC MEDICATIONS

Relative contraindications
  Maternal cardiac disease
  Mild pregnancy-induced hypertension
  Mild vaginal bleeding
  Hyperthyroidism
  Fetal distress
  Nonlethal fetal anomaly
  Mild intrauterine growth retardation
Absolute contraindications
  Fetal maturity
  Severe pregnancy-induced hypertension
  Eclampsia
  Severe vaginal bleeding
  Chorioamnionitis
  Fetal demise
  Lethal fetal anomaly
  Severe intrauterine growth retardation

marily have beta-2-adrenergic effects, which include the decrease in uterine myometrial activity; they also often have undesired beta-1-adrenergic effects, which include increases in cardiac stroke volume and heart rate.

(1) **Ritodrine (Yutopar) 0.050 to 0.350 mg/min IV** or **5 to 10 mg IM every 2 to 4 hours** or **20 mg PO every 2 to 4 hours** or

(2) **Terbutaline (Brethine) 0.01 to 0.08 mg/min IV** or **0.25 to 0.50 mg IM or SC every 3 to 4 hours** or **2.5 to 5.0 mg PO every 2 to 4 hours**

The tocolytic beta-adrenergic medication should be administered intravenously with an infusion pump, and the dosage given should be the lowest recommended. The dosage is then increased every 15 to 30 minutes until uterine contractions are obliterated or until untoward maternal side effects occur. The serum levels of the drugs correlate closely with maternal heart rate. Some have advocated using a maternal pulse rate of 90 to 105 beats/min as an indication of an adequate drug dose. The dose should not be increased once the maternal heart rate has increased to 130 beats/min or the systolic blood pressure has decreased to <80 mm Hg. Once the uterine contractions have been halted, the infusion should be continued for 12 to 24 hours. The IV dose should then be decreased and intramuscular (IM) or subcutaneous (SC) therapy started 30 minutes before IV therapy is discontinued. If tocolysis continues to be successful, IM or SC therapy is continued for 12 to 24 hours before changing to oral therapy. If uterine contractions do not return when the patient is on oral therapy, the patient can then be discharged home and allowed to ambulate, although she should be advised to avoid strenuous physical activity and prolonged periods of time on her feet. Because semen contains prostaglandins, which stimulate uterine contractions, and it has been found that uterine contractions occur with orgasm, it is also recommended that patients not engage in sexual intercourse.

(3) Maternal side effects caused by beta-adrenergic tocolytic drugs include the following:

    (a) Nausea

    (b) Emesis

    (c) Restlessness

    (d) Agitation

    (e) Paralytic ileus and dermatitis (rare)

(4) Potential complications of beta-adrenergic medications include the following:

    (a) Pulmonary edema

        Pulmonary edema is the most common complication. It usually takes place 30 to 60 hours after the

initiation of treatment and can occur even after the intravenous route of administration has been discontinued. The cause of pulmonary edema is unclear, but predisposing factors are excessive IV hydration, multiple gestation, persistent maternal heart rate >130 beats/min, corticosteroid administration, anemia, infection, and underlying maternal cardiac disease.
- (b) Hypotension
- (c) Cardiac insufficiency
- (d) Cardiac arrhythmia
- (e) Myocardial ischemia
- (f) Hyperglycemia
    The administration of beta-adrenergic drugs can cause hyperglycemia, which is usually of no consequence in the nondiabetic patient but can result in ketoacidosis in diabetic patients.
- (g) Hypokalemia
    Hypokalemia is associated with hyperglycemia. Hypokalemia usually results only from intravenous administration of the beta-adrenergic drug and is transient, commonly resolving by 24 hours. Supplemental potassium is rarely needed.
- (h) Maternal death
- (5) Precautionary steps to be taken when a patient is treated with a beta-adrenergic tocolytic include the following:
    - (a) Obtain baseline maternal weight.
    - (b) Obtain baseline laboratory tests.
        - [1] Serum potassium
        - [2] Serum glucose
        - [3] Complete blood count (CBC)
        - [4] Urinalysis
    - (c) Repeat laboratory tests every 6 to 12 hours.
    - (d) Record intake and output.
    - (e) Limit fluid intake to 1500 to 2500 ml per 24 hours.
    - (f) Auscultate lungs for evidence of pulmonary edema every 6 to 12 hours.
- (6) Contraindications to the use of beta-adrenergic tocolytics, in addition to the contraindications listed in Table 21–3, include the following:
    - (a) Maternal cardiac arrhythmia
    - (b) Maternal cardiac disease
    - (c) Diabetes mellitus
    - (d) Uncontrolled hypertension
    - (e) Thyrotoxicosis

b. Magnesium sulfate
  Although the mechanism of action is unclear, magnesium sulfate depresses myometrial contractility.

(1) **Magnesium sulfate 4.0 to 6.0 g IV over 20 minutes as a loading dose and 1.0 to 3.0 g/hr IV as the maintenance dose** or

(2) **Magnesium gluconate or magnesium oxide 0.5 to 2.0 g PO every 2 to 4 hours**

Magnesium sulfate should be administered intravenously with an infusion pump, and the initial dose should be the lowest dose recommended. The dose should be increased every 15 to 30 minutes until uterine contractions are obliterated or untoward maternal side effects occur. The optimal dose of magnesium sulfate should be continued IV for approximately 24 hours. The patient should then be given an IM or SC beta-adrenergic medication followed by an oral beta-adrenergic tocolytic or oral magnesium gluconate or magnesium oxide. Magnesium has a depressant effect on the central nervous system and also has a competitive antagonistic role with calcium. Inhibition of myometrial contractility takes place at a serum magnesium level of 5 to 8 mg/dl. Loss of deep tendon reflexes occurs at a serum magnesium level of 9 to 13 mg/dl, and respiratory depression takes place at a serum level ≥ 14 mg/dl.

(3) Maternal side effects caused by magnesium sulfate include the following:

    (a) Hot flashes

    (b) Headache

    (c) Nausea

    (d) Dizziness

    (e) Nystagmus

    (f) Dryness of the mouth

    (g) Lethargy

    (h) Urticarial eruptions

(4) Potential complications from magnesium sulfate include the following:

    (a) Pulmonary edema

        As with beta-adrenergic tocolytics, the mechanism of pulmonary edema is unclear, and the use of a corticosteroid, often given to accelerate fetal lung maturity, increases the risk of this complication.

    (b) Hypocalcemia

    (c) Hypotension

    (d) Respiratory depression and arrest

    (e) Fetal and neonatal depression

        When the maternal serum level of magnesium is in the therapeutic range, approximately 50% of fetuses have a nonreactive nonstress test, and 80% do not have sustained respiratory movements on biophysical profile testing.

    (f) Cardiac depression and arrest

(5) Precautionary steps that should be taken when a patient is being treated with magnesium sulfate include the following:

(a) Obtain baseline maternal weight.

(b) Monitor deep tendon reflexes.

(c) Obtain baseline serum magnesium and calcium.

(d) Repeat laboratory tests every 6 to 12 hours, or as indicated by the clinical status.

(e) Record intake and output.

Because magnesium is excreted by the kidneys, urine output should be monitored as an indicator of renal function.

(f) Limit fluid intake to 1500 to 2500 ml per 24 hours.

(g) Auscultate lungs for evidence of pulmonary edema every 6 to 12 hours.

(h) Keep readily available a 10% solution of calcium gluconate to treat respiratory and cardiac arrest caused by magnesium toxicity; if needed, administer 10 ml (1 g) IV of calcium gluconate 10% solution over 10 minutes.

(6) Contraindications to the use of magnesium sulfate for tocolysis, in addition to those listed in Table 21–3, include the following:

(a) Hypocalcemia

(b) Myasthenia gravis

(c) Renal failure

c. **Prostaglandin synthesis inhibitors**

Because prostaglandins stimulate myometrial contractility, antiprostaglandin agents can be effective in the treatment of preterm labor.

(1) **Indomethacin, 100-mg rectal suppository, as a loading dose followed by 25 mg PO every 6 hours**

Indomethacin inhibits the synthesis of prostaglandins by inhibiting the enzyme cyclooxygenase. It is not used for more than approximately 48 hours because of the risk of oligohydramnios. This complication is a result of decreased fetal urine output.

(2) Maternal side effects caused by indomethacin include the following:

(a) Nausea

(b) Emesis

(c) Headaches

(d) Dizziness

(e) Depression

(f) Psychosis

(3) Potential complications associated with indomethacin use include the following:

(a) Postpartum hemorrhage

    (b) Oligohydramnios

    (c) Premature closure of the ductus arteriosus, resulting in pulmonary hypertension in the fetus

  (4) Contraindications to the use of indomethacin for to-colysis, in addition to the contraindications listed in Table 21–3, include the following:

    (a) Asthma

    (b) Oligohydramnios

    (c) Coronary artery disease

    (d) Renal failure

    (e) Hepatic failure

    (f) Gastrointestinal bleeding

d. Calcium antagonists

Calcium channel blockers such as nifedipine inhibit the movement of calcium ions through cell membranes, resulting in inhibition of smooth muscle contractility.

  (1) **Nifedipine 10 mg sublingual, repeat after 20 minutes if necessary, and 10 to 20 mg every 4 to 6 hours as the maintenance dose**

  (2) Maternal side effects caused by nifedipine include the following:

    (a) Vasodilatation

    (b) Flushing

    (c) Nausea

    (d) Headaches

  (3) Potential complications associated with nifedipine use include the following:

    (a) Hypotension

    (b) Liver toxicity

  (4) Contraindications to the use of nifedipine for tocolysis, in addition to those listed in Table 21–3, include the following:

    (a) Maternal liver disease

    (b) Maternal hypotension

4. Corticosteroids

Antepartum corticosteroid therapy should be considered for women in preterm labor with gestational ages of 24 to 34 weeks. The major benefits derived from corticosteroid therapy are decreased morbidity from respiratory distress syndrome and intraventricular hemorrhage and decreased neonatal mortality. Although the maximum benefits occur 24 hours after initiation of treatment, some benefits can be gained after less than 24 hours. Therefore, corticosteroids should be administered unless delivery is imminent.

Celestone Soluspan solution 2 ml IM, repeat dose in 24 hours (1 ml of Celestone contains 3 mg of betamethasone sodium and 3 mg of betamethasone acetate)

The effects of treatment last for 7 days; therefore, a repeat dose should be administered if the fetus remains undelivered and the patient is still undergoing treatment for preterm labor.

5. **Maternal transport**

The extremely preterm infant who is delivered in a facility with specialized intensive perinatal and neonatal services has a greater chance of survival and a lower incidence of both short-term and long-term morbidity than the infant who is transported to such a facility after birth. Therefore, if the patient is initially admitted to a medical facility where these services are not available, she should be transported before delivery to the proper facility as soon as she has been stabilized.

6. **Management during labor**

If efforts to halt preterm labor have failed and delivery is anticipated, management of the patient requires recognition that preterm labor and delivery are associated with a higher incidence of complications including fetal distress, malpresentation, and birth trauma. The following steps should be taken:

a. Initiate continuous electronic fetal heart rate monitoring.
b. Notify the anesthesiologist and pediatric or neonatal team of the patient's condition.
c. Provide adequate anesthesia to ensure a controlled delivery.
d. Have available the proper personnel and equipment for an emergency cesarean section.
e. Consider the use of low forceps and an episiotomy to reduce resistance and trauma to the fetal head, especially with prolonged second stage of labor.
f. Decide on the route of delivery for the preterm fetus by using the same guidelines that would normally apply to the term fetus.

   Cesarean section should be performed for the frank breech infant with an estimated weight <1500 g because of the increased morbidity associated with vaginal delivery of these infants.

■ BACKGROUND AND DEFINITION

Shoulder dystocia: An obstetrical emergency that occurs when the anterior shoulder does not deliver either spontaneously or with downward traction and episiotomy after delivery of the head. The incidence of shoulder dystocia is 0.2 to 2.0%.

■ CLINICAL PRESENTATION

Recoil of the fetal chin into the perineum immediately after delivery of the head, also referred to as the "turtle sign," is seen.

■ PHONE CALL

Degree of Urgency

Shoulder dystocia is an obstetrical emergency, and the patient should be seen immediately.

■ ELEVATOR THOUGHTS

What are factors that contribute to shoulder dystocia?

The best management of shoulder dystocia is prevention. Even though risk factors for shoulder dystocia have been identified, the use of these risk factors to predict shoulder dystocia has been unsuccessful.

- Maternal diabetes mellitus
  Maternal diabetes is associated with a twofold to sixfold increase in the incidence of shoulder dystocia, compared with nondiabetic pregnant women.
- Maternal obesity
  The incidence of shoulder dystocia is 5.1% if the maternal weight is greater than 250 lb.
- Fetal macrosomia
  Shoulder dystocia occurs more frequently in infants with birth weights of >4000 g (8 lb 13 oz). Even in nondiabetic women, a birth weight of >4500 g is associated with a 4 to 23% incidence of shoulder dystocia. However, between 40 and 50% of all cases of shoulder dystocia occur with birth weights <4000 g.

- Postdate pregnancy
- Oxytocin administration

   Fetal macrosomia often causes abnormal labor and requires the administration of oxytocin, which is associated with a higher risk of shoulder dystocia.

- Prolonged second stage of labor

   The incidence of shoulder dystocia increases to 4.6% when the second stage of labor is prolonged. A prolonged second stage of labor is defined as >2 hours for a nulliparous patient or >1 hour for a multiparous patient.

- Midpelvic or high-pelvic operative delivery with forceps or vacuum extraction

These factors are cumulative. The combination of maternal diabetes and fetal macrosomia is probably the most significant, resulting in a 20 to 50% incidence of shoulder dystocia. The incidence of shoulder dystocia with an infant weighing >4000 g and delivered by midpelvic operative delivery after a prolonged second stage of labor is 23%.

What types of traumatic neonatal injuries are associated with shoulder dystocia?
- Fracture of the clavicle
- Fracture of the humerus
- Phrenic nerve injuries
- Brachial plexus injuries or Erb palsy

   Brachial plexus injuries result from excessive downward traction and lateral extension of the fetal head in an attempt to deliver the anterior shoulder. Such injuries occur in 10 to 20% of infants whose deliveries are complicated by shoulder dystocia. Fortunately, 80 to 90% of infants with this injury recover completely. Brachial plexus injuries can occur without shoulder dystocia and can even occur during cesarean delivery. Furthermore, because these injuries have been observed in the absence of excessive traction of the fetal head, it is felt that some cases of brachial plexus injuries occur in utero from the forces of labor.

■ MAJOR THREAT TO FETAL LIFE

- Fetal asphyxia

   The perinatal mortality rate from shoulder dystocia is as high as 33% and results primarily from asphyxia due to cord compression, which is a result of obstructed delivery.

■ MAJOR THREAT TO MATERNAL LIFE

- Maternal postpartum hemorrhage from uterine atony or lacerations of the cervix, vagina, or vulva

■ BEDSIDE

Quick Look Test

Does the patient appear to have adequate anesthesia?

The maneuvers used to manage shoulder dystocia can be uncomfortable and, furthermore, may require patient cooperation. Therefore, an anesthesiologist should be called immediately if anesthesia does not appear to be adequate.

Vital Signs

Vital signs are normal.

Selective History and Chart Review

1. Before delivery, a patient's chart should be reviewed to determine whether she has any antepartum risk factors for shoulder dystocia, namely diabetes, fetal macrosomia, excessive maternal weight gain, or postterm pregnancy.
2. The labor records should also be reviewed for intrapartum risk factors such as the use of oxytocin, prolonged second stage of labor, and a high fetal station requiring midpelvic operative delivery.

Selective Physical Examination

Pelvic

External genitalia and vagina	"Turtle sign" with the fetal chin pulled back into the perineum after delivery of the fetal head

Orders

Have the nurse call immediately for assistance from another obstetrician and/or another labor and delivery nurse, an anesthesiologist, and the pediatric or neonatal team.

■ DIAGNOSTIC TESTING

Shoulder dystocia is diagnosed at the time of delivery based on the clinical findings. There are no diagnostic tests that can be used to accurately predict when shoulder dystocia will occur. Ultrasound examination for estimating fetal weight has not generally been accurate. Only 60% of cases of macrosomia are diagnosed by ultrasound examination.

■ MANAGEMENT

Even though most cases of shoulder dystocia cannot be predicted, it is reasonable to consider cesarean section for diabetic patients with fetal macrosomia, especially when the estimated fetal weight is >4500 g.

When shoulder dystocia is encountered, management should consist of some or all of the following steps. Even when appropriate steps are employed and maneuvers performed, neonatal injury might still occur.

1. **Immediate call for additional help**
   Assistance should be requested from another obstetrician or a labor and delivery nurse, an anesthesiologist, and the pediatric or neonatal team.
2. **Cutting of a generous episiotomy**
3. **Sharp flexion of the hips or McRoberts maneuver**
   The McRoberts maneuver consists of removing the patient's legs from the stirrups and flexing the hips sharply so that the knees are brought back against the patient's chest. This maneuver straightens the sacrum, rotates the pubic symphysis toward the patient's head, and decreases the angle of pelvic inclination. The cephalad rotation of the pelvis will, it is hoped, free the anterior shoulder from behind the pubic symphysis.
4. **Suprapubic pressure**
   An assistant should apply suprapubic pressure with the palm of the hand or a closed fist downward toward the floor, while the delivering physician applies downward traction to the fetal head. Suprapubic pressure is applied in an attempt to dislodge the anterior shoulder from behind the pubic symphysis. It is important for the assistant to be elevated on a stand or a lift in order to apply sufficient pressure downward. Furthermore, it is important that the assistant does not apply fundal pressure.
5. **Shoulders rotated to an oblique diameter**
   This maneuver is accomplished by placing a hand behind the anterior shoulder of the fetus and pushing forward toward the anterior surface of the chest, so that the shoulders are now in an oblique orientation instead of an anterior-posterior orientation (Fig. 22–1).
6. **Corkscrew maneuver or Woods' maneuver**
   Woods' maneuver is performed by placing a hand behind the posterior fetal shoulder and pushing forward to rotate the shoulders 180° in a corkscrew fashion (Fig. 22–2). This maneuver is performed to rotate the anterior shoulder from behind the pubic symphysis.
7. **Delivery of the posterior shoulder**
   To perform this maneuver, a hand is placed along the

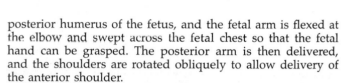

Figure 22-1 □ Rotation of the shoulder to an oblique diameter. (From Plauche WC, Morrison JC, O'Sullivan M: Surgical Obstetrics. Philadelphia, WB Saunders Co, 1992, p 319.)

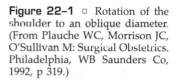

posterior humerus of the fetus, and the fetal arm is flexed at the elbow and swept across the fetal chest so that the fetal hand can be grasped. The posterior arm is then delivered, and the shoulders are rotated obliquely to allow delivery of the anterior shoulder.

8. **Abduction of the shoulders or Rubin's maneuver**

    Rubin's maneuver is performed by pushing both shoulders toward the fetal chest, resulting in abduction of the shoulders (Fig. 22–3). This decreases the shoulder-to-shoulder diameter and allows the anterior shoulder to be freed from behind the pubic symphysis.

9. **Deliberate fracture of the clavicle**

    This maneuver is performed by pressing the anterior clavicle against the ramus of the pubis. Fracture of the clavicle frees the anterior shoulder from behind the pubic symphysis. Clavicular fractures heal rapidly without any serious sequelae.

Figure 22-2 □ Corkscrew or Woods' maneuver. (From Plauche WC, Morrison JC, O'Sullivan M: Surgical Obstetrics. Philadelphia, WB Saunders Co, 1992, p 319.)

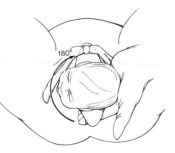

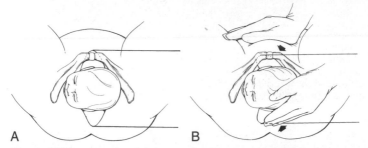

Figure 22-3 □ *A*, The shoulder-to-shoulder diameter is maximal, with the anterior shoulder trapped by the symphysis. *B*, Abduction of the shoulders by Rubin's maneuver. (From Plauche WC, Morrison JC, O'Sullivan M: Surgical Obstetrics. Philadelphia, WB Saunders Co, 1992, p 320.)

10. Cephalic replacement or Zavanelli's maneuver

This maneuver is performed by first administering a tocolytic drug such as **terbutaline 0.25 mg SC.** The fetal head is then rotated back to an occiput anterior (OA) or occiput posterior (OP) position. The head is then flexed and slowly pushed back into the vagina. Delivery is then accomplished by cesarean section. In some cases, general anesthesia is necessary to perform this maneuver because of patient discomfort.

■ BACKGROUND AND DEFINITIONS

Physical trauma occurs in approximately 1 of 12 pregnancies. Trauma can be **blunt trauma** or **penetrating trauma**. The most common cause of blunt trauma in pregnant patients is motor vehicle accidents, which account for almost two-thirds of all trauma sustained by pregnant women. Motor vehicle accidents are followed in frequency by falls and direct assaults to the abdomen. Domestic violence is occurring with increasing frequency. The prevalence of violence against pregnant women is as high as 20%. Gunshot and knife wounds are the most common types of penetrating trauma. Because of the protective effect of the uterus, penetrating wounds to the abdomen result in injury to other intra-abdominal organs in only 19% of pregnant patients. However, the fetus is vulnerable to direct injury from penetrating trauma. Trauma to the uterus is rare in the first trimester, because the uterus is still protected by the bony pelvis. Beyond the first trimester, the uterus begins to rise out of the pelvis and is therefore much more vulnerable to trauma.

■ CLINICAL PRESENTATION

The clinical presentation depends on the severity and the type of trauma. In addition to the signs and symptoms that result directly from the trauma, placental abruption may occur. Abruption rarely occurs with minor trauma but may be encountered in 40 to 50% of women who sustain severe trauma. If placental abruption has developed, the following signs and symptoms may be present:

Vaginal bleeding
Hypovolemic shock, sometimes out of proportion to the amount of visible bleeding
Coagulopathy
Uterine pain and tenderness
Uterine irritability
Fetal distress
Fetal demise

■ PHONE CALL

Questions

1. What is the type and the severity of trauma sustained by the patient?

2. What is the gestational age of the pregnancy?
3. What are the patient's vital signs?

Degree of Urgency

In severe cases or if the severity of the trauma is unknown or unclear, the patient should be seen immediately.

■ ELEVATOR THOUGHTS

What are the possible obstetrical complications of trauma?
- Blunt trauma
    Placental abruption
    Uterine rupture
    Direct fetal injury
    Rupture of membranes
- Penetrating trauma
    Uterine trauma
    Direct trauma to the fetus or placenta

■ MAJOR THREAT TO FETAL LIFE

- Direct fetal trauma
- Placental abruption
- Prematurity
- Uterine rupture
- Maternal shock
- Maternal death

Minor trauma that is not life threatening is associated with a 1 to 5% pregnancy loss rate. Major trauma that is life threatening is associated with a 40 to 50% loss rate. Direct fetal trauma occurs in fewer than 1% of all cases of trauma sustained by pregnant women.

■ MAJOR THREAT TO MATERNAL LIFE

- Hypovolemic shock
    Both blunt and penetrating trauma can result in significant intra-abdominal and retroperitoneal hemorrhage. Rupture of the spleen is the most common cause of intraperitoneal hemorrhage after blunt trauma.
- Visceral injuries
    The maternal mortality rate from penetrating trauma is less than 9%. This is lower than the mortality rate for nonpregnant patients, because the pregnant uterus shields other ab-

dominal organs. In contrast, penetrating trauma to the uterus results in a perinatal mortality rate of 41 to 71%.

■ BEDSIDE

Quick Look Test

Does the patient have life-threatening injuries?

Does the patient appear to be in hypovolemic shock?

Does the patient have uterine contractions or uterine tenderness?

Vital Signs

In patients who have experienced severe trauma, bleeding could result in hypovolemic shock with hypotension and tachycardia. Furthermore, the patient might have postural hypotension. Changes in blood pressure (BP) and pulse should be measured when the patient is assisted in sitting or standing from a supine position. A fall in systolic or diastolic BP >15 mm Hg or a rise in pulse >15 beats/min is evidence of hypovolemia.

Selective History and Chart Review

1. What is the gestational age of the fetus?
2. What is the nature of the trauma sustained by the patient?
3. Has the patient sustained penetrating trauma, and could the uterus have been injured directly?

Selective Physical Examination

Abdominal	Bruising is usually seen with blunt trauma.
	Uterus is tender in placental abruption and uterine rupture.
	Uterine contractions and irritability are present in placental abruption.
Pelvic	
External genitalia and vagina	Vaginal bleeding may be present.
Cervix	Bleeding may be present.
	Pooling of fluid if membranes are ruptured
Uterus and adnexa	Tender in placental abruption and uterine rupture
	Irritable with or without contractions in placental abruption

Orders

If the patient has sustained severe trauma, the following should be ordered.

1. Start a large-bore IV and administer crystalloids.
2. Provide supplemental oxygen by nasal cannula or mask.
3. Crossmatch 2 to 4 units of blood.
4. Displace the uterus off the midline with a hip roll or by turning the patient to one side.
5. Obtain a complete blood count (CBC).
6. Obtain coagulation studies: prothrombin time (PT), partial thromboplastin time (PTT), platelet count, fibrinogen, and fibrin split products.
7. Obtain a chemistry panel.
8. Perform urinalysis.
9. Insert urethral catheter.
10. Record intake and output.
11. Listen for fetal heart tones and begin continuous electronic fetal monitoring (fetal heart tones are not usually heard until the gestational age is >10 weeks).
12. Begin electronic uterine monitoring if the gestational age is >20 weeks.
13. Give the patient nothing by mouth (NPO status) in case surgery becomes necessary.

■ DIAGNOSTIC TESTING

1. **Ultrasound examination**

   Ultrasound examination is useful for determining gestational age, diagnosing placental abruption, and confirming fetal viability. The finding of a retroplacental blood clot is evidence of abruption. Placental location does not influence the risk of abruption. Amniotic fluid volume can also be estimated. A very low amniotic fluid volume is found in patients with ruptured membranes. Intra-abdominal fluid caused by bleeding can also be found by ultrasound examination.
2. **Computed tomography (CT) of the abdomen**

   CT scan of the abdomen and uterus may be helpful in delineating the degree of injury. CT scan usually exposes the fetus to 3 to 4 rad.
3. **Electronic fetal heart rate monitoring in patients with gestational ages >20 weeks**

   Fetal heart rate monitoring is useful in predicting placental abruption secondary to trauma. The finding of fetal tachycardia and/or late decelerations is suggestive of fetal compromise secondary to placental abruption. If uterine contractions either are absent or occur at a frequency of less than once every 10 minutes after 4 hours of fetal monitoring, placental abruption is extremely unlikely. Fetal monitoring should be performed for approximately 4 to 6 hours. Fetal monitoring should be continued if uterine contractions, uterine tenderness or irritability, vaginal bleeding, abnormalities in the fetal heart rate tracing, rupture of membranes, or severe maternal injuries are present. Abruption associated with trauma usually presents within 24 hours after the trauma.

4. **Peritoneal lavage**

Open peritoneal lavage is safe and sensitive and can be helpful in diagnosing intraperitoneal hemorrhage. Instead of blind needle insertion, sharp dissection should be performed at the umbilicus and carried down to the peritoneum, which is opened under direct visualization. Peritoneal lavage does not need to be performed if it is obvious that intraperitoneal bleeding is present. Indications for peritoneal lavage include the following findings:

   a. **Unexplained or equivocal abdominal signs or symptoms suggestive of intraperitoneal bleeding**
   b. **Altered sensorium**
   c. **Unexplained shock**
   d. **Major thoracic injury**
   e. **Multiple major orthopedic injuries**

The interpretation of diagnostic peritoneal lavage for blunt trauma in pregnancy is summarized in Table 23–1.

5. **Kleihauer–Betke stain of maternal blood**

Bleeding from the fetal to the maternal circulation occurs in 10 to 30% of trauma cases. The presence of fetal red blood cells in the maternal circulation can be documented by Kleihauer–Betke staining of maternal blood. This test is done by acid elution treatment, after which fetal red blood cells rich in hemoglobin F stain darkly and maternal cells poor in hemoglobin F stain lightly.

■ MANAGEMENT

The initial treatment of trauma in the pregnant patient should be identical to that in the nonpregnant patient. The top priority is the complete assessment and stabilization of the patient. Pregnancy should place very few restrictions on the diagnostic and resuscitative procedures necessary to achieve these goals. There are, however, several important considerations specific to pregnancy.

1. **Normal physiological changes of pregnancy**
   a. **Increased blood volume**

The pregnant patient normally has a 35 to 40% increase in total blood volume when she is near term. Therefore, the

Table 23-1 □ **INTERPRETATION OF RESULTS OF DIAGNOSTIC PERITONEAL LAVAGE* AFTER BLUNT TRAUMA**

Positive†
    Grossly bloody lavage fluid
    RBC count >100,000/mm³
    WBC count >175/dl
    Amylase >175/dl
    Lavage fluid identified in Foley catheter
Indeterminate‡
    RBC count >50,000/mm³ but <100,000/mm³
    WBC count >100/mm³ but <500/mm³
    Amylase >75/dl but <175/dl
Negative
    RBC count <50,000/mm³
    WBC count <100/mm³
    Amylase <75/dl

*Peritoneal lavage performed with 1 L of Ringer's lactate solution.
†Positive lavage (any one criterion) suggests need for surgical exploration.
‡Recommendations are to repeat lavage.
Modified from Rothenberger DA, Quattlesbaum FW, Zabel J, et al: Diagnostic peritoneal lavage for blunt trauma in pregnant women. Am J Obstet Gynecol 1977;129:479.

pregnant patient will have had significantly greater blood loss than the nonpregnant patient for a similar degree of shock. For this reason, larger amounts of blood and fluid will be needed for replacement in pregnant patients.

b. Increased heart rate

The heart rate in pregnant patients normally increases by approximately 15%; therefore, this finding should not be interpreted as a sign of shock.

c. Decreased blood pressure

Maternal blood pressure usually falls, in particular in the second trimester, and should not be interpreted as a sign of shock.

d. Compression of the inferior vena cava causing decreased venous return to the heart

When the patient is supine, compression of the inferior vena cava by the pregnant uterus decreases blood return to the heart, resulting in hypotension. This can be corrected with lateral displacement of the uterus, by tilting the patient partly to one side with a towel roll or wedge placed underneath the patient's hip.

e. Displacement of the bowel into the upper abdomen

As the uterus enlarges, the bowel is pushed up into the upper abdomen. As a result, trauma to the upper abdomen often injures both small and large intestines. Furthermore, paracentesis or peritoneal lavage is more risky in the patient with an advanced pregnancy.

f. **Decreased gastrointestinal motility and delayed stomach emptying**

Decreased gastrointestinal motility and delayed emptying of the stomach result in a greater risk of aspiration during intubation.

g. **Mild elevation in white blood cell count**

Pregnancy is normally associated with a mild leukocytosis. Therefore, a mild elevation in white blood cells may not be an indication of sepsis in the pregnant patient.

h. **Hypercoagulable state**

Pregnancy is normally a hypercoagulable state. Serum fibrinogen is normally 350 to 400 mg/dl in pregnancy; therefore, a lower level that would be considered normal in the nonpregnant patient could be an early sign of disseminated intravascular coagulation in the pregnant patient.

2. **Fetal–maternal hemorrhage**

Trauma results in some degree of fetal–maternal hemorrhage in 10 to 30% of cases. However, the amount of the hemorrhage is <15 ml in >90% of cases. The Kleihauer–Betke stain of maternal blood can be used to estimate the amount of fetal–maternal hemorrhage. To prevent Rh isoimmunization, patients who are Rh negative should receive Rh immunoglobulin if the Rh factor of the father is positive or unknown. One ampule of 300 μg of Rh immunoglobulin should be administered intramuscularly for every 30 ml of whole blood that is estimated to have been transfused. Rh immunoglobulin should be administered within 72 hours of fetal–maternal hemorrhage.

3. **Fetal radiation exposure from radiographic procedures**

There is no increase in teratogenesis or risk of childhood malignancy if the fetus is exposed to <10 rad (0.1 Gy) of radiation. By using the proper precautions, such as shielding of the uterus, most radiological procedures can be performed with a fetal radiation exposure of <1 rad. The fetal dose of radiation is approximately the same as the ovarian dose, which has been estimated for common radiological procedures (Table 23–2).

4. **Tetanus toxoid prophylaxis**

Tetanus toxoid prophylaxis should be administered with the same indications as used in nonpregnant patients. If the patient has had a tetanus toxoid booster in the last 10 years, no additional toxoid is needed. If it has been more than 10 years since a booster or if the immunization history is unknown, the patient should receive 250 units of tetanus antitoxin intramuscularly.

5. **Perimortem cesarean delivery**

If survival of the pregnant trauma patient is doubtful, peri-

Table 23-2 □ ESTIMATED OVARIAN RADIATION EXPOSURE FROM COMMON RADIOLOGICAL PROCEDURES*

Procedure	Estimated Ovarian Dose (millirad)	Average Number of Films per Examination
Chest examination		
Radiography	8	1.4
Fluoroscopy	71	
Upper gastrointestinal series		
Total	558	4.4
Radiography	360	
Fluoroscopy	198	
Barium enema		
Total	805	3.5
Radiography	439	
Fluoroscopy	366	
Intravenous or retrograde pyelography	407	5.0
Abdominal radiographs	289	1.7
Lumbar spine radiographs	275	2.5
Pelvic radiographs	41	1.5

*Ovarian dose approximates fetal exposure.

Adapted from Penfil RL, Brown ML: Genetically significant dose to the United States population from diagnostic medical roentgenology. Radiology 1968;90:209.

mortem cesarean section should be considered if the pregnancy has reached a viable gestational age, usually >25 weeks. It should be remembered that a cesarean section, and especially the blood loss associated with the operation, will further compromise the patient. After 10 to 20 minutes have elapsed since the loss of maternal vital signs, survival of the fetus is unlikely. Therefore, if cesarean section is planned, it should usually be performed after 4 to 6 minutes of cardiopulmonary resuscitation.

PATIENT-RELATED GYNECOLOGICAL PROBLEMS: THE COMMON CALLS

ABNORMAL UTERINE BLEEDING

■ BACKGROUND AND DEFINITIONS

The normal menstrual interval averages 28 days, with a normal range of 21 to 35 days. The normal duration of bleeding is 4 to 5 days, with a normal range of 3 to 7 days. The average blood loss during menses is 35 ml, with a normal range of 20 to 80 ml.

Menorrhagia: Prolonged or excessive bleeding that occurs at regular intervals; also referred to as **hypermenorrhea**

Metrorrhagia: Bleeding that occurs at irregular intervals

Menometrorrhagia: Prolonged or excessive bleeding that occurs at irregular intervals

Polymenorrhea: Bleeding that occurs regularly but at intervals of <21 days

Oligomenorrhea: Bleeding that occurs regularly but at intervals of >35 days

Hypomenorrhea: Bleeding that occurs regularly but in small amounts

Dysfunctional uterine bleeding (DUB): Abnormal bleeding from the uterine endometrium that is unrelated to any anatomical lesion of the uterus. More than 80% of all cases of DUB are due to a disruption of normal ovarian function and anovulation. Therefore, the term **anovulatory bleeding** is used synonymously with DUB. During anovulatory cycles, the failure of ovulation results in an absence of progesterone production, so that the endometrium is exposed to prolonged unopposed estrogen stimulation. Chronic estrogen stimulation results in an overgrowth of endometrium that then breaks down and bleeds. The remaining 20% of DUB cases are associated with ovulatory cycles but with dysfunction of the corpus luteum and abnormal but not absent progesterone production. Bleeding that results from pregnancy, uterine leiomyomata, uterine malignancy, polyps, or coagulopathy is not considered DUB.

■ CLINICAL PRESENTATION

Vaginal bleeding or spotting at times other than when menses is expected or for a longer duration than expected

Heavy bleeding
Passage of blood clots

■ PHONE CALL

Questions

1. How severe is the patient's bleeding?
2. What are the patient's vital signs?

Degree of Urgency

The degree of urgency depends on the degree of bleeding. Patients with prolonged heavy bleeding and signs of hypovolemic shock should be seen immediately. Likewise, patients with bleeding and a positive pregnancy test should be seen immediately.

■ ELEVATOR THOUGHTS

What are causes of abnormal uterine bleeding?
- Dysfunctional bleeding
    Anovulatory bleeding
    Dysfunction of the corpus luteum
- Pregnancy complications
    Spontaneous abortion
    Ectopic pregnancy
    Molar pregnancy
- Uterine lesions
    Leiomyomata
    Endometrial polyps
    Atrophic endometrium
    Adenomyosis
    Endometrial hyperplasia
    Endometrial carcinoma
- Lower genital tract lesions
    Cervical polyp
    Cervical carcinoma
    Vaginal malignancy
    Vulvar malignancy
- Infection
    Pelvic inflammatory disease
    Vaginitis
    Cervicitis
    Endometritis

- Systemic conditions
    Coagulopathies
        von Willebrand's disease
        Thrombocytopenic purpura
    Endocrine disorders
        Polycystic ovary syndrome
        Thyroid disease
        Adrenal disorders
        Hyperprolactinemia
    Liver disease
        Decreased synthesis of coagulation factors
        Impaired metabolism of estrogen
    Renal disease
        Impaired excretion of both estrogen and progesterone
    Obesity
- Use of hormonal medications
    Oral contraceptive pills
    Intrauterine device
    Nonpill hormonal contraception
        Norplant implant system
        Depo-Provera
    Postmenopausal estrogen and/or progestin replacement
    therapy

■ MAJOR THREAT TO LIFE

- Hypovolemic shock
    Abnormal uterine bleeding is rarely severe enough to be
    life threatening.

■ BEDSIDE

Quick Look Test

Does the patient appear to be in hypovolemic shock?

What are the patient's vital signs?

Vital Signs

Vital signs are usually normal. If the patient has had heavy
bleeding, she may have hypotension and tachycardia. The patient
might have postural hypotension. Changes in blood pressure (BP)
and pulse should be measured when the patient is assisted in
sitting or standing from a supine position. A fall in systolic or
diastolic BP >15 mm Hg or a rise in pulse >15 beats/min is
evidence of hypovolemia.

Selective History and Chart Review

1. What is the patient's age?

    Women in the reproductive age group can have bleeding secondary to pregnancy complications. Furthermore, throughout the entire reproductive age range, especially at both extremes, anovulation is a common cause of abnormal uterine bleeding. In adolescent patients with persistent bleeding severe enough to require hospital admission, coagulopathy accounts for approximately 20% of cases. In postmenopausal patients, abnormal uterine bleeding is commonly caused by hormone replacement therapy. Uterine malignancy and endometrial atrophy are other causes in this age group.

2. What is the nature of the abnormal uterine bleeding?

    The amount, duration, interval, and frequency of the bleeding should be ascertained.

3. When was the patient's last normal menstrual period?

4. Is the patient taking any hormonal medication such as hormonal contraception or postmenopausal hormone replacement?

5. If the patient is of reproductive age, is she using contraception? If so, what type?

    Use of contraception would make pregnancy-related causes of bleeding unlikely. The use of an intrauterine device (IUD) may be associated with menorrhagia or at least an increase in flow over what had been normal for the patient.

6. Is the patient pregnant? If so, what is the gestational age of the fetus?

7. Has the patient had bleeding from the gums, prolonged bleeding after minor cuts, or easy bruisability suggestive of a coagulopathy?

8. Does the patient complain of pain in association with the bleeding?

9. Does the patient have a history of any gynecological disorders?

    It should be determined whether the patient has a history of fibroid tumors, abnormal cervical cytology, polycystic ovary syndrome, gynecological malignancy, genital infection, or prior episodes of abnormal uterine bleeding.

10. Does the patient have a history of medical conditions that may cause abnormal bleeding, such as coagulopathy, thyroid disease, or hepatic disease?

11. Does the patient engage in strenuous physical activities?

    Rigorous exercise can be a cause of chronic anovulation and DUB.

12. Has the patient had significant psychological or emotional stress or an eating disorder?

    These are common causes of anovulation and DUB.

Selective Physical Examination

General	Obesity often associated with anovulatory bleeding
	Hirsutism and other signs of virilization associated with chronic anovulation and polycystic ovary syndrome
Dermatological	Ecchymotic lesions in patients with coagulopathy
Abdominal	Abdominal mass in patients with uterine leiomyoma
Pelvic	
External genitalia and vagina	Discharge and erythema in patients with vaginitis
	Bleeding lesion in patients with trauma or malignancy
Cervix	Tender with purulent discharge in patients with cervicitis
	Friable cervix that bleeds to the touch in patients with cervicitis
	Bleeding lesion in patients with cervical malignancy
	Cervical os may be dilated with protruding tissue in patients with spontaneous abortion
Uterus and adnexa	Enlarged and often irregular in patients with leiomyomata
	Tender in patients with endometritis
	Adnexal tenderness with a palpable mass may be a tubal pregnancy

Orders

1. Obtain a complete blood count (CBC).
2. Perform a urine pregnancy test in patients of reproductive age.
3. Obtain coagulation studies in adolescent patients: platelet count, bleeding time, prothrombin time (PT), and partial thromboplastin time (PTT).
4. Start IV if the patient is bleeding heavily or appears to be in hypovolemic shock.

■ DIAGNOSTIC TESTING

1. **Complete blood count (CBC)**

2. **Urine pregnancy test (hCG)**

   Urine pregnancy test should be performed in all patients of reproductive age.

3. **Coagulation studies: platelet count, bleeding time, PT, and PTT**

   Coagulation studies should be obtained, especially in adolescent patients.

4. **Serum prolactin**

   Serum prolactin is often elevated in patients with chronic anovulation.

5. **Serum androgens: testosterone and dehydroepiandrosterone sulfate**

   Serum androgens can be elevated in patients with chronic anovulation or polycystic ovary syndrome and should be measured, especially if there are signs of virilization.

6. **Thyroid function tests**

7. **Liver function tests**

8. **Ultrasound examination**

   Ultrasound examination of the pelvis can detect uterine leiomyomata. Furthermore, the endometrial thickness can be determined by sonography. Endometrial thickness >20 mm is associated with increased risk of endometrial polyps, hyperplasia, and adenocarcinoma. Polycystic ovaries can also be detected by ultrasound examination.

9. **Cervical culture**

   Cervical cultures should be obtained if cervicitis is suspected.

10. **Cervical Pap smear (if one has not been performed within the last year).**

11. **Endometrial sampling**

    Endometrial sampling should be performed in all women with abnormal bleeding, especially postmenopausal women, if premalignant or malignant disease of the endometrium is suspected. Endometrial hyperplasia, especially with atypia, is a premalignant finding, and adenocarcinoma is the most common malignancy of the endometrium. Endometrial sampling can also confirm the diagnosis of DUB or anovulatory bleeding. In these patients, the endometrium is disordered and proliferative because it has been exposed only to estrogen; secretory endometrium, on the other hand, has been exposed to progesterone that is produced by the corpus luteum after ovulation.

    a. **Endometrial biopsy**

       Endometrial biopsy is performed as an office procedure without the need for anesthesia. However, this procedure provides only a sample of endometrium and not the entire endometrium.

    b. **Office endometrial aspiration**

       Office endometrial aspiration with a small suction curette usually provides more tissue than endometrial biopsy.

c. **Dilatation and curettage**

Dilatation and curettage while under anesthesia can be both diagnostic and therapeutic because of the greater amount of endometrium obtained. This procedure can also be performed along with hysteroscopy.

12. **Hysteroscopy**

Hysteroscopy allows direct visualization of the entire endometrial cavity. Furthermore, operative hysteroscopy can be performed to remove lesions such as polyps and submucosal leiomyomata.

■ MANAGEMENT

Anatomical and Medical Causes of Uterine Bleeding

The management of specific anatomical causes of abnormal uterine bleeding, such as spontaneous abortion, ectopic pregnancy, and leiomyomata, is discussed in other chapters. The management of patients with abnormal uterine bleeding caused by medical conditions such as thyroid disease, genital tract infection, and liver dysfunction depends on the correction of these medical conditions.

Dysfunctional or Anovulatory Uterine Bleeding

The goals of the management of DUB are to prevent endometrial hyperplasia and to restore normal menstrual bleeding. This can be accomplished by the following treatment options.

1. **Combination oral contraceptive pills**

Combination oral contraceptive pills containing 30 to 35 μg of estrogen can be administered in the following manner:

a. **1 pill PO daily starting on day 5 of the menstrual cycle and continuing for 21 days, followed by a hiatus of 7 days. This cycle is then repeated. This is the standard regimen used for contraception.**

For acute and heavy bleeding, the following alternative regimen can be used:

b. **1 pill PO three times per day for 7 days, followed by a hiatus of 7 days, and then two standard cycles of 1 pill PO each day for 21 days, followed by a hiatus of 7 days**

In both regimens, normal menstrual bleeding is expected during the 7-day hiatus.

2. **Progesterone**

Progesterone is administered to replace the progesterone that is not produced endogenously because of the absence of ovulation. Progesterone can be administered either orally or intramuscularly. With either route, limited withdrawal bleeding is expected after progesterone administration as a result of progesterone withdrawal.

   a. **Medroxyprogesterone 2.5 to 10 mg PO daily for 10 to 14 days each month** or
   b. **Progesterone, in oil, 50 to 100 mg IM each month**
3. **Combination estrogen and progesterone therapy**

   For patients with acute, heavy, and prolonged bleeding, estrogen should be administered to stabilize the endometrium before progesterone is given. Estrogen can be given orally, or for extremely heavy bleeding it can be administered intravenously.

   a. **Conjugated estrogen 1.25 to 2.5 mg PO four times per day** or
   b. **Conjugated estrogen 25 mg IV every 4 hours**

   Either of the above regimens is continued until bleeding subsides. Then, the following oral regimen of estrogen and progesterone is administered to produce withdrawal bleeding:

   c. **Conjugated estrogen 2.5 mg PO daily for 3 weeks, followed by both conjugated estrogen 2.5 mg PO and medroxyprogesterone 10 mg PO daily for 7 to 10 days, followed by a hiatus to allow withdrawal bleeding**

The choice of treatment regimen depends on the severity and duration of the bleeding and on the age of the patient, which in turn determines the appropriate maintenance regimen. Younger patients who have chronic and recurrent bleeding of light to moderate amounts and who desire contraception should have oral contraceptive pills given as described previously. After treatment of the bleeding, these patients can be prescribed a standard regimen of oral contraceptive pills. Patients who have light to moderate bleeding and do not need contraception may be given progesterone alone. Patients who have acute and heavier bleeding and who are in the perimenopausal years should be given a combination of estrogen and progesterone therapy. After treatment of bleeding, these patients may continue taking estrogen and progesterone in the usual doses given for postmenopausal hormone replacement.

25 | BARTHOLIN'S ABSCESS

■ BACKGROUND AND DEFINITIONS

Bartholin's glands: Bilateral round, lobulated glands, approximately 1 cm in diameter, located in the posterior lateral aspect of the vestibule. Also referred to as **major vestibular glands,** they secrete lubrication during intercourse, but their major function is unclear.

Bartholin's cyst: This cyst results from obstruction and subsequent distention of the duct of the Bartholin's gland secondary to trauma and/or infection.

Bartholin's abscess: An abscess that develops from an infection of Bartholin's cyst. It is more accurately referred to as **Bartholin's duct abscess.**

■ CLINICAL PRESENTATION

Vulvar enlargement, usually unilateral
Acute vulvar pain
Dyspareunia
Difficulty sitting or walking

Bartholin's cysts without the formation of an abscess are usually asymptomatic unless they are significantly enlarged. They can range from 1 to 8 cm in diameter and are usually unilateral.

■ PHONE CALL

Questions

1. Does the patient appear to be seriously ill?
2. What are the patient's vital signs?
Bartholin's abscess can result in cellulitis, and in rare cases, synergistic bacterial gangrene and sepsis can occur.

Degree of Urgency

Uncomplicated Bartholin's abscess is rarely life threatening, but because of the intense discomfort that is associated with this condition, the patient should be seen as soon as possible. If sepsis or bacterial gangrene is suspected, the patient should be seen immediately.

■ ELEVATOR THOUGHTS

What is the differential diagnosis of Bartholin's abscess?
- Vulvar hematoma
- Sebaceous cyst
- Epithelial inclusion cyst
- Mesonephric cyst
- Gartner's duct cyst
- Skene's duct cyst
- Perineal hernia
- Enterocele
- Ischiorectal abscess
- Hydrocele of the round ligament
- Lipoma
- Fibroma
- Metastatic carcinoma
- Adenocarcinoma of Bartholin's gland
    Adenocarcinoma of the Bartholin's gland is found most often in postmenopausal women. There is a history of inflammation in approximately 10% of the cases. Even though this malignancy makes up only 5% of vulvlar malignancies, it should not be overlooked. Adenocarcinoma of the Bartholin's gland can be misdiagnosed as a recurrent abscess.

■ MAJOR THREAT TO LIFE

- Synergistic bacterial gangrene
- Sepsis

■ BEDSIDE

Quick Look Test

How ill does the patient appear?

Does the patient appear to be having pain?
    Significant discomfort is associated with Bartholin's abscess, ischiorectal abscess, and vulvar hematoma, whereas other conditions in the differential diagnosis are not associated with excessive pain.

Vital Signs

Vital signs are usually normal. The patient may have a fever if she has extensive cellulitis. A patient with septic shock will be hypotensive and tachycardic.

Selective History and Chart Review

1. Has the patient had a prior Bartholin's abscess on the same side?

   Bartholin's abscesses can be recurrent. Furthermore, a recurrent abscess in a postmenopausal patient should raise suspicion for adenocarcinoma of Bartholin's gland.

2. Has the patient had any recent trauma, especially "saddle injuries," in the area affected?

   A vulvar hematoma should be suspected if there is a positive history of local trauma.

3. Does the patient have a history of diabetes mellitus?

   Diabetes mellitus is associated with a higher risk of bacterial gangrene.

Selective Physical Examination

Pelvic

External genitalia and vagina	Unilateral, tense enlargement of the vulva
	Severe tenderness
	Diffuse erythema
	Yellow-green or bronze discoloration with crepitation in bacterial synergistic gangrene
Cervix	Normal
Uterus and adnexa	Normal

Orders

1. Have available the equipment necessary for an incision and drainage procedure.

   At the minimum, this would include a scalpel, local anesthetic, a hemostat or similar clamp, and a catheter such as a Word catheter.

2. Have available the material needed to culture the abscess fluid.

■ DIAGNOSTIC TESTING

The diagnosis of Bartholin's abscess can usually be made based on the physical examination. Usually, no specific diagnostic tests are necessary.

■ MANAGEMENT

1. Incision and drainage

Incision and drainage is the initial step in the management of all Bartholin's abscesses and symptomatic Bartholin's cysts.

This procedure can be performed easily if the abscess is pointing. If the abscess is not pointing, the patient can be instructed to use warm compresses on the abscess and to return in several days. An incision should then be made where the abscess is pointing, with a no. 11 scalpel; the abscess should then be drained by both manual expression and the use of a sterile clamp to break up any loculations within the abscess cavity. The abscess fluid should be sent for culture and sensitivity testing. Organisms most commonly recovered are listed in Table 25-1. Any patient with a positive culture should be treated with the appropriate antibiotics.

2. **Accompanying procedure**

Incision and drainage alone are usually not adequate management. Bartholin's abscesses treated this way have a recurrence rate of 68 to 75%. Therefore, initial incision and drainage should be accompanied by one of the following procedures.

a. **Placement of an indwelling catheter**

The goal in the placement of an indwelling catheter into the abscess cavity is to develop a permanent fistula between the duct and the vaginal mucosa. A Word catheter is commonly used. This catheter has an inflatable balloon at the distal tip to keep the catheter in the abscess cavity. After incision and drainage, the catheter is placed into the abscess cavity, and the balloon is filled, by syringe, with 2 to 3 ml of saline in a way similar to the filling of a Foley catheter balloon. The catheter should be kept in place for a minimum of 3 weeks before removal to allow the fistula tract to become epithelialized. The patient should be seen weekly during this time; if necessary, additional saline can be infused into the balloon if it appears to be deflating spontaneously. To decrease the risk of the catheter's falling out prematurely, the initial incision into the abscess cavity should be <2 cm long. The recurrence rate after use of an indwelling catheter is 3 to 17%.

b. **Marsupialization**

As with the placement of an indwelling catheter, the goal of marsupialization is the development of a permanent com-

---

**Table 25-1 ▫ ORGANISMS COMMONLY RECOVERED
FROM BARTHOLIN'S ABSCESSES**

Escherichia coli	*Proteus* spp.
Neisseria gonorrhoeae	*Pseudomonas* spp.
Chlamydia trachomatis	*Klebsiella* spp.
Bacteroides spp.	*Clostridium* spp.
Enterococcus spp.	*Staphylococcus aureus*

munication, in this case a stoma, between the duct and the vaginal mucosa. Marsupialization should not be performed in the presence of acute inflammation, and therefore it should not be used for an acute Bartholin's abscess. Instead, it can be used in the patient with an uninfected Bartholin's cyst or a chronic or recurrent Bartholin's abscess. The initial incision should be made in the vagina and should be made long enough to ensure patency of the stoma. After drainage of the cyst, the inner lining of the cyst is everted and approximated to the vaginal mucosa with interrupted sutures of 2-0 absorbable suture. This creates a "buttonhole" appearance. The recurrence rate after marsupialization is 10 to 24%.

c. **Excision of the cyst**

Total removal of the cyst is rarely necessary. As with marsupialization, this procedure is usually performed on patients with symptomatic, uninfected cysts or chronic or recurrent abscesses, but not on patients with acute abscesses. Excision of the cyst is indicated in the postmenopausal patient with a recurrent cyst, especially when there is induration of the base of the cyst, because of the risk of adenocarcinoma of Bartholin's gland. Excision of Bartholin's cyst is usually accompanied by significant blood loss and should be performed in the operating room.

26 | ECTOPIC PREGNANCY

■ BACKGROUND AND DEFINITIONS

Ectopic pregnancy: Pregnancy that implants somewhere other than the endometrial lining of the uterus

Tubal pregnancy: Ectopic pregnancy that implants in the fallopian tube, usually in the ampullary portion of the tube

The incidence of ectopic pregnancy is increasing. Ectopic pregnancies occur at a rate of approximately 20 per 1000 reported pregnancies or 1 of every 50 pregnancies. This incidence is a fourfold increase over that reported in 1970. Earlier detection of ectopic pregnancies has resulted in a steady decrease in the mortality rate, which is now fewer than 5 deaths per 10,000 cases. Ectopic pregnancies account for approximately 9% of all pregnancy-related deaths.

Although there are several implantation sites for ectopic pregnancies, nearly 98% of all ectopic pregnancies implant in the fallopian tubes (Fig. 26–1). **Interstitial** or **cornual pregnancies** are the second most common type of ectopic pregnancies and are caused by implantation of the embryo in the interstitial or intramyometrial portion of the fallopian tube. **Cervical** and **ovarian pregnancies** are rare. **Abdominal pregnancies** are the rarest of

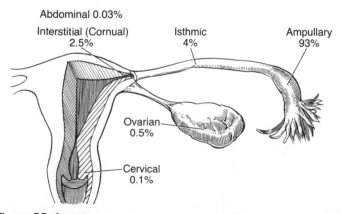

Abdominal 0.03%

Interstitial (Cornual) 2.5%   Isthmic 4%   Ampullary 93%

Ovarian 0.5%

Cervical 0.1%

Figure 26–1 □ Sites for ectopic pregnancy implantation. (From Copeland LJ: Textbook of Gynecology. Philadelphia, WB Saunders Co, 1993, p 244.)

ectopic pregnancies and are believed to be caused by tubal abortion in which the embryo is aborted into the peritoneal cavity and reimplantation occurs on the gastrointestinal tract or pelvic side wall. Because the incidence of these ectopic pregnancies is so low compared with tubal pregnancies, the terms "tubal pregnancy" and "ectopic pregnancy" are often used synonymously.

■ CLINICAL PRESENTATION

Abdominal pain
Pelvic pain
Vaginal bleeding
Palpable adnexal mass
Hypovolemic shock

The classic presentation is the triad of abdominal or pelvic pain, vaginal bleeding, and the finding of an adnexal mass.

■ PHONE CALL

Questions

1. **What are the patient's vital signs?**
2. **Does the patient appear to be in hypovolemic shock?**
   Intra-abdominal bleeding from a ruptured tubal pregnancy must be ruled out in any patient of reproductive age who presents with hypovolemic shock.
3. **Is the patient having heavy vaginal bleeding?**
   Patients with tubal pregnancies usually do not have heavy vaginal bleeding. Vaginal hemorrhage is more suggestive of spontaneous abortion.

Degree of Urgency

Because intra-abdominal bleeding from a ruptured tubal pregnancy is life threatening, the patient should be seen immediately.

■ ELEVATOR THOUGHTS

What are risk factors for tubal pregnancy?
- History of pelvic inflammatory disease
  Pelvic inflammatory disease, especially when caused by *Chlamydia trachomatis*, increases the risk of tubal pregnancy. Of those patients who conceive after a history of pelvic inflammatory disease or salpingitis, 4 to 5% will have an ectopic pregnancy.

- Tubal reconstructive surgery
  Up to 20% of pregnancies occurring after tubal reconstructive surgery are tubal pregnancies.
- Tubal sterilization
  Up to 75% of pregnancies resulting from failure of tubal sterilization are tubal pregnancies.
- Reversal of tubal sterilization
- History of infertility
  Even in the absence of tubal disease, a prior history of infertility increases the risk of tubal pregnancy.
- Use of ovulation-inducing drugs
- In vitro fertilization and embryo transfer
- Use of intrauterine device (IUD)
  Unless complicated by salpingitis, use of the IUD does not increase the risk of tubal pregnancy. However, if an IUD user becomes pregnant, that pregnancy has a greater chance of being a tubal pregnancy than it would in a non-IUD user. This is because the IUD offers better protection against intrauterine pregnancy than it does against tubal pregnancy. Up to 10% of pregnancies that occur in IUD users are tubal.
- Previous tubal pregnancy
  Patients with one tubal pregnancy have a recurrence rate of up to 15 to 20%.
- History of ruptured appendix
- In utero exposure to diethylstilbestrol (DES)
- Smoking

■ BEDSIDE

Quick Look Test

Does the patient appear to be in hypovolemic shock?
The patient who is in hypovolemic shock and in whom a tubal pregnancy is suspected must undergo immediate surgical intervention even if all diagnostic tests have not been performed.

Vital Signs

A patient in hypovolemic shock from a ruptured tubal pregnancy will be hypotensive and tachycardic. The patient might have postural hypotension. Changes in blood pressure (BP) and pulse should be measured when the patient is assisted in sitting or standing from a supine position. A fall in systolic or diastolic BP >15 mm Hg or a rise in pulse >15 beats/min is evidence of hypovolemia.

Selective History and Chart Review

1. When did the patient's last menstrual period begin?

   Almost all patients with tubal pregnancies present in the first trimester of pregnancy. Patients with interstitial or cornual pregnancies typically present later in the first trimester than those with tubal pregnancies do because the interstitial portion of the tube is more distensible than the rest of the tube.

2. Has the patient had any recent episodes of syncope or lightheadedness?

   Such episodes would suggest hypovolemia from bleeding.

3. Has the patient had unilateral abdominal or pelvic pain?

   Pain is one part of the triad that represents the classic presentation of ectopic pregnancy.

4. Has the patient passed any tissue through the vagina?

   Although patients with tubal pregnancies can pass decidual tissue (also referred to as a **decidual cast**) through the vagina, spontaneous abortion should be suspected in patients who pass a significant amount of tissue.

5. Does the patient have any of the risk factors listed above?

Selective Physical Examination

Abdominal	Tenderness, usually unilateral
	Distended, if there is a significant hemoperitoneum
Pelvic	
External genitalia and vagina	Normal, except for vaginal bleeding
Cervix	Bleeding through the cervical os
	Cervical os usually closed
Uterus and adnexa	Uterus of normal size or is slightly enlarged
	Unilateral adnexal tenderness
	Unilateral adnexal mass

Orders

1. Obtain a complete blood count (CBC).
2. Perform a rapid urine qualitative pregnancy test to confirm the presence of a pregnancy.
3. Measure serum quantitative human chorionic gonadotropin (hCG).
4. Obtain the blood type and Rh factor.
5. Type and crossmatch 2 units of blood if the patient appears to be in hypovolemic shock.
6. Start IV infusion.

7. Insert urethral catheter.
8. Record intake and output.
9. Place the patient on bedrest, and give nothing by mouth (NPO).

■ DIAGNOSTIC TESTING

1. **Rapid urine pregnancy test**
   The currently available rapid urine pregnancy tests are monoclonal enzyme–linked immunoassays that are sensitive in the range of 15 to 25 mIU/ml.
2. **Serum human chorionic gonadotropin (hCG)**
   Serum hCG rises exponentially in the first trimester of a normal intrauterine pregnancy (Fig. 26–2). The interpretation of serum hCG is complicated by the existence of two reference standards, the Second International Standard (Second IS) and the International Reference Preparation (IRP). The use of serum hCG in the diagnosis of ectopic pregnancies is based on the following two principles:
   a. **When serum hCG values reach a certain level defined by the discriminatory zone, a gestational sac should be detectable by ultrasound examination in a normal intrauterine pregnancy.**

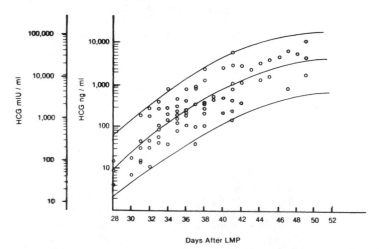

Figure 26–2   □   Rise in serum hCG in normal intrauterine pregnancies. (Modified from Pittaway DE, Reish RL, Wentz AC: Doubling times of human chorionic gonadotropin in early viable intrauterine pregnancies. Am J Obstet Gynecol 1985;152:299.)

When the serum hCG exceeds 6500 mIU/ml (IRP), a gestational sac should be detectable by transabdominal ultrasound examination. If transvaginal ultrasound examination is performed, a gestational sac should be detected when the serum hCG exceeds 2000 mIU/ml (IRP) or 1000 mIU/ml (Second IS).

b. **Because ectopic pregnancies are abnormal pregnancies, they produce an abnormal rise in serum hCG.**

In the early first trimester of a normal intrauterine pregnancy, serum hCG doubles every 1.5 to 3.5 days. In the first trimester, serum hCG should rise by ≥66% every 48 hours. If serial measurements of serum hCG demonstrate an abnormal rise or a fall, either an ectopic pregnancy or an abnormal intrauterine pregnancy should be suspected. However, almost 15% of patients with normal first-trimester pregnancies have abnormal rises in serum hCG levels. Furthermore, approximately 17% of patients with ectopic pregnancies have normal rises in hCG.

3. Ultrasound examination

Ultrasound examination rarely confirms the diagnosis of a tubal pregnancy. The finding of a complex adnexal mass is suggestive, although not diagnostic, of a tubal pregnancy. The only ultrasound finding that is diagnostic of a tubal pregnancy is a fetus with cardiac activity in the adnexa. In most cases, ultrasound examination is useful because it rules out the presence of a normal intrauterine pregnancy, based on the hCG discriminatory zone and ultrasound findings listed in Table 26–1.

4. Serum progesterone

A single serum progesterone level ≥25 ng/ml is highly suggestive of a normal intrauterine pregnancy. Among women with spontaneous abortion or ectopic pregnancy, 85 to 90% have a progesterone level <10 ng/ml. Therefore, a serum progesterone level <5 ng/ml is a strong indication of an abnormal pregnancy. Unfortunately, this test cannot distinguish be-

Table 26–1 □ SONOGRAPHIC FINDINGS IN NORMAL FIRST TRIMESTER PREGNANCIES

| | Gestational Age at Detection (weeks) | |
Ultrasound Finding	Transabdominal Examination	Transvaginal Examination
Gestational sac	6	5
Yolk sac	6	5
Fetus	7	6
Fetal cardiac activity	7	6

tween an ectopic pregnancy and an abnormal intrauterine pregnancy.

5. **Culdocentesis**

Culdocentesis is performed to detect blood in the peritoneal cavity. A 20- or 22-gauge spinal needle attached to a 20-ml syringe is placed transvaginally through the posterior vaginal fornix into the posterior cul-de-sac (Fig. 26–3). A positive culdocentesis is defined by the finding, on aspiration, of free-flowing and nonclotting blood. This is an indication of intraperitoneal bleeding or hemoperitoneum, but it does not determine the cause of the bleeding. In addition to a tubal pregnancy, a hemorrhagic corpus luteum cyst is a common gynecological cause of a positive culdocentesis. A negative culdocentesis is defined by the finding of straw-colored peritoneal fluid. If no fluid is obtained, the test is nondiagnostic.

6. **Dilatation and curettage**

When serum hCG rises abnormally or falls, dilatation and curettage is helpful in distinguishing between an abnormal intrauterine pregnancy and a tubal pregnancy. If chorionic villi are seen by direct visual inspection of the specimen or are found on pathological evaluation, an intrauterine pregnancy is confirmed. This finding virtually precludes the diagnosis of tubal pregnancy, although the incidence of coexistent intrauter-

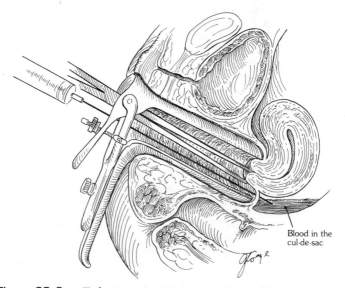

Blood in the
cul-de-sac

Figure 26–3 □ Technique of culdocentesis. (From Hacker NF, Moore JG: Essentials of Obstetrics and Gynecology, 3rd ed. Philadelphia, WB Saunders Co, 1998, p 494.)

ine and tubal pregnancy is actually much higher than was once thought and may be as high as 1 in 3000 pregnancies.

7. **Diagnostic scheme**

Early diagnosis of tubal pregnancy not only decreases mortality and morbidity but also allows for more conservative management that preserves tubal function. A diagnostic scheme for ectopic pregnancy is illustrated in Figure 26–4. The following are key points of the diagnostic scheme:

a. **Any patient with a suspected ectopic pregnancy should first have a rapid urine pregnancy test.**

A negative urine pregnancy test rules out the diagnosis of ectopic pregnancy.

b. **If the patient has a positive urine pregnancy test but is hemodynamically unstable, portable ultrasound examination should be performed. If ultrasound is not immediately available, culdocentesis should be performed.**

If the culdocentesis is positive, the patient should undergo either laparotomy or laparoscopy immediately.

c. **If the patient has a positive urine pregnancy test and is hemodynamically stable, ultrasound examination should be performed.**

Transabdominal ultrasound examination should be performed first. If an intrauterine gestational sac is not found, then a transvaginal ultrasound examination should be performed. The finding of an intrauterine gestational sac usually excludes the diagnosis of ectopic pregnancy. On the other hand, the finding of a complex adnexal mass and fluid in the pelvic cavity is highly suggestive of a tubal pregnancy with a hemoperitoneum, and either surgical or medical treatment should be initiated.

d. **If an intrauterine gestational sac is not found on transvaginal ultrasound examination, serum hCG should be measured to determine whether the patient is in the discriminatory zone.**

If the serum hCG exceeds 2000 mIU/ml (IRP) or 1000 mIU/ml (Second IS), an ectopic pregnancy or abnormal intrauterine pregnancy should be suspected.

e. **If the serum hCG is below the discriminatory zone, it should be measured again in 48 hours.**

If there has been at least a 66% increase in serum hCG, a repeat ultrasound examination should be planned and the patient can be monitored expectantly. If a 66% increase has not been achieved or if the serum hCG falls, then either an ectopic pregnancy or an abnormal intrauterine pregnancy should be suspected.

f. **Dilatation and curettage can be used to distinguish between an abnormal intrauterine pregnancy and an ectopic pregnancy.**

If villi are seen on visual examination of the specimen,

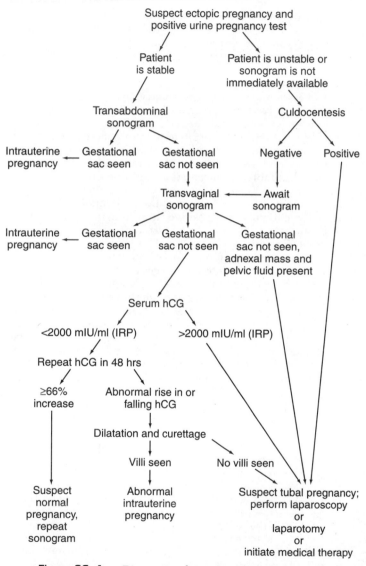

Figure 26–4 □ Diagnostic scheme for ectopic pregnancy.

an abnormal intrauterine pregnancy is confirmed. If villi are not seen, then frozen-section examination can be performed by a pathologist. If villi still are not detected, the patient should be treated for an ectopic pregnancy.

■ MANAGEMENT

The management of a tubal pregnancy can be conservative, with the goal of preserving tubal function, or nonconservative, in which tubal function is sacrificed. The type of management used depends on the patient's desire to preserve fertility, the status of the affected fallopian tube, and the status of the contralateral tube. Conservative management may not be possible in a patient with active hemorrhage from a ruptured fallopian tube. A greater attempt at conservative management should be made if the contralateral tube has already been removed or severely damaged in a patient who desires to maintain her fertility. In a patient who has a tubal pregnancy after undergoing tubal sterilization, conservative management is usually not appropriate. Conservative management can be either surgical or medical. Both conservative and nonconservative surgical management can be performed via laparoscopy. Laparoscopy has the advantages of a shorter hospitalization and a faster postoperative convalescence for the patient, compared with laparotomy.

1. **Conservative management**
   a. **Surgical management**
      (1) **Segmental tubal resection or partial salpingectomy**
      The segment of fallopian tube containing the ectopic pregnancy is removed, with an attempt made to preserve as much of the uninvolved tube as possible. Partial salpingectomy can be performed via laparotomy (Fig. 26–5) or via laparoscopy (Fig. 26–6). This allows for the possibility of tubal reanastomosis to restore tubal patency at a future time.
      (2) **Linear salpingostomy**
      With this procedure, on the antimesenteric surface over the tubal pregnancy, an opening in the tube is made with a scalpel, electrocautery, or laser beam, and then the tubal pregnancy is removed (Fig. 26–7). A vasoconstrictive agent is often used before the salpingostomy. A dilute solution of 20 units (1 ml) of vasopressin in 50 ml of injectable saline can be injected with a spinal needle into the serosa of the fallopian tube at the planned incision site. After the salpingostomy and removal of the tubal pregnancy, bleeding sites are coagulated and the tubal incision is left to heal by secondary

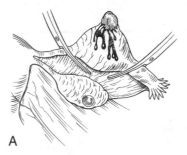

A

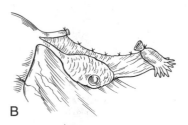

B

Figure 26–5 □ Segmental resection of tubal pregnancy via laparotomy. *A,* Kelly clamps are placed across the fallopian tube and the mesosalpinx. *B,* The tube and mesosalpinx are sutured. (From Keye WR, Chang RJ, Rebar RW, Soules MR: Infertility, Evaluation and Treatment. Philadelphia, WB Saunders Co, 1995, p 489.)

Figure 26–6 □ Segmental resection of tubal pregnancy via laparoscopy. *A,* The tube is elevated and a pretied suture is looped around the ectopic pregnancy. *B,* The segment of fallopian tube containing the pregnancy is excised and removed, leaving the two stumps secured by the suture. (From Keye WR, Chang RJ, Rebar RW, Soules MR: Infertility, Evaluation and Treatment. Philadelphia, WB Saunders Co, 1995, p 491.)

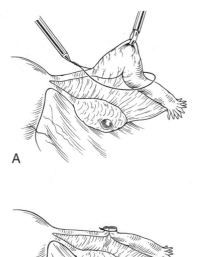

A

B

intention. Following the procedure, serum pregnancy tests should be performed until the results are negative. A negative pregnancy test is good evidence that the entire tubal pregnancy was removed.

b. **Medical management with methotrexate therapy**

Medical therapy with methotrexate is successful when treating the patient who is stable and in whom the diagnosis of tubal pregnancy has been made early. Methotrexate

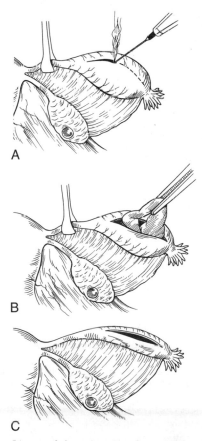

Figure 26-7 □ Linear salpingostomy via laparoscopy. *A,* After the fallopian tube is secured with a Babcock clamp, an incision is made in the antimesenteric border of the tube over the ectopic pregnancy. *B,* The pregnancy is then removed with the forceps. *C,* The incision is left open to heal. (From Keye WR, Chang RJ, Rebar RW, Soules MR: Infertility, Evaluation and Treatment. Philadelphia, WB Saunders Co, 1995, p 488.)

is a folic acid antagonist that interferes with the synthesis of DNA. Trophoblastic tissue is sensitive to methotrexate because of its rapid growth. The drug can be administered on an outpatient basis. The advantages of medical therapy include decreased cost, the lack of surgical and anesthetic risks, reduced tissue trauma, and less adhesion formation than results from surgery.

(1) Criteria for the use of methotrexate therapy in the patient with a tubal pregnancy are as follows:
  (a) Desire for preservation of fertility
  (b) Patient stable with no active bleeding
  (c) Tubal pregnancy unruptured
  (d) Size of tubal pregnancy <3.5 cm in diameter
  (e) Absence of fetal cardiac activity by ultrasound examination
  (f) Peak value of hCG <15,000 mIU/ml (IRP)
      Methotrexate can be administered to patients with serum hCG levels >15,000 mIU/ml, but there may be a higher treatment failure rate.

(2) A suggested protocol for methotrexate therapy is as follows:
  (a) Obtain baseline laboratory studies.
      [1] Complete blood count (CBC)
      [2] Platelet count
      [3] Blood urea nitrogen (BUN)
      [4] Serum creatinine
      [5] Asparate transaminase (AST)
  (b) Administer methotrexate 50 mg/m² IM (day 1).
  (c) Obtain serum hCG on day 4 and repeat on day 7.
  (d) If there is not a decrease of ≥15% in serum hCG between day 4 and day 7, repeat a dose of methotrexate 1 week after the first dose.
  (e) Repeat serum hCG weekly until the level falls to <15 mIU/ml.
  (f) Repeat course of methotrexate if hCG plateaus or increases. Alternatively, surgery can be considered. Surgery should be performed if there are signs or symptoms of rupture of the tubal pregnancy.

Serum hCG usually rises immediately after treatment and peaks on day 4. Patients should be warned that there is a 20% incidence of lower abdominal pain approximately 5 to 10 days after treatment and that 5 to 15% of patients experience rupture of the fallopian tube, making surgery necessary. Side effects of methrotrexate therapy such as stomatitis, gastritis, dermatitis, pleuritis, bone marrow suppression, and elevation in liver enzymes occur in fewer than 5% of cases.

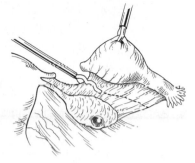

Figure 26–8 □ Total salpingectomy via laparoscopy. (From Keye WR, Chang RJ, Rebar RW, Soules MR: Infertility, Evaluation and Treatment. Philadelphia, WB Saunders Co, 1995, p 491.)

      (3) Contraindications to methotrexate therapy are as follows:
        (a) Poor patient compliance
        (b) History of active liver or renal disease
        (c) Active peptic ulcer disease
        (d) White blood cell count $<30,000/mm^3$
        (e) Platelet count $<100,000/mm^3$
        (f) Abnormal serum creatinine
        (g) Abnormal serum AST

2. Nonconservative management
  a. Total salpingectomy
     This procedure removes the entire fallopian tube and therefore precludes future tubal function (Fig. 26–8). Total salpingectomy is appropriate management if the patient does not want to preserve tubal function or if the extent of damage to the tube makes normal function extremely unlikely. Total salpingectomy should also be considered if the patient had a previous tubal pregnancy in the same tube.

■ BACKGROUND AND DEFINITIONS

Gonorrhea: Infection caused by *Neisseria gonorrhoeae*, a gram-negative diplococcus that has a predilection for columnar and pseudostratified epithelium of the genital tract. This infection involves primarily the endocervical canal and transformation zone of the cervix. In 80% of infected women, the urethra is also infected. Approximately 15 to 20% of women with gonorrhea develop pelvic inflammatory disease (PID) (discussed in Chapter 29). Among women who have undergone a hysterectomy, the urethra is the primary site of infection. Skene's glands or the paraurethral glands and Bartholin's glands can also become infected. In pediatric and postmenopausal patients, gonorrhea can also cause vaginitis. Gonorrhea in pregnant women has been associated with a higher risk of spontaneous abortion, premature rupture of membranes, chorioamnionitis, and preterm delivery. Nongenital gonorrheal infections in women include pharyngeal infection and disseminated gonorrhea.

The incubation period of gonorrhea is 3 to 5 days, and transmission is primarily by sexual contact. Women are more vulnerable to infection than men. The risk of transmission from an infected male to a female after a single sexual contact is 80 to 90%, whereas the risk of transmission from an infected female to a male is 20 to 25%. Forty to 60% of women with gonorrhea are asymptomatic. Almost 50% of gonorrhea isolates are resistant to penicillin, tetracycline, and spectinomycin.

> **Disseminated gonorrhea** has two stages: (1) an initial bacteremic stage manifested by systemic symptoms and skin lesions from gonococcal emboli, and (2) a later, arthritic stage usually involving the knees, ankles, or wrist joints.

Chlamydial infections: The most prevalent sexually transmitted infections in the United States, caused by *Chlamydia trachomatis*, an obligatory intracellular bacterium. The prevalence of these infections is 3% in asymptomatic women and as high as 33% in women who present to sexually transmitted disease clinics. Fifteen serotypes of *C. trachomatis* have been identified. Serotypes D, E, F, G, H, I, J, and K are responsible for urethritis, cervicitis, infection of Bartholin's gland, endometritis, PID, perihepatitis, and perinatal infections; and serotypes L1, L2, and L3 are responsible for lymphogranuloma venereum (discussed in Chapter 36).

The incubation period is 6 to 14 days. As with gonorrhea, many women are asymptomatic. Approximately 40 to 60% of women with gonorrhea have concomitant chlamydial infection.

■ CLINICAL PRESENTATION

The clinical presentations of gonorrhea and chlamydial infections are similar:
Mucopurulent cervical and vaginal discharge
Dysuria
Abnormal vaginal bleeding
Erythema of the cervix
Cervical friability
Pelvic discomfort
Pharyngitis
Symptoms associated with PID:
    Abdominal pain
    Pelvic pain
    Fever and chills
    Perihepatitis or Fitz-Hugh–Curtis syndrome
    Nausea
    Vomiting
    Anorexia

Clinical presentation associated with disseminated gonococcal infection:
Fever and chills
Skin lesions characterized by erythematous macules that become pustules with hemorrhagic base and necrotic center, most commonly found on the fingers and palm of the hand
Tenosynovitis
Polyarthralgias
Hepatitis
Myocarditis
Pericarditis
Meningitis

■ PHONE CALL

Questions

1. **What are the patient's vital signs?**
2. **What symptoms does the patient have?**
    The presence of fever and severe pain is suggestive of

PID, tubo-ovarian abscess (TOA), or disseminated gonorrhea.

Degree of Urgency

Most cases of sexually transmitted disease caused by *N. gonorrhoeae* and *C. trachomatis* are uncomplicated and are not life threatening. However, the severely ill patient should be seen immediately because of the possibility of ruptured TOA or disseminated gonorrhea.

■ ELEVATOR THOUGHTS

What are the risk factors for gonorrhea and chlamydial infection?
- Young age; highest incidence in women 20 to 24 years of age
- Lower socioeconomic class
- Young age at time of first intercourse
- Multiple sexual partners
- Partner with multiple sexual partners
- Failure to use barrier-method contraception

■ MAJOR THREAT TO LIFE

- Ruptured TOA
- Gonococcal meningitis
- Gonococcal endocarditis

Gonorrhea and chlamydial infection are rarely life threatening. However, overwhelming sepsis from a ruptured TOA and certain complications of disseminated gonorrhea can be fatal.

■ BEDSIDE

Quick Look Test

Does the patient appear severely ill?
PID, TOA, or disseminated gonorrhea should be suspected in a patient who appears to be extremely ill.

Vital Signs

Vital signs are usually normal in a patient with uncomplicated gonorrhea or chlamydial infection. The finding of a fever suggests PID or disseminated gonorrhea. Hypotension with a systolic

blood pressure of <60 mm Hg and tachycardia are usually found in the patient with a ruptured TOA.

Selective History and Chart Review

1. How long has the patient had symptoms of a sexually transmitted infection?
2. What risk factors does the patient have for gonorrhea or chlamydial infection?
3. Has the patient had a prior gonococcal or chlamydial infection?
4. Is the patient sexually active? If so, what does she use for contraception?
5. Does the patient's sexual partner have any symptoms suggestive of a sexually transmitted infection?
6. When was the patient's last menstrual period?

Selective Physical Examination

Dermatological	Erythematous macules with a diameter of 1 to 5 mm that become pustules with a hemorrhagic base and a necrotic center, most commonly found on the fingers and palm of the hand in a patient with disseminated gonorrhea
Abdominal	Tenderness to palpation, sometimes with guarding and rebound tenderness in PID
	Rigid and board-like with ruptured TOA
Pelvic	
External genitalia and vagina	Mucopurulent discharge
Cervix	Mucopurulent discharge through the cervical os
	Tender to cervical motion
	Erythematous
	Friable and bleeding
Uterus and adnexa	Adnexal tenderness in PID
	Adnexal mass if TOA is present
Extremities	Tenosynovitis and arthritis, most commonly involving the knees in patients with disseminated gonorrhea

Orders

1. Obtain a complete blood count (CBC) with differential.
2. Obtain erythrocyte sedimentation rate (ESR).

3. Start IV in the severely ill patient.
4. Insert a urethral Foley catheter in the severely ill patient.
5. Record intake and output in the severely ill patient.
6. Perform a urine pregnancy test if the patient has missed a menstrual period or is unsure when her last menses began.

■ DIAGNOSTIC TESTING

Diagnostic tests for uncomplicated gonorrhea and chlamydial infections are listed here. Diagnostic tests for patients with suspected PID or TOA are discussed in Chapter 29.

1. **Gonorrhea**
   a. **Endocervical culture**
      An endocervical culture using selective media containing antibiotics has a sensitivity of 80 to 90% from a single culture.
   b. **Gram stain**
      A Gram stain showing gram-negative intracellular diplococci has a sensitivity of 50 to 70% and a specificity of 97%. A Gram stain can also be performed on joint effusion in patients with disseminated gonorrhea.
   c. **Blood culture**
      A blood culture is positive in approximately 25% of patients with disseminated gonorrhea.
   d. **Aspiration and culture of joint effusion**
      A culture of joint effusion is positive in 20 to 30% of patients with disseminated gonorrhea.
2. **Chlamydial infection**
   a. **Endocervical culture**
      A specimen of as many cervical epithelial cells as possible should be obtained to optimize the sensitivity of the culture. A rayon- or cotton-tipped applicator with a plastic or metal shaft should be used.
   b. **Enzyme-linked immunosorbent assay**
      Enzyme-linked immunosorbent assays (ELISAs) such as Chlamydiazyme have a sensitivity of 90% and a specificity of 97%.
   c. **Fluorescence-labeled monoclonal antibody testing**
      Detection tests, such as MicroTrak, that use monoclonal antibodies have a sensitivity of 89% and a specificity of 98%.

■ MANAGEMENT

1. **Uncomplicated gonorrhea in nonpregnant patients**
   a. Administer one of the following antibiotics:

      (1) **Ceftriaxone 125 mg IM once** or
      (2) **Cefixime 400 mg PO once** or
      (3) **Ciprofloxacin 500 mg PO once** or
      (4) **Ofloxacin 400 mg PO once** or
      (5) **Spectinomycin 2 g IM once**

   b. Because of the high frequency of a coexistent chlamydial infection, also administer

      (1) **Doxycycline 100 mg PO two times per day for 7 days** or
      (2) **Azithromycin 1 g PO once**

2. Uncomplicated gonorrhea in pregnant patients

   a. Administer one of the following antibiotics:

      (1) **Ceftriaxone 250 mg IM once** or
      (2) **Cefixime 400 mg PO once** or
      (3) **Spectinomycin 2 g IM once**

   b. Because of the high frequency of a coexistent chlamydial infection, also administer one of the following:

      (1) **Erythromycin base 500 mg PO four times per day for 7 days** or
      (2) **Azithromycin 1 g PO once** or
      (3) **Amoxacillin 500 mg PO three times per day for 7 days**

3. Gonococcal bacteremia and arthritis

   a. Administer one of the following antibiotics:

      (1) **Ceftriaxone 1 g IV daily** or
      (2) **Ceftizoxime 1 g IV every 8 hours** or
      (3) **Cefotaxime 1 g IV every 8 hours**

   b. For patients allergic to β-lactam drugs, initial therapy may consist of one of the following:

      (1) **Ciprofloxacin 500 mg IV every 12 hours** or
      (2) **Ofloxacin 400 mg IV every 12 hours** or
      (3) **Spectinomycin 2 g IM every 12 hours**

   c. All of these regimens should be continued for 24 to 48 hours after there is clinical improvement. Then one of the following agents should be administered for a full week:

      (1) **Cefixime 400 mg PO two times per day** or
      (2) **Ciprofloxacin 500 mg PO two times per day** or
      (3) **Ofloxacin 400 mg PO two times per day**

4. Gonococcal meningitis and endocarditis

   a. Administer one of the following antibiotics:

      (1) **Ceftriaxone 1 to 2 g IV daily for at least 10 to 14 days** or
      (2) **Penicillin G at least 10 million units IV daily for at least 10 days** or
      (3) **Chloramphenicol 4 to 6 g IV daily for at least 10 days**

5. *C. trachomatis* in nonpregnant patients

   a. Administer one of the following antibiotics:

      (1) **Azithromycin 1 g PO once** or
      (2) **Doxycycline 100 mg PO two times per day for 7 days** or

(3) **Erythromycin 500 mg PO four times per day for 7 days** or

(4) **Erythromycin ethylsuccinate 800 mg PO four times per day for 7 days** or

(5) **Ofloxacin 300 mg PO two times per day for 7 days**

6. *C. trachomatis* **in pregnant patients**

a. Administer one of the following antibiotics:

(1) **Erythromycin 500 mg PO four times per day for 7 days** or

(2) **Amoxicillin 500 mg PO three times per day for 10 days** or

(3) **Erythromycin base 250 mg PO four times per day for 14 days** or

(4) **Erythromycin ethylsuccinate 800 mg PO four times per day for 7 days** or

(5) **Erythromycin ethylsuccinate 400 mg PO four times per day for 14 days** or

(6) Azithromycin 1 g PO once

7. **Lymphogranuloma venereum** (see Chapter 35)

a. Administer one of the following antibiotics:

(1) **Doxycycline 100 mg PO two times per day for 21 days** or

(2) **Erythromycin 500 mg PO four times per day for 21 days**

■ BACKGROUND AND DEFINITIONS

Gestational trophoblastic neoplasia (GTN): A spectrum of diseases that result from the abnormal proliferation of trophoblastic tissue associated with pregnancy. GTN is a constellation of diseases with benign hydatidiform mole at one end of the spectrum and malignant choriocarcinoma at the other (Table 28–1). All forms of GTN are associated with abnormally high serum levels of human chorionic gonadotropin (hCG).

Hydatidiform mole: The benign and most common form of GTN. Approximately 85 to 90% of all GTNs are hydatidiform moles, also referred to as **molar pregnancies.** The incidence of molar pregnancies ranges from 1 in 1500 to 1 in 2000 pregnancies among white women in the United States, to 1 in 800 pregnancies among Asian women in the United States, to 1 in 85 to 200 pregnancies among Asian women in Asia. Molar pregnancies appear grossly as multiple vesicles that have the appearance of a bunch of grapes. Hydatidiform moles do not metastasize, but embolization or deportation of vesicles can occur, most commonly to the lungs.

Complete moles make up the majority (60 to 75%) of molar pregnancies and have a 46 XX karyotype. In complete moles, there is an absence of fetal tissue, except in the rare instance of a twin pregnancy in which one of the twin gestations is a molar pregnancy.

Partial moles or incomplete moles make up 25 to 40% of molar pregnancies and are distinguished by the coexistence of a pregnancy confirmed by the presence of normal villi or products of conception. When a fetus is present, fetal demise usually occurs. Most partial moles have a triploid karyotype, usually

Table 28–1 □ CLASSIFICATION OF GESTATIONAL TROPHOBLASTIC NEOPLASIA

Benign disease
  Hydatidiform mole
    Complete mole
    Partial mole or incomplete mole
Malignant disease (may be metastatic or nonmetastatic)
  Invasive mole or chorioadenoma destruens
  Choriocarcinoma

69 XXY; the next most common karyotype is trisomy, most commonly trisomy 16.

After treatment by surgical evacuation, both complete and partial moles can result in persistent GTN in the form of invasive mole or choriocarcinoma. The risk of persistent GTN is 15 to 20% with complete moles and decreases to 5 to 7% with partial moles.

Invasive moles or **chorioadenoma destruens:** A form of GTN that is locally invasive into the myometrium of the uterus. Approximately 5 to 10% of all GTNs are invasive moles. They can cause rupture of the uterus and hemorrhage by penetrating through the entire thickness of the myometrium. The diagnosis of invasive mole is usually made by pathological evaluation of the uterus after hysterectomy is performed for continued bleeding or persistently elevated serum hCG. Metastasis to the vagina and the lungs can occur.

Choriocarcinoma: The malignant form of GTN. Approximately 3 to 5% of all GTNs are choriocarcinomas. Of all patients who develop choriocarcinoma, 50% have had a preceding molar pregnancy, 15% have had a preceding term pregnancy, and 25% have had a preceding spontaneous abortion, therapeutic abortion, or ectopic pregnancy. Choriocarcinoma progresses rapidly and metastasizes hematogenously to the brain, lungs, liver, kidneys, gastrointestinal tract, and lower genital tract (Table 28–2).

■ CLINICAL PRESENTATION

- Complete hydatidiform mole
  - Vaginal bleeding, initially painless, in the first or early second trimester of pregnancy
  - Uterine contractions
  - Passage of vesicles
  - Excessive nausea or hyperemesis gravidarum
  - Pelvic pain from theca-lutein cysts

Table 28–2 □ SITES AND FREQUENCY OF
METASTATIC CHORIOCARCINOMA

Site	Frequency (%)
Lungs	60–90
Vagina	40–50
Vulva or cervix	10–15
Brain	5–15
Liver	5–15

Symptoms of preeclampsia before 24 weeks of gestational age in 5 to 10% of patients:

Hypertension

Edema

Proteinuria

Central nervous system (CNS) symptoms: headache, mental confusion, dizziness, drowsiness

Visual symptoms: blurred vision, scotomata, flashes of light, diplopia, blindness

Gastrointestinal symptoms: epigastric pain, vomiting, hematemesis

Renal symptoms: anuria, oliguria, hematuria

Symptoms of hyperthyroidism in 2 to 7% of patients:

Nervousness

Tremulousness

Anorexia

Uterus large for dates in 50% of patients

Absence of fetal heart tones or palpable fetal parts

Dyspnea in patients with pulmonary embolization of vesicles

- Partial hydatidiform mole—Same as the presentation for complete mole except for the following:

Uterus large for dates in only 11% of patients

Uterus small for dates in 66% of patients

Fetal heart tones and fetal parts may be present

Symptoms usually manifest later than with complete moles, often in the late first trimester or second trimester

- Invasive mole or chorioadenoma destruens

Hemorrhage

Sudden onset of heavy vaginal or intra-abdominal bleeding may result from penetration through the myometrium and rupture of the uterus

Symptoms of metastasis:

Vaginal bleeding from vaginal metastasis

CNS symptoms from brain metastasis

- Choriocarcinoma—Most patients with choriocarcinoma have symptoms of metastasis:

Vaginal bleeding from vaginal metastasis

Symptoms of lung metastasis:

Hemoptysis

Cough

Dyspnea

Symptoms of brain metastasis:

Headaches

Dizziness

Syncopal episodes

■ PHONE CALL

Questions

1. Is the patient bleeding? If so, how heavily?
2. What are the patient's vital signs?
3. Does the patient appear to be short of breath or dyspneic?

Degree of Urgency

Patients who have heavy vaginal bleeding or suspected intra-abdominal hemorrhage should be seen immediately. Patients with severe preeclampsia or hyperthyroidism also should be seen immediately.

■ ELEVATOR THOUGHTS

What is the differential diagnosis of molar pregnancy?
- Spontaneous abortion
- Ectopic pregnancy

What are risk factors for molar pregnancy?
- Young maternal age (<15 years)
- Advanced maternal age (>40 years)
- Prior molar pregnancy
- Prior spontaneous abortion
- Diet with vitamin A deficiency
- Asian ethnicity

■ MAJOR THREAT TO LIFE

- Hemorrhage
- Metastatic disease
- Complications of preeclampsia
    Disseminated intravascular coagulation (DIC)
    Eclampsia
    Stroke

■ BEDSIDE

Quick Look Test

Does the patient appear to be in hypovolemic shock?
  Hypovolemic shock can result from blood loss due to either vaginal bleeding or intra-abdominal bleeding.

Does the patient appear to have any respiratory difficulties?
Dyspnea and hemoptysis are suggestive of either pulmonary metastasis or embolization of vesicles.

Does the patient appear to be hyperthyroid?
Hyperthyroidism is found in 2 to 7% of patients and results either from the high levels of hCG, which has thyroid-stimulating activities, or from an elevated level of T_4, which is found in 25 to 50% of patients.

Vital Signs

Hypotension and tachycardia can occur in a patient with significant blood loss. Postural hypotension may be present. Changes in blood pressure (BP) and pulse should be measured when the patient is assisted in sitting or standing from a supine position. A fall in systolic or diastolic BP >15 mm Hg or a rise in pulse >15 beats/min is evidence of hypovolemia. Tachycardia alone may result from hyperthyroidism.

Selective History and Chart Review

1. Has the patient had a normal pregnancy recently?
   GTN that develops after a normal pregnancy is almost always a choriocarcinoma and not a hydatidiform mole or an invasive mole.
2. When was the patient's last menstrual period?
3. Has the patient had a prior molar pregnancy?
4. Has the patient had a previous ultrasound examination demonstrating the presence of fetal parts or a viable fetus?
   This finding would be diagnostic of a partial mole. The finding of a viable fetus is an indication for amniocentesis for karyotype determination of the fetus.

Selective Physical Examination

General	Tremulousness, diaphoresis, anxiety, and nervousness if the patient is hyperthyroid
Pulmonary	Wheezing and rhonchi may be present due to embolization of vesicles
Abdominal	Enlarged uterus with a complete mole; small for gestational age with a partial mole
	Absence of fetal parts on palpation or fetal heart tones on auscultation unless there is a partial mole with a viable fetus

Pelvic

External genitalia and vagina	Vaginal bleeding usually present
	Spontaneous passage of vesicles sometimes present
	Polypoid vaginal lesion may be present if there has been vaginal metastasis from choriocarcinoma
Cervix	Cervix may be dilated, with bleeding and protruding vesicles
Uterus	Uterus is large for dates in one-half of patients with complete moles but may be appropriate or even small for dates with partial moles
Adnexa	Bilateral ovarian theca-lutein cysts may be present

Orders

1. Give nothing by mouth (NPO status) in preparation for surgical evacuation.
2. Obtain a serum hCG.
3. Obtain a complete blood count (CBC) with differential.
4. Obtain coagulation studies: platelet count, prothrombin time (PT), and partial thromboplastin time (PTT).
5. Obtain thyroid function tests: total thyroxine (T_4), triiodothyronine (T_3) resin uptake, and thyroid-stimulating hormone (TSH).
6. Type and crossmatch blood.
7. Obtain chest radiographs, posteroanterior and lateral.
8. Obtain an electrocardiogram (ECG).
9. Start IV.
10. Record input and output.

■ DIAGNOSTIC TESTING

1. Ultrasound examination

Ultrasound examination is the diagnostic test of choice for hydatidiform moles. The finding of a "snowstorm" pattern in a gestation of more than 14 weeks is diagnostic of a hydatidiform mole. This ultrasound finding in a pregnancy of less than 14 weeks' gestation may also be consistent with a spontaneous abortion. Ultrasonography can detect bilateral theca-lutein cysts, which are found in almost 25% of patients with hydatidiform moles and are caused by stimulation of the ovaries by elevated hCG levels. The concurrent finding of fetal parts or a viable fetus is diagnostic of a partial mole.

Table 28–3 □ HUMAN CHORIONIC GONADOTROPIN
LEVELS IN NORMAL PREGNANCIES

Gestational Age (weeks)	Serum hCG (mIU / ml)
4	100
6	1000–10,000
7	10,000–50,000
9	50,000–100,000
20	10,000–20,000

2. **Serum human chorionic gonadotropin**
   Serum hCG levels are elevated above those obtained in normal pregnancies (Table 28–3). A level significantly >100,000 mIU/ml is highly suggestive of a molar pregnancy or a multiple gestation.
3. **Thyroid function tests**
   In 25 to 50% of patients, T_4 is elevated above the normal levels found in pregnancy.
4. **Chest radiography**
   A chest radiograph may detect embolization of vesicles in patients with hydatidiform mole and lung metastasis in patients with either invasive mole or choriocarcinoma.
5. **Electrocardiogram**
   An ECG may reveal cardiac rhythm abnormalities such as supraventricular tachycardia associated with hyperthyroidism.

■ MANAGEMENT

Management of hydatidiform moles is threefold, as follows: (1) Treatment of medical complications such as preeclampsia and hyperthyroidism, (2) surgical evacuation of the uterus, and (3) posttreatment surveillance of hCG levels.

1. **Treatment of medical complications**
   a. **Preeclampsia**
      The definitive treatment for preeclampsia is surgical evacuation of the uterus. Before this, management of preeclampsia includes prevention of eclamptic seizures by the administration of magnesium sulfate and treatment of severe hypertension.
      (1) **Magnesium sulfate 2 to 4 g IV over 5 minutes as a loading dose, followed by 1.0 g/hr IV as the maintenance dose** or
      (2) **Magnesium sulfate 2 to 4 g IV over 2 to 4 minutes, concurrently with 10 g IM as the loading dose, followed by 5 g IM every 4 hours**

Side effects of magnesium sulfate include flushing and nausea. More serious complications resulting from magnesium toxicity include respiratory depression and cardiac arrest. If respiratory or cardiac arrest develops, the magnesium sulfate infusion should be discontinued and calcium gluconate should be administered as follows:

(3) **Calcium gluconate (10% solution), 10 ml (1 g) IV over 3 minutes**

b. **Hyperthyroidism**

The treatment of hyperthyroidism consists of administration of antithyroid drugs such as propylthiouracil or methimazole and a beta-adrenergic blocker such as propranolol.

(1) Antithyroid medication

(a) **Propylthiouracil (PTU) 100 to 150 mg PO every 8 hours** or

(b) **Methimazole (Tapazole) 20 to 30 mg PO every 12 hours**

(2) Beta-adrenergic blocker

(a) **Propranolol (Inderal) 10 to 40 mg two to three times per day**

2. **Surgical evacuation of the uterus**

a. **Suction dilatation and curettage**

Suction dilatation and curettage should be performed in an operating room with a 10- to 12-mm curette. Intravenous oxytocin should be administered after the procedure has begun. Severe blood loss may necessitate blood transfusion. After suction curettage, sharp curettage should be performed to ensure that all tissue has been evacuated. The major complications of the procedure are uterine perforation and hemorrhage. If the uterus is larger than 14 weeks' size, the use of ultrasound guidance should be considered to decrease the risk of uterine perforation. In patients with a partial mole and a dead fetus of more than 13 weeks' gestation, dilatation and evacuation may be required in addition to suction curettage. Even though the risk of Rh isoimmunization after suction dilatation and curettage for a molar pregnancy is unclear, anti–D immune globulin (RhoGAM) should be administered to Rh-negative patients.

b. **Hysterotomy**

Hysterotomy may be indicated if equipment or training for suction dilatation and curettage and/or dilatation and evacuation is lacking.

c. **Hysterectomy**

In certain patients who do not desire future fertility, abdominal hysterectomy may be considered

3. **Posttreatment surveillance of hCG levels**

After surgical evacuation, patients should have serum hCG

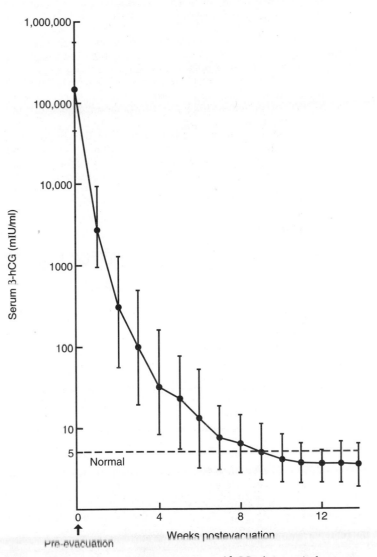

Figure 28–1 □ Normal regression curve of hCG after surgical evacuation of hydatidiform mole. (From Morrow CP, Kletzky OA, DiSaia PJ, et al: Clinical and laboratory correlates of molar pregnancy and trophoblastic disease. Am J Obstet Gynecol 1977;128:424.)

drawn weekly until the hCG level is negative for 3 consecutive weeks. Then serum hCG should be drawn monthly for 6 to 12 months. Figure 28–1 shows the normal regression curve for hCG after evacuation of a hydatidiform mole. During the period of surveillance, the patient must use contraception, preferably oral contraceptive pills. Otherwise, it will be impossible to distinguish between hCG from a new pregnancy and that from persistent and possibly metastatic disease. Approximately 80 to 85% of patients will have spontaneous regression and achieve a negative hCG. Approximately 15 to 20% of patients will demonstrate a plateau or rise in hCG. In these patients, a new pregnancy must first be ruled out. Then, staging and a metastatic workup should be performed. Patients with no metastatic disease should be treated with single-agent chemotherapy with methotrexate. Patients with metastatic disease will require combination therapy. MAC therapy, which includes methotrexate, actinomycin D, and cyclophosphamide, is a commonly used regimen.

■ BACKGROUND AND DEFINITIONS

Pelvic inflammatory disease (PID): Nonspecific term that refers to inflammation of the upper genital tract, which includes the uterus, the fallopian tubes, and the ovaries. This is in contrast to inflammation of the lower genital tract, which includes the cervix, the vagina, and the vulva. The term PID can refer to inflammation of the fallopian tubes (**salpingitis**), ovaries (**oophoritis**), uterine myometrium (**myometritis**), endometrium (**endometritis**), or broad ligament (**parametritis**). However, PID most commonly refers to **salpingitis.**

Pyosalpinx: A collection of pus in the fallopian tube, often encountered in acute salpingitis

Hydrosalpinx: A collection of sterile fluid in the fallopian tube, an end stage of pyosalpinx

Tubo-ovarian abscess (TOA): An abscess complex involving the tubes, the ovaries, and often the intestines. In a TOA, inflammation involves the stroma of the ovary, often resulting in destruction of the ovary.

There has been a steady increase in both the incidence of PID and the number of hospital admissions for PID. It is estimated that more than 1 million women are treated for PID each year in the United States. PID almost always results from infection ascending from the lower genital tract. It is usually a polymicrobial infection. Organisms that can cause PID are listed in Table 29–1.

The most serious immediate complication resulting from PID is formation of a TOA. The incidence of TOA formation in patients with PID is approximately 15%. The presence of a TOA may require surgical intervention if the abscess does not respond to antibiotic therapy or if the abscess ruptures. Rupture of a TOA

Table 29–1 □ ORGANISMS THAT CAN CAUSE PELVIC INFLAMMATORY DISEASE

Neisseria gonorrhoeae	*Peptostreptococcus* spp.
Chlamydia trachomatis	*Bacteroides fragilis*
Escherichia coli	*Mycoplasma hominis*
Peptococcus spp.	*Ureaplasma urealyticum*

constitutes a life-threatening emergency and has a mortality rate of 5 to 10%.

The major long-term sequelae resulting from PID include chronic pelvic and abdominal pain, infertility, tubal pregnancy, and recurrent PID. The incidence of chronic pelvic and abdominal pain after PID is approximately 20%. The incidence of tubal factor infertility is close to 12% after one episode of PID, increases to 25% after two episodes, and is approximately 50 to 60% after three episodes of PID. There is an increase of fourfold to eightfold in the risk of tubal pregnancy among patients with a history of PID. Approximately 50% of tubal pregnancies occur in tubes previously damaged by salpingitis. Recurrent PID is encountered in 15 to 25% of women with a history of PID.

■ CLINICAL PRESENTATION

Abdominal pain
Pelvic pain
Vaginal discharge
Abnormal vaginal bleeding
Fever
Chills
Nausea
Vomiting
Anorexia
Urinary symptoms

The frequencies of the above symptoms of PID are listed in Table 29–2.

■ PHONE CALL

Questions

1. What are the patient's vital signs?
2. Does the patient appear to be in shock?

Table 29–2 □ FREQUENCIES OF SYMPTOMS FOUND IN PATIENTS WITH PELVIC INFLAMMATORY DISEASE

Symptom	Frequency (%)
Lower abdominal or pelvic pain	99
Vaginal discharge	70
Irregular vaginal bleeding	40
Fever or chills	35
Urinary symptoms	20
Nausea or vomiting	10
Anorexia	10

The most serious complication resulting from PID is rupture of a TOA. These patients appear severely ill and can present in septic shock.

Degree of Urgency

PID is usually not life threatening unless it is complicated by ruptured TOA. If this complication is suspected, the patient should be seen immediately.

■ ELEVATOR THOUGHTS

What are the risk factors for PID?
- Younger age, <25 years
  Approximately 75% of all PID cases occur in women younger than 25 years of age.
- Young age at first intercourse
- Multiple sexual partners
  The risk of PID is increased fivefold in patients with multiple sexual partners.
- Partner with multiple sexual partners
- Single marital status
- Frequent intercourse with multiple partners
  The risk of PID is not increased with frequent intercourse with a single monogamous partner.
- Use of an intrauterine device (IUD)
  Women who have an IUD have a twofold to threefold increase in the risk of PID, especially in the first 3 months after IUD insertion.
- Transcervical instrumentation
  Any procedure that requires penetration of the cervical mucus barrier increases the risk of PID. Common procedures are dilatation and curettage, pregnancy termination, hysterosalpingogram, and IUD insertion. The incidence of PID after first-trimester pregnancy termination is approximately 1 in 200 cases.

What is the differential diagnosis of PID?
- Cervicitis
- Tubal pregnancy
- Adnexal mass with rupture or torsion
- Endometriosis
- Appendicitis
- Diverticulitis

■ MAJOR THREAT TO LIFE

- Sepsis from ruptured TOA
  This complication has a mortality rate of 5 to 10%.

■ BEDSIDE

Quick Look Test

How ill does the patient appear?

A patient who appears severely ill, with signs and symptoms of septic shock, should be suspected of having a ruptured TOA.

Vital Signs

Approximately 35% of patients with PID present with a fever. Hypotension with systolic blood pressure <60 mm Hg and tachycardia is usually found in patients with sepsis from a ruptured TOA.

Selective History and Chart Review

1. What risk factors for PID does the patient have?
2. Has the patient had prior episodes of PID?
3. How long has the patient had symptoms of PID?
4. Is the patient sexually active? If so, what does she use for contraception?
5. Does the patient's sexual partner have symptoms suggestive of a sexually transmitted disease?
6. When was the patient's last menstrual period?

Selective Physical Examination

Abdominal	Tenderness to palpation
	Guarding
	Rebound tenderness
	Rigid and board-like with ruptured TOA
Pelvic	
External genitalia and vagina	Purulent vaginal discharge
Cervix	Tender to cervical motion
	Purulent discharge through the cervical os
Uterus and adnexa	Adnexal tenderness
	Adnexal mass or fullness if TOA, pyosalpinx, or hydrosalpinx is present

Orders

1. Obtain a complete blood count (CBC) with differential.
2. Obtain erythrocyte sedimentation rate (ESR).
3. Start IV in the severely ill patient

4. Insert a urethral Foley catheter in the severely ill patient.
5. Record intake and output in the severely ill patient.
6. Perform a urine pregnancy test if the patient has missed a menstrual period or is unsure when her last menses began.

■ DIAGNOSTIC TESTING

1. Laparoscopy

Laparoscopy is the most accurate diagnostic procedure for PID. In patients with uncomplicated PID, the fallopian tubes appear erythematous, indurated, and edematous. An exudate is usually seen on the tubal surface or at the fimbriated end of the tube. A pyosalpinx or hydrosalpinx may be observed. Laparoscopy also confirms or rules out the presence of a TOA. Furthermore, laparoscopy helps in ruling out an adnexal mass and appendicitis, both of which are part of the differential diagnosis for PID. In practice, PID is usually diagnosed based on clinical presentation, with confirmation of the diagnosis by less invasive tests. Laparoscopy is usually reserved for the patient who has an unclear diagnosis or who fails to respond to antibiotic therapy.

2. Ultrasound examination

Ultrasound examination is crucial in detecting a TOA. Furthermore, it also detects pyosalpinx and hydrosalpinx, although it cannot distinguish between the two. Ultrasound examination is often helpful in obtaining more information about a pelvic mass when pelvic examination reveals one. Finally, ultrasound examination is helpful when a patient has too much tenderness to permit an adequate pelvic examination.

3. Laboratory tests

The following laboratory tests can be helpful in confirming the diagnosis of PID, but all of these tests are nonspecific:

a. Vaginal wet smear with normal saline

Microscopic examination of a wet smear of vaginal discharge reveals the presence of multiple white blood cells.

b. Gram stain of cervical discharge

The finding of >30 white blood cells per high-power field is highly suggestive of cervicitis. Furthermore, the presence of gram-negative intracellular diplococci is suggestive of *Neisseria gonorrhoeae* infection. However, Gram stain has only a 50 to 60% sensitivity for *N. gonorrhoeae* infection.

c. White blood cell count

Leukocytosis is defined by a white blood cell count >10,000 cells/mm^3. Fewer than 50% of patients with PID have leukocytosis.

d. **Erythrocyte sedimentation rate**

An elevated ESR >20 mm/hr is found in nearly 75% of patients with PID.

e. **C-reactive protein**

An elevated C-reactive protein concentration >2 mg/dl, like the white blood cell count and ESR, is a nonspecific indicator of infection and is only slightly more sensitive than the ESR.

f. **Testing for *N. gonorrhoeae* and *Chlamydia trachomatis***

Cervical culture is the best test for detection of *N. gonorrhoeae*, and rapid antigen detection tests such as Chlamydiazyme or MicroTrak are the most readily available tests for *C. trachomatis*. Positive testing may be helpful in supporting the diagnosis of PID. However, cervical cultures are diagnostic only for cervicitis.

g. **Culdocentesis**

Although it is nonspecific, culdocentesis can help to confirm the diagnosis of PID if purulent peritoneal fluid is obtained. In patients with PID, the white blood cell count of peritoneal fluid is usually >30,000 cells/mm^3.

h. **Endometrial biopsy**

An endometrial biopsy allows for the pathological diagnosis of endometritis. However, this test is not able to distinguish between endometritis alone and endometritis with salpingitis.

4. **Clinical criteria for the diagnosis of PID**

Because of the nonspecific nature of diagnostic tests other than laparoscopy, the following clinical criteria for the diagnosis of PID should be used. Patients must have all three of the following:

a. **Abdominal tenderness**
b. **Cervical motion tenderness**
c. **Adnexal tenderness**

In addition, patients might have one or more of the following:

d. **A positive Gram stain for gram-negative intracellular diplococci**
e. **A fever (>38°C or 100.4°F)**
f. **An elevated white blood cell count (>10,000 cells/mm^3)**
g. **Purulent fluid obtained from the peritoneal cavity by culdocentesis or laparoscopy**
h. **A pelvic abscess detected by either pelvic examination or ultrasonography**

■
MANAGEMENT OF PELVIC INFLAMMATORY DISEASE

PID can be treated with antibiotics on either an inpatient or an outpatient basis. Early and aggressive treatment can decrease the incidence of long-term sequelae such as infertility (Table 29–3).

**Table 29–3 □ INCIDENCE OF LONG-TERM SEQUELAE
OF PELVIC INFLAMMATORY DISEASE (PID)**

Sequelae	Incidence (%)
Chronic pelvic pain	20
Infertility	
One episode of PID	12
Two episodes of PID	25
Three episodes of PID	50–60
Tubal pregnancy	6–13
Recurrent PID	15–25

1. **Indications for hospitalization and treatment with parenteral antibiotics include the following:**
   a. Failure of outpatient therapy
   b. Nulliparity, especially in a young patient
   c. Pregnancy
   d. Presence of TOA
   e. Presence of gastrointestinal symptoms
   f. Peritonitis in the upper abdominal quadrants
   g. Presence of IUD
   h. Inability to rule out surgical emergencies such as appendicitis and ectopic pregnancy
   i. Patient is severely ill
   j. Patient is unreliable, and noncompliance with outpatient therapy and follow-up is suspected
   k. Patient intolerance of outpatient therapy
   l. Unclear diagnosis
2. **Inpatient treatment regimen for uncomplicated PID**
   a. Administer the following regimen:
      (1) **Cefoxitin 2 g IV every 6 hours or Cefotetan 2 g IV every 12 hours** plus
      (2) **Doxycycline 100 mg IV or PO every 12 hours**
   b. An alternative inpatient regimen is the following:
      (1) **Clindamycin 900 mg IV every 8 hours** plus
      (2) **Gentamicin 2 mg/kg IV loading dose followed by 1.5 mg/kg IV every 8 hours**
   c. Either of the above regimens is continued for at least 48 hours after there has been clinical improvement. The patient is then placed on one of the following antibiotics:
      (1) **Doxycycline 100 mg PO two times per day for 10 to 14 days** or
      (2) **Clindamycin 450 mg PO four times per day for 10 to 14 days**
3. **Outpatient treatment regimen for uncomplicated PID**
   a. Administer the following:

       (1) **Cefoxitin 2 g IM with probenecid 1 g PO or Ceftriaxone 250 mg IM**

  b. In addition, administer one of the following:

       (1) **Doxycycline 100 mg PO two times per day for 10 to 14 days** or

       (2) **Tetracycline 500 mg PO four times per day for 10 to 14 days** or

       (3) **Erythromycin 500 mg PO four times per day for 10 to 14 days**

4. **Alternative outpatient regimen**

  a. Administer the following:

       (1) **Ofloxacin 400 mg PO two times per day for 14 days** plus

       (2) **Clindamycin 450 mg PO four times per day for 14 days** or

       (3) **Metronidazole 500 mg PO two times per day for 14 days**

■ MANAGEMENT OF PELVIC INFLAMMATORY DISEASE WITH TUBO-OVARIAN ABSCESS

Initial management of a TOA consists of the administration of IV antibiotics including an agent that provides anaerobic coverage such as clindamycin or metronidazole. Patients with an abscess larger than 8 cm in diameter have a higher incidence of treatment failure. Patients in whom antibiotic therapy fails require either drainage or surgical excision.

1. **Antibiotic therapy**

  a. **Inpatient antibiotic regimen**

       (1) **Clindamycin 900 mg IV every 8 hours** plus

       (2) **Gentamicin 2 mg/kg IV loading dose followed by 1.5 mg/kg IV every 8 hours**

  b. **Alternative inpatient antibiotic regimen**

       (1) **Metronidazole 15 mg/kg IV loading dose over 1 hour followed by 7.5 mg/kg IV every 6 hours** plus

       (2) **Gentamicin 2 mg/kg IV loading dose followed by 1.5 mg/kg IV every 8 hours**

Either of the above regimens is continued for at least 48 hours after there has been clinical improvement. The patient can then be discharged on one of the following antibiotic regimens:

  c. **Postdischarge antibiotic regimen**

       (1) **Doxycycline 100 mg PO two times per day for 10 to 14 days** or

       (2) **Clindamycin 450 mg PO four times per day for 10 to 14 days**

2. **Drainage of abscess**

If there is no clinical improvement after 72 hours of IV antibiotics, surgical drainage should be considered.

a. **Posterior colpotomy**

Transvaginal drainage of a TOA can be considered if the abscess fulfills the following three requirements:

(1) Abscess is midline

(2) Abscess dissects the rectovaginal septum and is adherent to the cul-de-sac peritoneum

(3) Abscess is fluctuant and cystic

b. **Radiographically guided drainage**

Fluoroscopically guided drainage can be performed by interventional radiologists. An indwelling catheter can be left in the abscess cavity for irrigation and continued drainage.

3. **Surgical excision**

In patients in whom antibiotic therapy and attempts at drainage fail and those who have rupture of a TOA, laparotomy is indicated with excision of the abscess.

a. **Unilateral salpingo-oophorectomy**

If preservation of fertility is desired, conservative surgery with unilateral salpingo-oophorectomy is indicated.

b. **Total abdominal hysterectomy with bilateral salpingo-oophorectomy**

If preservation of fertility is not desired or if the severity of the infection makes conservative surgery ill-advised, total hysterectomy and bilateral salpingo-oophorectomy should be performed. In a patient with a ruptured TOA, the case is contaminated and consideration should be given to leaving the surgical incision open.

■ BACKGROUND AND DEFINITIONS

The adnexa comprise the fallopian tubes, ovaries, and round ligaments. Pelvic masses commonly arise from the adnexa and are referred to as **adnexal masses**. Pelvic masses can also arise from the uterus or from organs other than the reproductive organs, such as the bladder and the gastrointestinal tract. The differential diagnosis of an adnexal mass is vast and depends on the patient's age. Adnexal masses are uncommon in the premenarchal or postmenopausal patient, and when they are encountered an ovarian neoplasm should be suspected. In contrast, adnexal masses are commonly found in women in the reproductive age range because of the frequency of **functional or physiological cysts**. These cysts result from the process of ovulation and usually resolve spontaneously. A large variety of nonneoplastic and neoplastic ovarian masses, both benign and malignant, are found in women of all age groups. The most common pelvic masses not involving the adnexa are **leiomyomata**, or **fibroids**. Leiomyomata are benign tumors that originate from smooth muscle cells in the myometrium of the uterus. Approximately 10 to 25% of white women and 30 to 50% of black women have leiomyomata.

■ CLINICAL PRESENTATION

Pelvic pain
Abdominal pain
Abdominal distention
Dyspareunia
Vaginal bleeding
Urinary frequency
Gastrointestinal symptoms
   Nausea
   Dyspepsia
   Obstipation
   Painful bowel movements

■ PHONE CALL

Questions

1. **How much pain is the patient experiencing?**
   In patients with severe pain, torsion of an adnexal mass,

tubal pregnancy, hemorrhagic ovarian cyst, and tubo-ovarian abscess should be suspected.

2. What are the vital signs, and is the patient unstable?

A ruptured tubo-ovarian abscess or a ruptured tubal pregnancy with intra-abdominal bleeding should be suspected in the patient who is unstable and has a pelvic mass.

Degree of Urgency

In most cases, a pelvic mass is not life threatening. If the patient is in severe pain, has a positive pregnancy test, or is unstable, she should be seen immediately.

■ ELEVATOR THOUGHTS

What is the differential diagnosis of the pelvic mass?

Table 30–1 lists the differential diagnosis of the pelvic mass.

1. **Ovarian masses**
   a. **Functional or physiological cysts**
      (1) Follicular cysts
          Follicular cysts are the most common cystic masses

Table 30–1 □ **DIFFERENTIAL DIAGNOSIS OF THE PELVIC MASS**

Source	Ultrasound Characteristics	
	Cystic	*Solid or Complex*

Ovaries	Functional cyst
	Endometrioma
	Neoplasm
	  Benign
	  Malignant
		Neoplasm
		  Benign
		  Malignant

Fallopian tubes	Hydrosalpinx Tubo-ovarian abscess Pyosalpinx Paratubal cyst	Neoplasm Tubo-ovarian abscess Tubal pregnancy
Uterus		Intrauterine pregnancy Uterine anomaly Leiomyoma Adenomyosis Sarcoma
Bowel	Ileus	Appendiceal abscess Diverticular abscess Neoplasm Stool
Bladder and kidneys	Distended bladder	Pelvic kidney

found in the ovary. They result from either failure of the mature follicle to ovulate or failure of an immature follicle to resorb or undergo atresia. Most follicular cysts are asymptomatic and range in diameter from several millimeters to 8 cm.

(2) Corpus luteum cysts

Corpus luteum cysts are approximately 4 cm in diameter and result from hemorrhage into the corpus luteum 2 to 3 days after ovulation. Because these cysts may rupture and result in intra-abdominal bleeding, they can mimic tubal pregnancies. Rupture usually occurs late in the menstrual cycle and is associated with acute pain, which usually lasts less than 24 hours but may be present for up to 1 week.

(3) Theca-lutein cysts

Theca-lutein cysts develop from overstimulation of the ovaries by human chorionic gonadotropin (hCG). They are encountered in patients with molar pregnancies and in those who have undergone ovulation induction for infertility.

b. **Endometriomas**

Endometriomas can develop in patients with endometriosis involving the ovaries. These cysts are filled with old blood that has the appearance of chocolate, so endometriomas are also called "chocolate cysts."

c. **Ovarian neoplasms** (Table 30–2)

(1) Benign neoplasms

(2) Malignant neoplasms

2. **Tubal masses**

a. **Tubal pregnancy**

b. **Pyosalpinx**

c. **Hydrosalpinx**

d. **Tubo-ovarian abscess**

e. **Paratubal cyst**

Paratubal cysts are found adjacent to the fallopian tubes. They are predominantly cystic and are asymptomatic unless they undergo torsion. Paratubal cysts found at the fimbriated ends of the tube are also referred to as hydatid cysts of Morgagni.

3. **Uterine masses**

a. **Leiomyomata (fibroids)**

b. **Intrauterine pregnancy**

c. **Adenomyosis of the uterus**

d. **Uterine sarcoma**

e. **Congenital anomaly of the uterus**

(1) Bicornuate uterus

(2) Rudimentary uterine horn

(3) Didelphic uterus

Table 30-2 □ **HISTOGENETIC CLASSIFICATION OF OVARIAN NEOPLASMS**

Origin	Frequency (%)	Tumor Types
Celomic epithelium	75–80	Serous tumor Mucinous tumor Endometrioid tumor Clear cell or mesonephroid tumor Brenner tumor Carcinosarcoma or mixed mesodermal tumor Undifferentiated carcinoma

Germ cell	10–15	Teratoma
		  Mature teratoma
		    Solid adult teratoma
		    Dermoid cyst
		    Struma ovarii
		    Malignant neoplasm arising from mature cystic teratoma
		  Immature teratoma
		Dysgerminoma
		Embryonal carcinoma
		Endodermal sinus tumor
		Choriocarcinoma
		Gonadoblastoma

Specialized gonadal stroma	3–5	Granulosa–theca cell tumors
		  Granulosa cell tumor
		  Thecoma
		Sertoli-Leydig cell tumors
		  Arrhenoblastoma
		  Sertoli cell tumor
		Gynandroblastoma
		Lipid cell tumor

Nonspecific mesenchyme	≤1	Fibroma Hemangioma Leiomyoma Lipoma Lymphoma Sarcoma
Metastatic to ovary	4–8	Gastrointestinal tract (Krukenberg's tumor) Breast Uterine endometrium Lymphoma

4. Masses from the gastrointestinal tract
   a. Appendiceal abscess
   b. Diverticular abscess
   c. Stool or gas in the sigmoid colon
5. Masses from the kidneys and the urinary tract
   a. Distended bladder
   b. Pelvic kidney
6. Miscellanous masses
   a. Abdominal wall abscess, seroma, or hematoma
   b. Retroperitoneal neoplasm

What are potential complications associated with an adnexal mass?

1. **Torsion**

   An adnexal mass that is freely mobile on a pedicle can undergo spontaneous torsion. Torsion can be intermittent, resulting in crampy, colicky pain that is episodic. Torsion can also compromise the vascular supply and cause ischemic damage to the ovary or fallopian tube.

2. **Rupture of cyst**

   Rupture can result in resolution of the cyst. However, in certain cysts, rupture can lead to further complications such as intraperitoneal dissemination of disease with malignant ovarian cysts or chemical peritonitis with a dermoid cyst. Rupture of a tubo-ovarian abscess causes peritonitis and sepsis and is life threatening.

3. **Hemorrhage**

   Bleeding into a cyst results in distention of the cyst and increased pain. Rupture of the cyst and intraperitoneal bleeding severe enough to lead to hypovolemic shock can result. This is most commonly found in a ruptured hemorrhagic corpus luteum cyst. Bleeding from an adnexal mass may also be caused by a ruptured tubal pregnancy, as discussed in Chapter 26.

■ MAJOR THREAT TO LIFE

- Hypovolemic shock from rupture and hemorrhage of an adnexal mass
- Sepsis secondary to ruptured tubo-ovarian abscess
- Sepsis secondary to ruptured abdominal abscess from appendicitis or diverticulitis
- Ovarian malignancy

■ BEDSIDE

Quick Look Test

Does the patient appear to be severely ill?

Rupture of a tubal pregnancy, a hemorrhagic cyst, or a tubo-ovarian abscess should be suspected in a patient who appears to be severely ill with either severe pain or unstable vital signs.

Vital Signs

Vital signs are normal unless the patient is in shock from rupture of a tubal pregnancy, a hemorrhagic cyst, or a tubo-ovarian abscess. A patient in hypovolemic shock will be hypotensive and tachycardic and might have postural hypotension. Changes in blood pressure (BP) and pulse should be measured in the supine, sitting, and standing positions. A fall in systolic or diastolic BP >15 mm Hg or a rise in pulse >15 beats/min when the patient is assisted into the sitting or standing position from the supine position is evidence of hypovolemia.

Selective History and Chart Review

1. Does the patient have a history of a chronic pelvic mass?

   Chronic pelvic masses include leiomyomata, hydrosalpinges, and endometriomas.
2. Is the patient premenarchal or postmenopausal?

   Adnexal masses are more likely to be neoplastic in these patients, compared with women in the reproductive age group.
3. If the patient is of reproductive age, when was her last menstrual period?

   Women who have missed a menstrual period should have intrauterine and ectopic pregnancies ruled out.
4. Is the patient using oral contraceptive pills?

   Oral contraceptive pills suppress ovulation, and therefore functional cysts are less likely although not totally precluded in pill users. Women who use contraceptive pills are also less likely to have either an intrauterine or an ectopic pregnancy, although neither is totally excluded.
5. Does the patient have a history of pelvic inflammatory disease (PID)?

   The patient with a history of PID who has a pelvic mass should be suspected of having a pyosalpinx, a hydrosalpinx, or a tubo-ovarian abscess.
6. Does the patient have a history of pelvic endometriosis?

   An endometrioma should be suspected in these patients.
7. Does the patient have a history of weight loss and vague abdominal symptoms such as anorexia, dyspepsia, distention, nausea, and dull pain or discomfort?

   These symptoms can be caused by ovarian malignancy.
8. Does the patient have abnormal vaginal bleeding?

   Abnormal bleeding in a patient with a pelvic mass is

suggestive of intrauterine pregnancy, ectopic pregnancy, uterine leiomyoma, and uterine sarcoma.

Selective Physical Examination

Abdominal	Mass with or without tenderness may be palpable
	Distention from the mass or hemorrhage
	Ascites may be present in ovarian malignancy
Pelvic	
External genitalia and vagina	Vaginal bleeding in ectopic pregnancy, intrauterine pregnancy, uterine fibroids, or sarcoma
Cervix	Cervical motion tenderness may be present with PID or tubo-ovarian abscess
Uterus	Enlarged with or without tenderness in leiomyomata, sarcoma, or intrauterine pregnancy
Adnexa	Mass may be palpable, either unilateral or bilateral, with or without tenderness
	Fixed and nonmobile adnexa is suggestive of endometrioma, PID, or ovarian malignancy

Orders

1. Obtain a complete blood count (CBC) with differential.
2. Perform a urine pregnancy test for patients of reproductive age.
3. Start IV in the patient who appears severely ill.
4. Have the patient keep her bladder full for ultrasound examination.
5. Keep the patient NPO (nothing by mouth) if surgery is anticipated.

■ DIAGNOSTIC TESTING

1. Ultrasound examination

Ultrasound examination confirms the presence of a pelvic mass and furthermore provides information concerning the size, bilaterality, origin, and consistency of the mass, whether cystic, solid, or complex. Ultrasonography is the method of choice in the radiological evaluation of an ovarian mass. Table 30–3 lists characteristics detected on clinical examination and ultrasound examination that are suggestive of benign and malignant masses.

Table 30–3 □ CHARACTERISTICS OF BENIGN
AND MALIGNANT ADNEXAL MASSES

Benign	Malignant
Cystic	Solid or complex
Unilateral	Bilateral
Smooth	Irregular
No ascites present	Ascites present
Slow growth or no growth	Rapid growth
Mobile	Fixed

2. Computed tomography

A computed tomography (CT) scan can sometimes supplement the information obtained by ultrasound examination. CT scan of the pelvis should be performed with contrast to opacify and therefore delineate the bowel. A CT scan is especially helpful in the evaluation of masses in the pelvic side wall. A CT scan is also helpful in staging pelvic malignancies, detecting peritoneal implants, and delineating pelvic abscesses during drainage procedures.

3. Magnetic resonance imaging

Magnetic resonance imaging (MRI) provides soft-tissue contrast resolution that is superior to that obtained by ultrasound examination or CT. It is especially helpful in the assessment of conditions that result in uterine enlargement, such as congenital anomalies of the uterus, leiomyomata, and adenomyosis. MRI can provide information on the size, number, and location of leiomyomata.

4. Intravenous pyelogram

An intravenous pyelogram (IVP) provides information concerning the kidneys and the bladder. A pelvic kidney can be diagnosed by IVP. Furthermore, displacement of the pelvic ureters by a pelvic mass is usually revealed by IVP, and this information is critical in patients who are about to undergo surgery.

5. Complete blood count with differential

A CBC with differential should be obtained to help with the diagnosis of masses associated with PID, such as a pyosalpinx or tubo-ovarian abscess. It can also detect anemia in those patients with intraperitoneal bleeding from any source.

6. Rapid urine pregnancy test

A pregnancy test should be obtained in all patients of reproductive age to rule out either intrauterine or ectopic pregnancy.

7. Serum cancer antigen-125

Cancer antigen-125 (CA-125) is a tumor marker for ovarian epithelial cancers. Unfortunately, CA-125 is nonspecific and is also elevated in adenocarcinoma of the uterus and colon, endometriosis, PID, inflammatory bowel disease, pregnancy, and hepatitis.

8. **Serum human chorionic gonadotropin and alpha-fetoprotein**
   Serum hCG and alpha-fetoprotein (AFP) are tumor markers in germ cell tumors of the ovaries. These tumors make up almost 20% of all ovarian neoplasms, and most occur in young women.

■ MANAGEMENT OF THE ADNEXAL MASS

Management of patients with tubal pregnancy and tubo-ovarian abscess is discussed in Chapters 26 and 29, respectively. Management of ovarian masses and other adnexal masses depends on the age of the patient, the severity of pelvic pain, and the consistency of the mass as demonstrated by radiographic examination.

1. **Expectant management**
   Expectant management should be considered in patients in the reproductive age group with a painless cystic mass less than 8 cm in diameter. These cysts are likely to be functional or physiological, and most resolve spontaneously within 2 months. Patients who frequently develop symptomatic functional cysts can be prescribed oral contraceptive pills to decrease the frequency of cyst formation. However, if the patient has a functional cyst already, treatment with oral contraceptive pills will not result in earlier resolution.

2. **Surgical management**
   a. **Laparoscopy and laparotomy**
      Surgical intervention with laparoscopy or laparotomy should be considered in the following clinical situations:
      (1) Persistent mass in any age group
      (2) Solid or complex mass in any age group
      (3) Cystic mass greater than 3 cm in diameter in a postmenopausal or premenarchal patient
      (4) Mass associated with severe pain
      (5) Mass associated with significant and persistent intra-abdominal bleeding
      (6) Mass suspected of being malignant based on symptoms, physical findings, radiological findings, and serum tumor markers.

■ MANAGEMENT OF LEIOMYOMATA

The management of the patient with leiomyomata depends on the severity of symptoms such as bleeding and pain, the desire for fertility, and the size of the leiomyomata.

1. **Expectant management**

Expectant management should be used in asymptomatic patients with an overall uterine size of 12 weeks of gestation or less and slow growth. Expectant management should be attempted even if the patient desires fertility because leiomyomata of this size rarely jeopardize fertility or result in spontaneous losses. Conservative management can also be used in asymptomatic patients who have an overall uterine size of more than 12 weeks if there is slow growth and the patient is not very symptomatic.

2. **Medical management**

   a. **Gonadotropin-releasing hormone (GnRH) agonist**

   The administration of a GnRH agonist such as the following results in a hypoestrogenic state similar to that found in menopause: **leuprolide acetate (Lupron) 3.75 mg IM each month** or **leuprolide acetate for depot suspension (Lupron Depot) 11.25 mg IM every 3 months.** GnRH administration results in a median reduction in uterine size of 50%. Unfortunately, within 12 weeks after cessation of therapy, there is often rapid regrowth of the leiomyomata. Patients treated with GnRH agonist should be warned to expect hypoestrogenic symptoms such as hot flashes and atrophic vaginitis. Furthermore, the risk of osteoporosis from the hypoestrogenic state limits the duration of treatment to 3 to 6 months. For these reasons, GnRH is not considered to be a primary treatment method for leiomyomata. GnRH treatment is used for the following purposes:

   (1) To decrease the symptoms of leiomyomata, especially bleeding, while the patient is awaiting surgery

   (2) To decrease the size of the leiomyomata to allow for greater ease of surgery and less intraoperative blood loss

   (3) To decrease the size and symptoms of leiomyomata in the perimenopausal patient with the hope that when menopause is reached, this decrease in uterine size and symptoms will be permanent

3. **Angiographic embolization**

This technique has been used for many years to control intractable pelvic bleeding, and it has recently been applied to the treatment of fibroids. Short-term results appear promising, but there are no long-term results available yet. The advantages of this technique are that it is nonsurgical and that it preserves the uterus and fertility.

4. **Surgical management**

   a. **Myomectomy**

   The major advantage of myomectomy is the preservation of fertility. This procedure can be performed via laparotomy, hysteroscopy, or laparoscopy. Myomectomy should be considered in any patient who has symptomatic or enlarging leiomyomata and who also wants to preserve her uterus. Myomectomy is indicated especially in patients in whom the leiomyomata are believed to be a cause of infertility or recurrent pregnancy losses.

b. **Hysterectomy**

Hysterectomy is the definitive treatment of leiomyomata in the patient who does not desire to preserve her fertility. Indications for hysterectomy include the following:

(1) An asymptomatic leiomyoma that is large or is growing rapidly
(2) Excessive bleeding caused by the leiomyoma
(3) Pelvic or abdominal pain caused by the leiomyoma

■ BACKGROUND AND DEFINITIONS

Dysmenorrhea: Painful menstruation; the pain is located in the lower abdomen and is frequently described as a painful, crampy sensation. It is often accompanied by nausea, vomiting, headaches, swelling, sweating, fatigue, or lightheadedness. The symptoms typically appear at or just before the onset of menses and can persist for days. Fifty to 75% of women have dysmenorrhea, although only 10 to 15% have dysmenorrhea that is severe enough to require bedrest and that interferes with routine daily life.

> **Primary dysmenorrhea:** Applies to women with no obvious pathological condition

> **Secondary dysmenorrhea:** Applies to women with pathological conditions that cause dysmenorrhea

Dyspareunia: Painful intercourse

Dyschezia: Painful bowel movements

Endometriosis: The presence and growth of endometrial glands and stroma in locations outside the endometrial cavity of the uterus. Endometriosis most often involves the ovaries, the cul-de-sac, the uterosacral ligaments, the rectosigmoid, and the posterior cervix. The classic symptoms of endometriosis include dysmenorrhea, dyspareunia, dyschezia, and infertility. The incidence of endometriosis in women of reproductive age is 10 to 15% and increases to 30 to 45% among women with infertility.

Adenomyosis: The presence and growth of endometrial glands and stroma in the uterine myometrium at a depth of ≥2.5 mm from the basal layer of the endometrium. The classic symptoms of adenomyosis include dysmenorrhea and menorrhagia, although some patients are asymptomatic. It is usually found in women 35 to 50 years old, and it has an incidence as high as 60% in that age group.

Pelvic congestion syndrome: Syndrome caused by pelvic varicosities that result in pelvic pain or heaviness that is worse during the premenstrual period, after prolonged standing, and after intercourse

Chronic pelvic pain: Pain that has remained unchanged in character and location for >6 months. Chronic pelvic pain may be difficult to evaluate and treat because the symptoms may be vague. Furthermore, there may be a significant psychogenic component to chronic pelvic pain even if an actual pathophysiological event initiated the pain before it became chronic. Pain that is acute is usually easier to evaluate and is more often associated with a pathophysiological event or condition.

■ CLINICAL PRESENTATION

Sharp, dull, colicky, crampy, or pressure-like pain
Localized or general pain
Pain with menses or ovulation
Associated symptoms
  Vaginal bleeding
  Gastrointestinal symptoms
    Nausea
    Vomiting
    Obstipation
    Dyschezia
    Anorexia
  Abdominal distention
  Fever
  Back pain
  Urinary symptoms such as frequency, urgency, and dysuria

■ PHONE CALL

Questions

1. **What are the patient's vital signs?**
2. **Is the patient having vaginal bleeding?**
      In patients of reproductive age who present with pain and vaginal bleeding a tubal pregnancy or spontaneous abortion should be suspected.

Degree of Urgency

Unless associated with a ruptured tubo-ovarian abscess, a ruptured tubal pregnancy, or intraperitoneal bleeding from a hemorrhagic cyst, pelvic pain is usually not life threatening. However, patients with significant pelvic pain or unstable vital signs should be seen immediately.

■ ELEVATOR THOUGHTS

What are causes of pelvic pain?
- Pelvic mass (see Chapter 30)
    Functional cyst of the ovary
    Ovarian neoplasm, benign or malignant

- Paratubal cyst
- Adnexal mass
- Ovarian remnant syndrome
- Endometriosis
- Adenomyosis
- Pelvic inflammatory disease (PID) (see Chapter 29)
    - Uncomplicated salpingitis
    - Pyosalpinx
    - Tubo-ovarian abscess
- Endometritis
- Cervicitis
- Uterine leiomyomata
- Pelvic adhesions
    - Prior pelvic surgery
    - Prior PID
- Tubal pregnancy (see Chapter 26)
- Spontaneous abortion (see Chapter 33)
- Pelvic congestion syndrome
- Dysmenorrhea
    - Primary
    - Secondary
- Pelvic organ prolapse
- Urological disorder
    - Urinary tract infection
    - Interstitial cystitis
    - Urethral syndrome
    - Renal or ureteral calculus
- Gastrointestinal disorder
    - Appendicitis
    - Diverticulitis
    - Cholelithiasis
    - Constipation
    - Gastric or duodenal ulcer
    - Inflammatory bowel disease
    - Irritable bowel syndrome
    - Bowel obstruction
    - Bowel neoplasm, benign or malignant
- Musculoskeletal disorder
    - Disk disease
    - Hernia
    - Low back pain
    - Nerve entrapment syndrome
    - Osteoporosis
    - Congenital abnormality of the spine
- Psychogenic disorder
    - Depression
    - Psychological stress

- Miscellaneous
  Sickle cell disease
  Porphyria
  Cocaine abuse

■ MAJOR THREAT TO LIFE

- Hypovolemic shock
  Ruptured tubal pregnancy
  Intra-abdominal bleeding from hemorrhagic ovarian cyst
- Sepsis from ruptured tubo-ovarian abscess

■ BEDSIDE

Quick Look Test

Does the patient appear to be unstable or in severe pain?
If the patient is unstable and in severe pain, a ruptured tubo-ovarian abscess, intra-abdominal bleeding from a ruptured tubal pregnancy, or a hemorrhagic ovarian cyst should be suspected.

Vital Signs

Vital signs are usually normal unless the patient has had significant bleeding or is in septic shock. This patient may be hypotensive, may be tachycardic, and may have postural hypotension. Changes in blood pressure (BP) and pulse should be measured when the patient is in the supine, sitting, and standing positions. A fall in systolic or diastolic BP >15 mm Hg or a rise in pulse >15 beats/min when the patient is assisted in sitting or standing from a supine position is evidence of hypovolemia. A patient with a fever should be suspected of having an infectious process such as PID, appendicitis, or diverticulitis.

Selective History and Chart Review

1. What is the quality, intensity, and location of the pain?
2. How long has the pain been present, and has any prior workup been performed?
3. When was the patient's last menstrual period?
   If the patient has missed a menstrual period, either intrauterine or ectopic pregnancy should be suspected.
4. What is the relationship between the pain and the menstrual cycle?
   Pain that is correlated with menses is suggestive of endometriosis, adenomyosis, or primary dysmenorrhea.

5. Is the pain exacerbated by intercourse, bowel movements, urination, or increased physical activity?

Pain that is worse with intercourse and bowel movements is suggestive of endometriosis, adhesions, or pelvic mass.

6. Is the pain associated with abnormal vaginal bleeding?

Pain associated with vaginal bleeding is suggestive of leiomyomata or adenomyosis. If the patient is pregnant, tubal pregnancy or spontaneous abortion should be ruled out.

7. Is there a history of PID?

Pelvic adhesions or hydrosalpinx can result from PID. Approximately 20% of patients with a history of PID have chronic pelvic pain.

8. Is there a history of infertility?

A history of infertility is consistent with endometriosis or pelvic adhesions from prior PID.

9. Has the patient had pelvic or abdominal surgery?

Previous surgery can result in pelvic pain from pelvic adhesions.

10. Is there a history of gastrointestinal or urological disease?

Selective Physical Examination

Abdominal	Tenderness to palpation
	Mass may be palpable
	Guarding may be present
	Rebound tenderness is suggestive of peritonitis
Pelvic	
External genitalia and vagina	Usually normal unless there is bleeding
Cervix	Tender to cervical motion and the presence of a purulent discharge, suggestive of PID
	Bleeding from the cervix in tubal pregnancy and spontaneous abortion
	Dilated with or without tissue protruding in spontaneous abortion
Uterus	Enlarged and irregular in patients with leiomyomata
	Uniformly enlarged and globular, tender around the time of menses in patients with adenomyosis
	Uterus often retroverted and fixed, with tenderness and scarring posterior to the uterus in patients with endometriosis. Tender nodularity of the utero-

	sacral ligaments is often palpable on rectovaginal examination.
	Tenderness in the parametrial area and pain on elevation of the uterus are suggestive of pelvic congestion syndrome.
Adnexa	Tender to palpation
	Mass may be palpable

Orders

1. Obtain a complete blood count (CBC) with differential.
2. Obtain an erythrocyte sedimentation rate.
3. Perform a rapid urine pregnancy test if the patient is of reproductive age.
4. Obtain a urinalysis.
5. Start an IV if the patient appears to be severely ill or the vital signs are unstable.
6. Keep the patient NPO (nothing by mouth) if surgery is anticipated.

■ DIAGNOSTIC TESTING

1. **Complete blood count with differential**

   A CBC with differential helps diagnose infection. Severe anemia is suggestive of bleeding from a ruptured tubal pregnancy or from a hemorrhagic ovarian cyst.
2. **Urinalysis**
3. **Urine pregnancy test**
4. **Ultrasound examination**

   Ultrasound examination detects pelvic masses such as uterine leiomyomata and adnexal masses as well as abdominal masses. Ultrasonography does not detect pelvic adhesions or pelvic endometriosis.
5. **Computed tomography**

   A computed tomography (CT) scan may provide additional information or clarify the ultrasound examination. Contrast enhancement should be used to opacify and identify the bowel. A CT scan is helpful in the evaluation of masses in the pelvic side wall. A CT scan can also detect pelvic abscesses and peritoneal implants and aid in staging pelvic malignancies.
6. **Magnetic resonance imaging**

   Magnetic resonance imaging (MRI) provides greater soft-tissue contrast resolution than either ultrasound examination or CT scan. Therefore, MRI is helpful in the diagnosis of conditions that cause pelvic pain and uterine enlargement, such as leiomyomata and adenomyosis. MRI can detect the size, number, and location of leiomyomata.

7. **Intravenous pyelogram**

An intravenous pyelogram (IVP) is helpful in evaluating the kidneys and the urinary tract. An IVP diagnoses pelvic kidneys.

■ MANAGEMENT

Management of pelvic pain depends on the severity and duration of the pain and on the physical, laboratory, and radiographic findings. Patients who have no physical, laboratory, or radiographic findings and who complain of only mild pain with recent onset should be followed conservatively. Patients with severe pain, pain of prolonged duration, or suspected pelvic pathology may require surgical intervention for diagnosis and possible treatment.

1. **Conservative management**
   a. **Nonsteroidal anti-inflammatory agents**
      (1) **Ibuprofen (Motrin, Nuprin, Advil) 600 to 800 mg three to four times per day with a maximum dosage of 3200 mg/day**
      (2) **Naproxen (Naprosyn, Anaprox) 500 mg two times per day with a maximum dosage of 1000 mg/day**
      Nonsteroidal anti-inflammatory agents are especially helpful in patients with primary or secondary dysmenorrhea.
   b. **Oral analgesics**
      (1) Low to intermediate potency
         (a) **Propoxyphene (Darvon) 65 mg PO every 3 to 4 hours**
         (b) **Acetaminophen with codeine (Tylenol with Codeine) 1 tablet PO every 4 hours**
         (c) **Hydrocodone (Vicodin) 1 to 2 tablets PO every 4 to 6 hours**
         (d) **Oxycodone (Percodan, Percocet) 1 tablet PO every 6 hours**
      (2) High potency
         (a) **Hydromorphine (Dilaudid) 2 to 4 mg PO every 4 to 6 hours or 1 to 2 mg IM every 4 to 6 hours**
         (b) **Meperidine hydrochloride (Demerol) 50 to 150 mg PO every 3 to 4 hours or 50 to 100 mg IM or SC every 4 hours**
         (c) **Morphine sulfate 10 to 30 mg PO every 4 hours or 5 to 20 mg IM every 4 hours or 2.5 to 15 mg IV every 4 hours**
   c. **Oral contraceptive pills**
      These are helpful in treating patients with dysmenorrhea and endometriosis and also suppress the formation of functional ovarian cysts by inhibiting ovulation.
   d. **Gonadotropin-releasing factor (GnRH) agonist**
      Administration of GnRH agonist results in the suppres-

sion of ovulation and in the establishment of a hypoestrogenic state similar to that found in menopause. GnRH agonist can be used in patients with pelvic pain secondary to endometriosis, adenomyosis, and uterine leiomyomata. Because ovulation is suppressed, the formation of functional ovarian cysts is also suppressed. Patients receiving GnRH agonist should be cautioned to expect hypoestrogenic symptoms such as hot flashes and atrophic vaginitis. Furthermore, the risk of osteoporosis from the hypoestrogenic state limits the duration of treatment to 3 to 6 months.

(1) **Leuprolide acetate (Lupron) 3.75 mg IM each month**
(2) **Nafarelin acetate (Synarel) 200-μg intranasal spray two times per day** (patients who do not achieve amenorrhea can be placed on 400 μg two times per day)

2. Surgical management

a. Laparoscopy

Laparoscopy is the definitive diagnostic test for evaluating patients with pelvic pain. In addition to providing a diagnosis, laparoscopy often allows certain therapeutic procedures to be performed, such as lysis of adhesions, cauterization or laser vaporization of endometrial implants, excision of ovarian or paratubal cysts, salpingostomy for removal of a tubal pregnancy, and even salpingo-oophorectomy. In patients with chronic pelvic pain, laparoscopy reveals no significant abnormalities in approximately 30% of cases.

b. Laparotomy

Laparotomy is indicated when the degree of pathology makes surgical treatment by laparoscopy unsafe or technically difficult. Hysterectomy for a large, fibroid uterus or excision of a large ovarian mass is usually performed by laparotomy. Patients with severe pelvic adhesions secondary to endometriosis or PID are often appropriate candidates for laparotomy. Laparotomy is indicated for patients with pelvic malignancies. Laparotomy is also indicated for patients with severe endometriosis.

3. Psychological evaluation and counseling

Patients with chronic pelvic pain and a negative workup after extensive diagnostic testing and diagnostic laparoscopy may benefit from psychological evaluation and counseling. A positive correlation has been found between a history of sexual abuse and chronic pelvic pain. Management of such patients is often most effective if it is provided by a multidisciplinary team comprising a gynecologist, a psychiatrist or psychologist, and an anesthesiologist who specializes in pain management.

4. Referral to urologist and/or gastroenterologist

If nongynecological causes of pelvic pain such as interstitial cystitis or irritable bowel syndrome are suspected, the patient should be referred to the appropriate specialist.

■ BACKGROUND AND DEFINITIONS

Sexual assault: Also referred to as **rape,** sexual assault is defined as any sexual act performed by one person on another without consent and performed with force, the threat of force on the victim or another person, or the inability of the victim to give appropriate consent. Sexual assault accounts for approximately 6% of all violent crimes. It has been determined that as many as 44% of women have been victims of sexual assault or attempted sexual assault, and half of these women have been sexually assaulted more than once. Furthermore, sexual assault is one of the most underreported crimes, and it has been estimated that 40 to 90% of cases go unreported. Fewer than 20% of rape victims seek medical attention, and only a minority present immediately after the assault. Women of all ages, ethnic origins, and socioeconomic classes can be victims of sexual assault. Very young women, very old women, and women with mental or physical handicaps are especially vulnerable. Almost 75% of victims know the assailant. Most cases involve persons of the same race.

Spousal rape: Sexual assault that occurs in a marriage

Date rape or acquaintance rape: Sexual assault that occurs during a date. Date rape is not usually reported, because the victim feels that she is partially responsible for the assault or even that she encouraged it. Rohypnol, also referred to as the "date rape drug," has been used on victims to diminish their ability to resist assault.

Statutory rape: Sexual intercourse with a female younger than a certain age, as specified by the laws of a particular state, regardless of whether consent is given

■ CLINICAL PRESENTATION

The clinical presentation of the victim of rape is highly variable. The patient may appear calm and in control, or she may appear with the complete loss of emotional control. She may appear to have depression, anxiety, or lability of mood. She may present with generalized complaints such as vague aches and pains, insomnia, and eating disturbances or with specific complaints referable to the genital area such as vaginal or rectal pain, itching, and discharge. The extent and severity of trauma are highly variable. Furthermore, injuries are often nongenital.

■ PHONE CALL

Questions

1. **How severe are the patient's physical injuries?**
2. **When did the alleged assault occur?**
   The amount of time that has passed between the alleged assault and patient's presentation determines how successful the effort to recover evidence for legal purposes will be and also determines the appropriate tests to obtain to screen for sexually transmitted diseases.

Degree of Urgency

The patient should be seen as soon as possible. If she has sustained severe physical trauma, she should be seen immediately.

■ ELEVATOR THOUGHTS

What are the components of the "rape trauma" syndrome?

The **rape trauma syndrome** described by Burgess and Holmstrom (Burgess AW, Holmstrom LL: Rape trauma syndrome. Am J Psychiatry 1974;131:981) is divided into two phases.

- **Disorganization or acute phase:** Lasts several days to many weeks and is composed of the following:
  - Fear of injury or death
  - Fear of being assaulted again
  - Humiliation and embarrassment
  - Guilt
  - Depression
  - Anger
  - Irritability
  - Difficulties in concentration
  - Anxiety
  - Thoughts of revenge
  - Generalized pain
  - Eating and sleeping disturbances
  - Vaginal pain, discharge, or itching
  - Rectal pain
- **Reorganization or delayed phase:** Lasts several months to years and is composed of the following:
  - Sexual aversion
  - Inability to attain orgasm
  - Vaginismus
  - Flashbacks
  - Nightmares
  - Insomnia

Paranoia
Phobias toward men and sex
Nonspecific gynecological and menstrual complaints

What are common misconceptions of rape?
- Rape is a crime of passion and the assailant is usually over-sexed or sexually frustrated.

  Rape is not a crime of passion but rather an act of violence in which the assailant wants to abuse, degrade, and control the victim.
- Rape is an indication of the victim's promiscuity.

  Rape victims are not more promiscuous than nonvictims. Furthermore, promiscuity does not justify rape.
- Certain victims deserve to be sexually assaulted because of their behavior, their manner of dress, or their state of intoxication.

  No one deserves to be raped, regardless of the circumstances. Victims do not encourage sexual assault.
- Women are raped because they do not resist sufficiently.

■ MAJOR THREAT TO LIFE

- Physical trauma

  As many as 40% of rape victims also suffer nongenital trauma. Approximately 1% require hospitalization for the trauma, and 0.1% have fatal injuries.

■ BEDSIDE

Quick Look Test

Does the patient appear to have sustained severe physical trauma?

What is the patient's state of mind?
One of the key aspects of sexual assault is that the victim has lost control to the assailant. One of the critical goals of health care providers is to restore control to the patient. This requires allowing the patient and her state of mind to dictate the pace of the history taking and the performance of the physical examination.

Vital Signs

Vital signs are usually normal. If signs of hypovolemic shock such as hypotension and tachycardia are present, intra-abdominal hemorrhaging secondary to trauma should be suspected.

Selective History and Chart Review

1. What was the time and the date of the assault?
2. What was the number of assailants?
3. What was the nature of the assault, and what acts were committed?
4. Did ejaculation occur? If so, where did it occur?
5. Was there any nongenital trauma?
6. Was there oral, vaginal, or rectal penetration?
7. Were any foreign objects used in the assault?
8. Has the patient already bathed or cleansed herself, changed her clothes, or brushed her teeth?
9. Does the patient have any pre-existing gynecological or medical conditions?
10. When was the patient's last menstrual period?
11. Is the patient using contraception?
12. When was the patient's last consensual intercourse?

Selective Physical Examination

General	Cuts, bruises, abrasions, and bite marks may be signs of extragenital trauma
Abdominal	Distention and tenderness are suggestive of intra-abdominal bleeding secondary to trauma
Pelvic	
External genitalia and vagina	Edema, erythema, and lacerations may be present in the areas of the urethra, vulva, rectum, or vagina
	Deep lacerations in the vagina and into the abdominal cavity may be present, especially if foreign objects were used in the assault
Cervix	Lacerations may be present from foreign objects
Uterus and adnexa	Usually normal, unless there is extensive trauma due to the use of foreign objects resulting in uterine laceration and broad ligament hematomas

Orders

1. Provide the patient with a private examination room.
2. Notify the appropriate social service worker or experts trained specifically to work with rape victims.
3. Notify the police of the alleged assault.
4. Obtain a urine pregnancy test to rule out pre-existing pregnancy.

5. Keep the patient from washing, to preserve evidence.

If the patient has suffered severe physical trauma, the following orders should be given:

1. Start a large-bore IV.
2. Type and crossmatch for 2 units of blood.
3. Obtain a complete blood count (CBC).
4. Obtain coagulation studies: platelet count, prothrombin time (PT), partial thromboplastin time (PTT), fibrinogen, and fibrin split products.
5. Obtain a chemistry panel.
6. Place a urethral catheter and obtain a urine specimen for urinalysis.
7. Keep the patient NPO (nothing by mouth) if surgery is anticipated.

■ DIAGNOSTIC TESTING

1. **Rapid urine pregnancy test**

   Pre-existing pregnancy should be ruled out. The pregnancy test should be repeated in 2 to 3 weeks if pregnancy is suspected.

2. **Testing for *Chlamydia trachomatis* (see Chapter 27)**

   Chlamydia is the sexually transmitted disease most likely to be acquired from sexual assault. Although culturing is the most sensitive test for chlamydia, it is expensive, time consuming, and not always available. Therefore, testing for chlamydia can be done by rapid antigen detection tests such as Chlamydiazyme or MicroTrak. Specimens should be obtained from any site of penetration or attempted penetration. Testing should be repeated in 2 to 3 weeks and again in 12 weeks.

3. **Cultures for *Neisseria gonorrhoeae* (see Chapter 27)**

   A rape victim's risk of acquiring gonorrhea is 6 to 12%. Obtain specimens from any site of penetration or attempted penetration. Cultures should be repeated in 2 to 3 weeks and again in 12 weeks.

4. **Vaginal smear for *Trichomonas vaginalis* (see Chapter 36)**

   A vaginal wet smear with normal saline should be performed to rule out *T. vaginalis*. The diagnosis of this sexually transmitted infection is easily made because of the finding of the motile *Trichomonas* protozoans. The organism has an ovoid body and a visible posterior flagellum, and it is usually found moving in circles in a jerky fashion. The vaginal smear should be repeated in 2 to 3 weeks and again in 12 weeks.

5. **Venereal Disease Research Laboratory (VDRL) test**

   Baseline serology results for syphilis should be obtained. The risk of acquiring syphilis from a sexual assault is estimated to be as high as 3%. Serology studies should be repeated in 2 to 3 weeks and again in 12 weeks.

6. **Serology for human immunodeficiency virus**

The risk of acquiring human immunodeficiency virus (HIV) from sexual assault is unknown. Baseline serology studies should be performed and repeated in 2 to 3 weeks and again in 6 months.

7. **Serology for herpes simplex virus**

Baseline serology results should be considered, and serology studies should be repeated in 2 to 3 weeks and again in 12 weeks.

8. **Serology for hepatitis B**

Baseline serology results should be considered, and serology studies should be repeated in 2 to 3 weeks and again in 12 weeks. Follow-up serology testing is not needed if hepatitis B virus vaccine was administered.

9. **Serology for cytomegalovirus**

Baseline serology results should be considered, and serology studies should be repeated in 2 to 3 weeks and again in 12 weeks.

■ MANAGEMENT

When the patient is a victim of sexual assault, the physician's responsibility is threefold: medical evaluation and treatment, documentation of injuries and collection of evidence for medical-legal reasons, and emotional support.

1. **Medical evaluation and treatment**
   a. **Examine thoroughly for injuries and treat injuries**
   b. **Screen for and treat sexually transmitted infections**
      These infections may not be detectable immediately. Nevertheless, baseline cultures and serology results should be obtained initially and repeated in 2 to 3 weeks and again in 12 weeks. Serology studies for HIV should be repeated in 3 to 6 months. Human papillomavirus (HPV) infection can be detected by the finding of genital warts or condylomata acuminata, by DNA hybridization testing, or by cytological smear of the cervix, which can show cellular changes suggestive of HPV infection.
   c. **Prophylactic antibiotics**
      An antibiotic regimen that covers the prevention of gonorrhea, chlamydia, and syphilis should be used.
      (1) **Ceftriaxone 125 mg IM** plus
      (2) **Metronidazole 2 g PO in a single dose** plus
      (3) **Doxycycline 100 mg PO two times per day for 7 days**
         In pregnant patients, doxycycline should be replaced

with **erythromycin 500 mg PO four times per day for 7 days.**

d. **Prevention of pregnancy**

In a victim not using contraception, the risk of pregnancy from a sexual assault is 2 to 4%. If it is possible that pregnancy may result from the sexual assault, pregnancy prevention should be offered with the "morning after" prophylaxis. A pregnancy test should be performed before treatment, to determine whether the victim is already pregnant.

(1) **50-μg or "medium-dose" combination birth control pill: 2 pills initially and repeated in 12 hours** or

(2) **30- to 35-μg or "low-dose" combination birth control pill: 4 pills initially and repeated in 12 hours** or

(3) **5 mg ethinyl estradiol PO every day for 5 days** or

(4) **20 to 30 mg conjugated estrogen PO every day for 5 days**

e. **Hepatitis B virus vaccination**

Hepatitis B immune globulin (0.06 ml/kg) IM and hepatitis B vaccine should be administered. Two more vaccinations for hepatitis B should be given, at 1 month and 6 months after the attack.

2. **Documentation of injuries and collection of evidence for medical-legal reasons**

a. **Obtain and record a detailed history.**

b. **Document and describe in detail all injuries.**

The terms "sexual assault" and "rape" are legal terms and therefore should not be used in the physician's diagnosis. Instead, the phase **"consistent with the use of force"** should be used. Drawings of injuries often provide additional information to the written description.

c. **Collect the patient's clothing if she did not change her clothing.**

d. **Collect fingernail scrapings.**

e. **Collect hair samples by combing the pubic hair.**

f. **Collect vaginal, rectal, and pharyngeal secretions for analysis for sperm or acid phosphatase.**

After ejaculation, motile sperm may be found in the vagina for up to 8 hours and in cervical mucus for up to 2 to 3 days. Nonmotile sperm may be detected in the vagina for up to 24 hours and in cervical mucus for up to 17 days. Acid phosphatase from seminal fluid can be detected in the vagina and in cervical mucus for up to 48 hours. Acid phosphatase should always be measured, because the assailant may have had a vasectomy.

3. **Emotional support**

a. **The physician should educate the patient concerning not** only what to expect from a medical standpoint but also what to expect in psychological and emotional recovery.

She should be reassured that she will recover from her physical injuries and that it is unlikely that reproductive function has been jeopardized by the assault.

b. **The patient should be allowed to express her anxieties and to ask questions concerning her injuries and her recovery.**

c. **Misconceptions should be corrected.**

Specifically, it should be emphasized that the patient is not to be blamed and that she did not deserve to be sexually assaulted.

d. **Experts who are trained specifically to work with victims of rape should be consulted to facilitate counseling and ongoing support.**

e. **A follow-up evaluation should be planned to reevaluate the patient's emotional state.**

Follow-up should be planned even if the patient initially appears to be calm and well controlled. This initial appearance is often just a defense mechanism and should not be interpreted as a sign that the patient does not need any emotional support.

■ BACKGROUND AND DEFINITIONS

Spontaneous abortion: The spontaneous loss of a pregnancy before 20 weeks of gestation, also referred to as "**miscarriage**" in lay terminology. This condition can be more accurately defined by the following terms, which describe the clinical findings:

Threatened abortion: Vaginal bleeding alone

Inevitable abortion: Vaginal bleeding plus cervical dilatation

Incomplete abortion: Spontaneous passage of some but not all fetal tissue

Completed abortion: Spontaneous passage of all fetal tissue

Blighted ovum: Ultrasonographic absence of a fetus within a normal gestational sac after 6 weeks of gestation; also referred to as anembryonic gestation

Missed abortion: Ultrasonographic absence of fetal cardiac activity after 7 weeks of gestation, without bleeding or passage of tissue

Septic abortion: Any clinical presentation of spontaneous abortion associated with clinical signs of infection

Habitual or recurrent abortion: History of three or more spontaneous abortions

Between 50 and 75% of pregnancies end in spontaneous abortion. A majority of these losses are not recognized because they occur before a missed period and therefore before pregnancy has been detected. Approximately 15 to 20% of diagnosed pregnancies undergo spontaneous abortion. Approximately one-third of pregnancy losses occurring before 8 weeks of gestation are due to a blighted ovum. Older women have higher incidences of spontaneous abortion than younger women. In approximately 50 to 60% of first-trimester and 30% of second-trimester spontaneous abortions, a fetal chromosomal abnormality is found. The distribution of chromosomal abnormalities found in aborted fetal tissue is as follows: 50% autosomal trisomy, 25% triploidy, 20% monosomy X (Turner's syndrome), and 5% translocation.

■ CLINICAL PRESENTATION

Vaginal bleeding
Uterine cramping
Passage of tissue through the vagina

■ PHONE CALL

Questions

1. **How heavy is the patient's vaginal bleeding?**
2. **What are the patient's vital signs?**
     Women undergoing spontaneous abortion can have bleeding significant enough to result in hypotension, tachycardia, and even shock. A fever is suggestive of septic abortion.
3. **Has the patient saved any tissue passed from the vagina?**

Degree of Urgency

Spontaneous abortion is usually not life threatening. However, a patient who is bleeding heavily, complaining of severe pelvic pain, or exhibiting signs or symptoms of shock should be seen immediately.

■ ELEVATOR THOUGHTS

What are some of the known causes of spontaneous abortion?
- Chromosomal abnormalities
- Infection
     Infections with *Treponema pallidum, Borrelia burgdorferi, Chlamydia trachomatis, Neisseria gonorrhoeae, Streptococcus agalactiae,* and *Listeria monocytogenes* have been associated with spontaneous abortion.
- Drugs
     Chemotherapeutic drugs such as aminopterin and methotrexate have been associated with spontaneous abortion. Other agents that have been associated with spontaneous abortion include certain anesthetic gases, heavy metals, and oral hypoglycemic agents. Alcohol intake, smoking, and caffeine use have also been implicated. However, for most of these agents, a causal relationship has not been definitely established.

What are other causes of vaginal bleeding in early pregnancy?
- Ectopic pregnancy
- Cervical polyps and other cervical lesions
- Friable cervix
- Incompetent cervix
- Vaginal lesion
- Molar pregnancy

What are possible causes of recurrent abortion?
- Anomalies of the reproductive tract

Structural anomalies of the uterus are especially common causes, accounting for up to 15% of recurrent abortions.
- Uterine fibroids
- Antiphospholipid syndrome
  Circulating antiphospholipid antibodies can cause recurrent abortion, thrombosis, and/or thrombocytopenia.
- Chromosomal abnormalities of the parents
- Luteal phase defect
  Low corpus luteum progesterone might cause recurrent losses.
- Infection
  Ureaplasma urealyticum infection of the endometrium and certain systemic viral infections might cause recurrent abortion.

■ MAJOR THREAT TO LIFE

- Hypovolemic shock
  Patients with spontaneous abortion and molar pregnancy can have vaginal bleeding significant enough to result in hypovolemic shock. In patients who exhibit signs and symptoms of shock without heavy vaginal bleeding, the diagnosis of tubal pregnancy with intraperitoneal bleeding should be considered.

■ BEDSIDE

Quick Look Test

Does the patient appear to be in shock?

Is the patient in significant pain?
  The presence of crampy, midline pain is consistent with uterine cramping associated with a spontaneous abortion. Unilateral pain would be suggestive of a tubal pregnancy.

Vital Signs

Patients may be mildly hypertensive and tachycardic because of pelvic pain from uterine cramping. Patients who have had significant vaginal bleeding will usually be hypotensive and tachycardic. Postural hypotension might be revealed by the finding of changes in blood pressure (BP) and pulse when the patient is assisted in sitting or standing from a supine position. A fall in systolic or diastolic BP >15 mm Hg or a rise in pulse >15 beats/min is evidence of hypovolemia.

Selective History and Chart Review

1. Has the patient had a positive pregnancy test?
2. When was the patient's last menstrual period?
3. Has the patient had a prior pelvic ultrasound examination confirming an intrauterine pregnancy, and what is the current gestational age of the fetus based on those fetal measurements?
4. How long has the patient been bleeding, and how severe has the vaginal bleeding been?
5. Has the patient passed any tissue through the vagina?
6. Does the patient have any risk factors for tubal pregnancy?
7. Does the patient have an intrauterine device (IUD)?

    In patients who are pregnant and bleeding and also have an IUD, the diagnosis of tubal pregnancy should be suspected because the IUD is more effective in preventing intrauterine pregnancies than ectopic pregnancies.

Selective Physical Examination

Abdominal	Mildly tender and soft; the uterus is usually not palpable on abdominal examination in a pregnancy of less than 12 weeks' gestation. At 16 weeks, the uterus is usually halfway between the pubic symphysis and umbilicus, and at 20 weeks, it is usually palpable at the level of the umbilicus.
Pelvic	
External genitalia and vagina	Blood-stained with or without tissue in the vagina
Cervix	Threatened abortion: bleeding without cervical dilatation
	Inevitable abortion: bleeding with cervical dilatation
	Incomplete abortion: bleeding with cervical dilatation and tissue present at the cervical os
	Missed abortion: normal cervix without bleeding
	Completed abortion: small amount of bleeding with closed cervical os
Uterus	Tender and enlarged
Adnexa	Adnexal mass and tenderness suggests a tubal pregnancy.

Orders

1. Perform a urine pregnancy test to confirm the diagnosis of pregnancy.
2. Obtain a complete blood count (CBC).
3. Test for blood type and Rh factor.
4. Start an IV if the patient is having heavy bleeding or if vital signs suggest significant blood loss.
5. Crossmatch blood if the bleeding is severe or if the patient is unstable.
6. If the patient passes tissue from the vagina, it should be collected and sent in a specimen bottle with formaldehyde solution for pathological evaluation.

■ DIAGNOSTIC TESTING

1. **Rapid qualitative urine or serum pregnancy test**

   A rapid urine pregnancy test can be helpful in all patients with suspected spontaneous abortion. Enzyme-linked immunosorbent assay pregnancy tests such as Icon, Quest, and Confidot are simple and quick tests that can be performed on both urine and blood. These tests can detect levels of beta subunit of human chorionic gonadotropin (hCG) as low as 20 mIU/ml. In a normal intrauterine pregnancy, serum hCG is approximately 100 mIU/ml at a gestational age of 4 weeks. Therefore, with these tests, a pregnancy can be diagnosed even before a menstrual period is missed. The test can remain positive for up to 1 month after spontaneous abortion. A negative test rules out an ongoing pregnancy or a recent spontaneous abortion.

2. **Pelvic ultrasound examination**

   Ultrasonographic findings in spontaneous abortion can include any of the following:

   a. **Fetus with absence of fetal cardiac activity**
   b. **Collapsed gestational sac with or without a fetus**
   c. **Empty gestational sac**

      The absence of a fetus in a gestational sac with a diameter of ≥3.0 cm is highly suggestive of a spontaneous abortion.

   d. **Absent gestational sac**

      An "endometrial stripe" is a bright longitudinal line found on ultrasound examination of the uterine cavity. The stripe results from approximation of the anterior and the posterior endometrial surfaces and is ultrasonographic evidence of an empty uterine cavity.

   Ultrasonographic milestones have been established for normal first-trimester pregnancies (Table 33–1). By transabdominal ultrasound examination, the gestational sac and yolk

Table 33–1 □ ULTRASONOGRAPHIC MILESTONES
IN NORMAL FIRST-TRIMESTER PREGNANCY

| | Gestational Age at Detection (weeks) | |
Ultrasonographic Finding	Transabdominal Examination	Transvaginal Examination
Gestational sac	6	5
Yolk sac	6	5
Fetus	7	6
Fetal cardiac activity	7	6

sac should be identified by a gestational age of 6 weeks. The fetus and fetal cardiac activity should be identified by a gestational age of 7 weeks. The vaginal transducer used for transvaginal ultrasound examinations can be placed closer to the uterus than the transabdominal transducer, and therefore the ultrasonographic milestones as detected transvaginally are reached 1 week earlier.

Because the gestational age of the fetus is sometimes unknown, ultrasonographic milestones have been established that correlate with serum hCG levels. In normal pregnancies, a gestational sac should be seen by transabdominal ultrasound examination when the serum hCG level is >6500 mIU/ml (International Reference Preparation). On transvaginal ultrasound examination, the gestational sac should be seen when the serum hCG is >2000 mIU/ml. These two serum hCG levels define what is commonly referred to as the "discriminatory hCG zones."

Whenever these ultrasonographic milestones cannot be identified at the corresponding gestational age or serum hCG levels, an abnormal pregnancy should be suspected. The abnormal pregnancy can be either an abnormal intrauterine pregnancy that has undergone or is about to undergo spontaneous abortion or an ectopic pregnancy. The differentiation between an abnormal intrauterine pregnancy and an ectopic pregnancy depends on the physical examination, serial serum hCG determination, and ultrasound examination. Evidence of an intrauterine pregnancy on ultrasound examination makes the likelihood of ectopic pregnancy extremely rare. The incidence of concurrent intrauterine pregnancy and tubal pregnancy is only 1 in 3000. When neither physical examination nor ultrasound examination is conclusive, serial serum hCG testing can be used to help distinguish between a spontaneous abortion and ectopic pregnancy.

3. **Serial serum human chorionic gonadotropin testing**
    Human chorionic gonadotropin is produced by the syncytio-

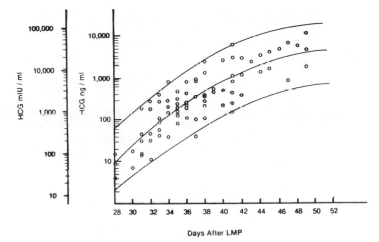

Figure 33–1 □ Rise in serum hCG in normal intrauterine pregnancies. (Modified from Pittaway DE, Reish RL, Wentz AC: Doubling times of human chorionic gonadotropin increase in early viable intrauterine pregnancies. Am J Obstet Gynecol 1985;152:299.)

trophoblast in the placenta, and serum levels rise exponentially in the first trimester (Fig. 33–1). A peak level of approximately 100,000 mIU/ml is reached at 9 weeks of gestation, and hCG levels then fall to a plateau of 10,000 to 20,000 mIU/ml, where they remain for the duration of the pregnancy. Even with normal pregnancies, there is a wide range of serum hCG levels at any given gestational age, and therefore it may be difficult to confirm the diagnosis of spontaneous abortion with only a single serum hCG determination (Table 33–2).

When serum hCG levels are measured serially several days apart, an abnormally rising serum hCG is diagnostic of an

Table 33–2 □ **HUMAN CHORIONIC GONADOTROPIN LEVELS IN NORMAL PREGNANCIES**

Gestational Age (weeks)	Serum hCG (mIU/ml)
4	100
6	1000–10,000
7	10,000–50,000
9	50,000–100,000
20	10,000–20,000

hCG = human chorionic gonadotropin.

abnormal pregnancy, either an ectopic pregnancy or a spontaneous abortion. In early pregnancy, with levels of serum hCG at <1200 mIU/ml, serum hCG normally doubles in 2 days. If there is not at least a 66% rise in serum hCG in 2 days, an abnormal pregnancy should be suspected. At serum hCG levels of 1200 to 6000 mIU/ml, the normal hCG doubling time is almost 3 days, and at levels of >6000 mIU/ml, the doubling time is approximately 4 days. A falling hCG in the first trimester of pregnancy is also suggestive of an abnormal pregnancy. A rapidly declining serum hCG is more suggestive of a completed or ongoing spontaneous abortion than of an ectopic pregnancy. The half-life of hCG is approximately 32 to 37 hours.

4. **Serum progesterone**

Women with normal intrauterine pregnancies almost always have a serum progesterone level of >25 ng/ml. Approximately 85 to 90% of women with spontaneous abortion or ectopic pregnancy have a serum progesterone of <10 ng/ml. Therefore, a serum progesterone level of <5 ng/ml is a strong indication of an abnormal pregnancy, although the level cannot differentiate between ectopic pregnancy and an abnormal intrauterine pregnancy.

5. **Complete blood count**

Bleeding from either a spontaneous abortion or an ectopic pregnancy can be significant enough to result in anemia. An elevated white blood cell count is suggestive of septic abortion.

6. **Blood Rh factor and antibody screen**

■ ADDITIONAL DIAGNOSTIC TESTING FOR SEPTIC ABORTION

In addition to the diagnostic tests listed above, the following tests may be helpful in diagnosing and managing a patient with suspected septic abortion:

1. **Serum chemistry including electrolytes**
2. **Urinalysis**
3. **Intrauterine culture and Gram stain**
4. **Blood cultures**
5. **Coagulation studies**
6. **Chest x-ray**

■ MANAGEMENT

1. **Threatened abortion**
   a. **Conservative management**

b. Instruct patient to avoid strenuous physical activity and intercourse
c. Instruct patient to return if bleeding, pelvic pain, or cramping increases

Bleeding occurs in approximately 20 to 30% of women during the first 20 weeks of gestation. Spontaneous abortion occurs in about 50% of these women. Although women with threatened abortion are often warned to avoid strenuous activity and intercourse and are sometimes even placed on bedrest, there is no evidence that these measures decrease the risk of subsequent pregnancy loss. Furthermore, although hormonal therapy with progestins and estrogens such as diethylstilbestrol (DES) has been attempted in the past, there is no medical therapy that decreases the likelihood of pregnancy loss in normal patients.

2. Inevitable abortion
   a. Conservative management allowing spontaneous evacuation of the uterus or
   b. Surgical evacuation of the uterus or
   c. Induction of uterine contractions with uterotonic agents
      (1) Prostaglandin E_2 20 mg suppository (Prostin) intravaginally every 4 hours or
      (2) Misoprostol (Cytotec) 200- to 800-μg tablet intravaginally every 12 hours

Patients who decide on conservative management should be warned to return to the hospital if they develop either severe or unremitting bleeding or pelvic pain. They should also be warned that suction curettage may still be necessary if not all of the fetal tissue is passed spontaneously. Suction curettage can be performed in an office or an emergency room and can be performed with either paracervical block or the use of intravenous drugs for sedation and analgesia. Some patients elect to have the procedure performed in an operating room under general anesthesia. Suction curettage should be performed with a sterile suction cannula with a diameter in millimeters that corresponds to the number of weeks of gestation based on uterine size. For example, a 7- or 8-mm cannula should be used if the uterus is palpated to be 8-week size, and an 11- or 12-mm cannula should be used if the uterus is palpated to be 12-week size. All tissue obtained by surgical evacuation should be submitted for pathological evaluation to confirm the diagnosis of spontaneous abortion.

Misoprostol is a prostaglandin E_1 analog that is not approved by the U.S. Food and Drug Administration for use in spontaneous abortion, even though its use for this indication is becoming common.

3. Incomplete spontaneous abortion
   a. Surgical evacuation of the uterus or

b. **Induction of uterine contractions with prostaglandin E_2 vaginal suppositories or misoprostol tablets intravaginally**

Women with incomplete spontaneous abortion usually have significant vaginal bleeding, which precludes conservative management. In some patients, speculum examination reveals fetal tissue protruding through the cervical os, and the abortion can be completed merely by grasping and removing the tissue. In the remaining patients, surgical evacuation by suction curettage is recommended for first-trimester pregnancies. For second-trimester pregnancies, dilatation and evacuation or medical induction of uterine contractions with prostaglandin E_2 or misoprostol can be performed as described for the management of inevitable abortion.

4. **Completed spontaneous abortion**
   a. **Serum hCG in several days** or
   b. **Rapid pregnancy test in several weeks**

   Women with completed spontaneous abortion have passed all fetal and placental tissue. The cervical os is usually closed, and bleeding is minimal. Therefore, no surgical intervention is necessary. If tissue is not available for pathological evaluation or if evaluation does not reveal evidence of fetal tissue, a quantitative serum hCG level could be obtained in a few days or weeks to confirm the diagnosis.

5. **Blighted ovum or missed abortion**
   a. **Surgical evacuation of the uterus by suction dilatation and curettage** or
   b. **Induction with prostaglandin E_2 vaginal suppositories or misoprostol tablets**

   Patients with either a blighted ovum or a missed abortion are usually asymptomatic. The cervical os is usually closed, and therefore cervical dilatation followed by suction curettage is recommended.

6. **Septic abortion**
   a. **Intravenous antibiotic therapy**
   b. **Surgical evacuation of the uterus**

   Septic abortion is a serious complication of spontaneous abortion with a fatality rate of approximately 0.5 per 100,000 women with spontaneous abortion. Organisms causing septic abortion include anaerobic bacteria (*Bacteroides* species, *Clostridium perfringens, Peptostreptococcus* spp.) and aerobic species (beta-hemolytic streptococcus, *Enterococcus faecalis, Escherichia coli, Pseudomonas* spp.). Broad-spectrum antibiotics that provide adequate coverage for these organisms should be administered intravenously immediately. No one specific antibiotic regimen has been shown to be superior to others in all patients. A popular regimen is the following combination:

(1) **Gentamicin 2.0 mg/kg IV loading dose followed by a maintenance dose of 1.5 mg/kg every 8 hours if renal function is normal** and

(2) **Clindamycin 900 mg IV every 8 hours**

Peak serum levels of antibiotics are usually attained 1 to 2 hours after administration, and the patient should then undergo surgical evacuation of the uterus. Postoperative care should include close monitoring of vital signs and urine output to detect septic shock.

7. **Rh-negative women**

All Rh-negative women who have had spontaneous abortions should receive Rh immune globulin if (1) they are nonimmunized, as documented by a negative antibody screen and (2) the Rh factor of the father is either positive or unknown.

In pregnancies with a gestational age of 12 weeks or less, the following should be given: **Rh immune globulin (MICRhoGAM) 50 µg IM within 72 hours of the spontaneous abortion**. After 12 weeks, a full dose of Rh immune globulin should be given as follows: **Rh immune globulin (RhoGAM) 300 µg within 72 hours of the spontaneous abortion**.

8. **All women with spontaneous abortion**

Almost all women who suffer pregnancy loss, even at an early gestational age, undergo a grieving process. Both parents should be treated with sympathy and compassion. Furthermore, they should be educated concerning the common occurrence of spontaneous abortions, and it should be emphasized that in almost all cases neither the patient nor her health care provider should be blamed for the loss. Information concerning support groups should be provided to both parents. After a single early spontaneous abortion, 80 to 90% of women have a successful outcome with the next pregnancy. In women who have had a previous successful pregnancy, the prognosis is even better.

■ BACKGROUND AND DEFINITION

Toxic shock syndrome (TSS): An acute, potentially fatal, multisystem illness caused by strains of *Staphylococcus aureus* that produce a toxin referred to as pyrogenic exotoxin or enterotoxin F. The incubation period for TSS is 1 to 4 days. Ninety to 95% of cases of TSS occur in women, and >95% of these cases occur in menstruating women. White women younger than 30 years of age are at greatest risk. The incidence of TSS in menstruating women is 6 to 7 per 100,000 per year. TSS that is not associated with menstruation can occur in women of any age. The fatality rate of TSS is 3 to 6%. In patients who survive, there is a 30% recurrence rate.

The following two conditions must be present for TSS to develop:

1. The patient must be colonized with a strain of *S. aureus* that produces the toxin.
2. There must be a portal of entry into the systemic circulation.

Toxins may enter into the systemic circulation through microulcerations that develop in the vagina secondary to trauma from tampons or tampon inserters. Almost 99% of cases of TSS associated with menstruation occur in women who use tampons. Women who use tampons during menstruation are 18 times more likely to develop TSS than women who do not use them. Women who used the Rely brand of tampons were almost 8 times more likely to develop TSS than women who use other brands of tampons. The use of high-absorbency synthetic materials in newer tampon products may predispose a patient to TSS because of an effect on the colonization rate of *S. aureus* or increased trauma to the vaginal wall. Patients who used the Rely brand of tampons were shown to have a 43% colonization rate for *S. aureus* compared with a colonization rate of 8% in users of other brands of tampons.

■ CLINICAL PRESENTATION

The following signs and symptoms are found in >90% of patients with TSS:

Fever ≥38.9° (102°F)

Hypotension

Shock
"Sunburn-like" skin rash with desquamation
Myalgias
Vomiting
Diarrhea

Other signs and symptoms that occur less frequently include the following:
Headache
Abdominal tenderness
Sore throat
Hyperemia of the pharynx and tongue
Conjunctivitis
Photophobia
Altered sensorium
Hyperemia of the vagina
Vaginal discharge
Arthralgia
Adnexal tenderness

■ PHONE CALL

Questions

1. How ill does the patient appear?
2. What are the vital signs?

Degree of Urgency

TSS is a potentially fatal disease, so patients should be seen immediately.

■ ELEVATOR THOUGHTS

What is the differential diagnosis of TSS?
- Streptococcal scarlet fever
    This infection is rare after the age of 10 years and is usually preceded by an upper respiratory infection. Serum antibodies to streptococcus such as antistreptolysin O are positive.
- Mucocutaneous lymph node syndrome (Kawasaki disease)
    This syndrome is usually encountered in pediatric patients <5 years of age. Furthermore, hypotension, shock, and adult respiratory distress syndrome (ARDS) are rarely present in this syndrome.
- Rubeola (measles)
- Rubella (German measles)
- Rocky Mountain spotted fever *(Ricksettsia rickettsii)*

This infection is caused by a gram-negative bacterium for which small rodents and occasionally larger mammals are the reservoir. Transmission to humans is by bites from multiple tick species.

- Leptospirosis

  This infection is caused by *Leptospira interrogans,* a spirochete found in domestic livestock, dogs, rodents, skunks, and foxes. Transmission is by contact with infected tissue, body fluids, or contaminated water. Those who work with animals, such as dairy or slaughterhouse workers, are at highest risk, although nearly 50% of cases are contracted during recreation in water contaminated by drainage from nearby farmland.

■ MAJOR THREAT TO LIFE

- ARDS
- Hypotensive shock
- Hemorrhage secondary to disseminated intravascular coagulation

■ BEDSIDE

Quick Look Test

Does the patient appear to be severely ill and in shock?

A patient in shock will usually appear distressed, ill, and apprehensive. She will appear pale and have cold and clammy skin.

Vital Signs

A patient with TSS will often be in hypotensive shock with a systolic blood pressure (BP) ≤90 mm Hg and tachycardia. Furthermore, the patient might have postural hypotension. Changes in BP and pulse should be measured when the patient is assisted in sitting or standing from a supine position. A fall in systolic or diastolic BP >15 mm Hg or a rise in pulse >15 beats/min is evidence of orthostatic hypotension.

Selective History and Chart Review

1. Has the patient menstruated recently?
2. Does the patient use tampons?
3. Does the patient have a history of TSS?

4. Has the patient suffered any type of trauma or surgical procedure that might provide a portal of entry for bacteria?
5. Has the patient had any recent exposure to livestock or engaged in any outdoor activities such as hiking and camping that would place her at risk for Rocky Mountain spotted fever or leptospirosis?

Selective Physical Examination

Dermatological	Sunburn-like macular rash
	Desquamation of the palms or soles
Head and neck	"Strawberry" tongue
	Hyperemia of the pharynx
	Conjunctivitis
Abdominal	Tenderness to palpation
Pelvic	
External genitalia and vagina	Hyperemia of the vagina
	Vaginal discharge
	Tampon or diaphragm may be found in the vagina
Cervix	Hyperemia of the cervix
Uterus and adnexa	Adnexal tenderness

Orders

1. Start IV.
2. Insert urethral catheter to monitor urine output.
3. Record intake and output.
4. Administer oxygen via face mask or nasal cannula.
5. Obtain a complete blood count (CBC) with differential.
6. Obtain a chemistry panel.
7. Obtain coagulation studies: prothrombin time (PT), partial thromboplastin time (PTT), platelet count, fibrinogen, and fibrin split products.
8. Obtain a urinalysis.

■ DIAGNOSTIC TESTING

There are no specific laboratory tests that are pathognomonic for TSS. Instead, the diagnosis is based on a constellation of physical findings and laboratory tests. The case definition proposed in 1982 by the Centers for Disease Control and Prevention for TSS is as follows:

1. **Fever (≥38.9°C or ≥102°F)**
2. **Diffuse macular rash**

3. Desquamation occurring 1 to 2 weeks after the onset of illness
4. Hypotension or orthostatic syncope
5. Involvement of three or more of the following organ systems:
   a. Gastrointestinal system (vomiting or diarrhea at onset of illness)
   b. Muscular system (myalgia, creatine phosphokinase level two times normal)
   c. Mucous membranes (vaginal, oropharyngeal, or conjunctival hyperemia)
   d. Renal system (blood urea nitrogen [BUN] or creatinine level at least two times normal or urinalysis with ≥5 white blood cells per high-power field in the absence of urinary tract infection)
   e. Hepatic system (total bilirubin, aspartate transaminase [AST], or alanine aminotransferase [ALT] two times normal level)
   f. Hematological system (platelets ≤100,000/mm³)
   g. Central nervous system (disorientation or alterations in consciousness without focal neurological signs in the absence of fever and hypotension)
6. Negative throat and cerebrospinal fluid cultures
7. Negative serological tests for Rocky Mountain spotted fever, leptospirosis, and rubeola

Tests that are often abnormal and therefore helpful in confirming the diagnosis of TSS are listed below along with the frequency with which abnormal findings are encountered.

1. **CBC with differential**
   a. Anemia (60%)
   b. Leukocytosis (60%)
2. **Coagulation studies**
   a. Thrombocytopenia (55%)
   b. Prolonged PT (55%)
   c. Prolonged PTT (50%)
3. **Blood chemistries**
   a. Hypoproteinemia (80%)
   b. Hypokalemia (80%)
   c. Elevated AST (75%)
   d. Hypocalcemia (70%)
   e. Elevated serum creatinine (65%)
   f. Hypophosphatemia (60%)
   g. Elevated lactate dehydrogenase (60%)
   h. Elevated creatine phosphokinase (CPK) (55%)
   i. Elevated BUN (55%)
   j. Hyponatremia (50%)
   k. Elevated ALT (50%)

4. Urinalysis
  a. Sterile pyuria (80%)
  b. Proteinuria (60%)
  c. Hematuria (60%)
5. Serological studies
  Acute and convalescent serological testing can rule out the following infections, which can present in a fashion similar to TSS:
  a. Rocky Mountain spotted fever
  b. Leptospirosis
  c. Rubeola
6. Cultures for *Staphylococcus aureus*
  If physical examination does not reveal an obvious site of entry, cultures should be obtained from the vagina, rectum, conjunctivae, oropharynx, and nares. Blood, urine, and cerebrospinal fluid can also be cultured.
7. Arterial blood gas
  a. Metabolic acidemia (80%)
  b. Hypoxemia
8. Chest radiograph
  a. Diffuse infiltrations consistent with ARDS
  b. Pulmonary edema

■ MANAGEMENT

1. Fluid resuscitation
  Aggressive fluid resuscitation is the initial step in the management of TSS. Patients can require >8 L of IV fluid per day.
2. Hemodynamic monitoring
  A pulmonary artery catheter (Swan-Ganz catheter) and arterial line will provide intensive hemodynamic monitoring that is necessary for the maintenance of cardiac output and blood pressure. Normal pulmonary artery catheter measurements are listed in Table 34–1.
4. Vasopressor therapy
  Dopamine, a vasoactive amine, has a positive inotropic effect resulting in increased myocardial contractility and heart rate. Furthermore, dopamine increases organ perfusion through vasodilation of the renal, mesenteric, coronary, and cerebral vasculatures. Dosage is as follows: **dopamine 5 μg/kg/min by IV infusion with the dose increased by 5 μg/kg/min increments to a maximum of 50 μg/mg/min.** The dose is monitored by Swan-Ganz catheter measurements of pulmonary artery and wedge pressure.
5. Respiratory support
  Oxygen should be administered by face mask or nasal cannula at a flow rate of 8 to 10 L/min. Arterial blood gas

Table 34–1 □ **NORMAL CENTRAL HEMODYNAMIC MEASUREMENTS IN NONPREGNANT AND PREGNANT PATIENTS**

Parameter	Nonpregnant	Pregnant
Cardiac output (L/min)	4.3 ± 0.9	6.2 ± 1.0
Heart rate (beats/min)	71 ± 10.0	83 ± 10.0
Systemic vascular resistance (dyne × cm × sec^{-5})	1530 ± 520	1210 ± 266
Pulmonary vascular resistance (dyne × cm × sec^{-5})	119 ± 47.0	78 ± 22
Colloid oncotic pressure (mm Hg)	20.8 ± 1.0	18.0 ± 1.5
Colloid oncotic pressure– pulmonary capillary wedge pressure (mm Hg)	14.5 ± 2.5	10.5 ± 2.7
Mean arterial pressure (mm Hg)	86.4 ± 7.5	90.3 ± 5.8
Pulmonary capillary wedge pressure (mm Hg)	6.3 ± 2.1	7.5 ± 1.8
Central venous pressure (mm Hg)	3.7 ± 2.6	3.6 ± 2.5
Left ventricular stroke work index (g × m × m^{-2})	41 ± 8	48 ± 6

From Clark SL, Cotton DB, Lee W, et al: Central hemodynamic assessment of normal term pregnancy. Am J Obstet Gynecol 1989;161:1439.

determination should be used to monitor the patient. Intubation may be necessary in the acutely ill patient.

6. **Beta-lactamase–resistant antistaphylococcal antibiotics**
   a. **Nafcillin sodium 500 to 1000 mg IV every 4 hours**
   b. **In patients who are allergic to penicillin, vancomycin should be administered: vancomycin hydrochloride 500 mg IV every 4 hours**
7. **Treatment of coagulopathy**
   a. **Platelets**
      Platelets should be transfused for a platelet count of <20,000/mm³. Each unit of platelets should increase the platelet count by 5000/mm³ to 10,000/mm³.
   b. **Fresh frozen plasma**
      Fresh frozen plasma (FFP) is transfused for coagulopathy due to clotting factor deficiency, manifested by a PT or PTT that is >1.5 times normal. Each unit of FFP increases any clotting factor by 2 to 3%. The usual initial dose is 2 units, and each unit has a volume of 200 to 250 ml.
   c. **Cryoprecipitate**
      Cryoprecipitate is transfused for coagulopathy due to deficiency of factor VIII, von Willebrand's factor, factor XIII, fibrinogen, or fibronectin. Cryoprecipitate is concentrated from FFP, and each bag has a volume of 10 to 15 ml. Each bag contains at least 150 mg of fibrinogen.

■ BACKGROUND AND DEFINITIONS

Vulvar lesions and ulcers can be placed into one of the following four categories:

Infectious lesions: Many are caused by sexually transmitted diseases

Vulvar nonneoplastic epithelial disorders: Formerly referred to as vulvar dystrophies; the most common of these disorders are lichen sclerosus, squamous cell hyperplasia, and vulvar vestibulitis

Vulvar malignancies: Most often encountered in postmenopausal women; the most common vulvar malignancy is squamous cell carcinoma

Vulvar trauma: Can be a result of sexual assault, vaginal delivery, or saddle-injury falls

■ CLINICAL PRESENTATION

Vulvar pain
Vulvar bleeding
Itching or burning
Inguinal lymphadenopathy
Vulvar rash, papule, or nodule
Vulvar vesicles or ulcer, with or without pain
Dyspareunia

■ PHONE CALL

Questions

1. **What is the patient's age?**
   Vulvar lesions and ulcers caused by sexually transmitted diseases are more common in younger patients who are sexually active, especially with multiple partners. Vulvar nonneoplastic epithelial disorders and malignancy are encountered more commonly in older patients.
2. **What are the patient's symptoms, and how severe are those symptoms?**
   Severe vulvar pain is usually associated with genital

herpes, chancroid, and granuloma inguinale. Vulvar itching is usually associated with yeast vulvovaginitis, scabies, pediculosis pubis, vulvar nonneoplastic epithelial disorders, and vulvar malignancy.

3. **Has the patient suffered any trauma?**

Trauma from falls can result in vulvar trauma such as "saddle injuries." Vulvar trauma can also be caused by sexual assault.

Degree of Urgency

Vulvar lesions and ulcers may be extremely uncomfortable but are rarely life threatening. Therefore, patients do not usually need to be seen immediately.

■ ELEVATOR THOUGHTS

What are causes of vulvar lesions and ulcers?
1. **Infection**
   a. **Genital herpes simplex virus (HSV)**

   Genital herpes is a sexually transmitted disease caused by HSV. HSV type 2 (HSV-2) causes approximately 85% of primary genital herpes, and HSV type 1 (HSV-1) is responsible for 15%. Genital herpes is endemic in the United States. The incidence of symptomatic disease is approximately 5% in women of reproductive age, and approximately 30% of women in the United States have HSV-2 antibodies. Genital herpes is a recurrent disease, and HSV-2 has a frequency of recurrence that is three to four times higher than that of HSV-1. Nearly 25% of recurrences are asymptomatic and manifested only by viral shedding. Primary infections are characterized by severe local pain with multiple lesions that progress from the vesicular to the ulcerative stages. Clinically, patients may experience prodromal symptoms consisting of mild paresthesia and burning. Inguinal lymphadenopathy is common, and the patient may have systemic symptoms such as fever, malaise, headaches, and myalgia. The incubation period is 3 to 7 days. Patients with primary infection can have lesions for 2 to 6 weeks. Patients with recurrent infection have milder local symptoms and rarely have systemic symptoms. The duration of recurrent infections is also shorter, usually 3 to 5 days. There is currently no cure for HSV infection.

   b. **Human papillomavirus (HPV)**

   More than 60 subtypes of HPVs have been described, and 21 have been implicated in genital disease. HPV infection is a sexually transmitted disease that results not only in lesions of the lower genital tract but also in premalignant or dysplastic changes. Condylomata acuminata, also referred to as venereal or genital warts, and low-grade dysplasia of the lower genital tract are usually associated with HPV subtypes 6, 11, 41, 42, 43, and 44. High-grade dysplasia and carcinoma are associated with HPV subtypes 16, 18, 31, 33, 35, 39, 45, 51, 52, and 56. HPV is highly contagious, with a transmission rate of 25 to 60%. The average incubation period is 3 months. HPV infection undergoes continuous remissions and recurrences. Although the visible lesions can be eradicated, there is no permanent cure for HPV.

There are three levels of HPV infection: clinical infection, subclinical infection, and latent infection.

(1) Clinical infection

This is manifested by the appearance of genital warts in the lower genital tract. Approximately one-third of patients with clinical infection have vulvar or external involvement alone; another one-third have both external as well as cervical and vaginal or internal involvement; and the remaining one-third have internal involvement alone.

(2) Subclinical infection

This is manifested by lesions that are visible only under the magnification of a colposcope or by cytological changes that are detectable by Pap smear.

(3) Latent infection

This is detected only by DNA hybridization testing, and no lesions are visible even under magnification.

c. Syphilis

Syphilis is a chronic sexually transmitted infection caused by an anaerobic spirochete, *Treponema pallidum*. It is moderately contagious, with a transmission rate of almost 10%. The incubation period is 10 to 90 days, with an average of approximately 3 weeks. The clinical course of syphilis is divided into primary, secondary, and tertiary phases.

(1) Primary syphilis

The manifestation of primary syphilis is the appearance of a hard, painless chancre. If untreated, the chancre resolves in 3 to 6 weeks, and hematogenous dissemination of the spirochete results in the secondary stage.

(2) Secondary syphilis

Secondary syphilis is a systemic disease that lasts 2 to 6 weeks and is characterized by lymphadenopathy, skin rash, and vulvar condylomata lata. If the patient is untreated, the secondary phase resolves, and the patient enters a latent phase in which there are usually no clinical manifestations. Latent syphilis lasts 2 to 20 years.

(3) **Tertiary syphilis**

Without treatment, approximately one-third of patients will develop tertiary syphilis, which consists of progressive damage to the central nervous system, cardiovascular system, and musculoskeletal system. Clinical manifestations of tertiary syphilis include tabes dorsalis, generalized paresis, aortic aneurysm, and gummata of soft tissues and bones.

d. **Chancroid**

Chancroid, also referred to as "soft chancre," is a highly contagious sexually transmitted disease caused by *Haemophilus ducreyi*, a gram-negative nonmotile bacillus. The incubation period is 3 to 5 days. The initial presentation includes vulvar pain and a papule that progresses in 2 to 3 days to a painful, tender ulcer. In 50% of women, a bubo characterized by acute and tender inguinal lymphadenopathy develops 7 to 10 days after the initial lesion. The bubo is unilateral in two-thirds of patients; if untreated, the bubo ruptures and a large ulcer forms.

e. **Granuloma inguinale**

Granuloma inguinale, also referred to as donovanosis, is caused by *Calymmatobacterium granulomatis*, a nonmotile gram-negative bacillus. It is not highly contagious, and repeated sexual contact or close nonsexual contact is necessary for transmission. The incubation period is 1 to 12 weeks. The initial manifestation is a painless papule or nodule that ulcerates and forms into enlarging, beefy-red granulation tissue. There is usually little lymphadenopathy. If untreated, lesions can coalesce and result in vulvar scarring and fibrosis.

f. **Lymphogranuloma venereum (LGV)**

LGV is a sexually transmitted infection caused by *Chlamydia trachomatis* serotypes L1, L2, and L3. The incubation period is 4 to 21 days. The clinical course of LGV can be divided into three phases: primary, secondary, and tertiary.

(1) **Primary LGV**

This is manifested by the appearance of a painless papular or vesicular lesion that may progress to an ulcer but heals within a few days.

(2) **Secondary LGV**

This develops 1 to 4 weeks after the primary lesion and is characterized by painful inguinal lymphadenopathy that is usually unilateral. Approximately 50% of patients have systemic symptoms such as fever, myalgias, and malaise. If untreated, the inguinal nodes become enlarged and progressively more tender. The nodes can become matted to each other and become adherent to the subcutaneous tissue and skin. If the femoral lymph nodes also become infected, the inguinal ligament forms a groove between the two groups of nodes. This "groove sign" is found in 10 to 20% of patients.

(3) **Tertiary LGV**

This is characterized by tissue destruction, scarring, and multiple draining sinuses arising from the lymph nodes.

g. **Molluscum contagiosum**

Molluscum contagiosum is caused by a pox virus and is transmitted both sexually and nonsexually by close physical contact. The incubation period is 2 to 7 weeks. The disease is only mildly contagious. The infection is usually asymptomatic, although some patients complain of pruritus. The characteristic lesion is a smooth papule, 2 to 5 mm in diameter, with an umbilicated center. The lesions are multiple and may number up to 20. The lesions are usually present for 6 to 9 months but can persist for several years.

h. **Scabies**

Scabies is caused by the mite *Sarcoptes scabiei* and is transmitted both sexually and nonsexually by close physical contact. The infection can be widespread throughout the entire body. The mite moves rapidly across the skin at a speed of 2.5 cm/min. The adult female mite digs burrows in the skin and deposits her eggs, which hatch in 3 to 4 days. The entire life span of the mite is 1 month. Clinical manifestations appear 4 to 6 weeks after infection. The primary presentation of scabies is a papular or vesicular rash and gradual onset of severe and intermittent itching, which is usually worse at night.

i. **Pediculosis pubis or crab lice**

Pediculosis pubis is transmitted both sexually and nonsexually by close contact or by fomites. It is caused by *Pthirus pubis*, the crab or pubic louse. The incubation period is 30 days. It is highly contagious, with a transmission rate of 95% after a single sexual encounter. The primary presentation of pubic lice is constant irritation and pruritus due to allergic sensitization to bites.

2. **Vulvar nonneoplastic epithelial disorders**

a. **Squamous cell hyperplasia**

Squamous cell hyperplasia was formerly referred to as "hyperplastic dystrophy." This lesion is associated with epithelial thickening and hyperkeratosis. However, the clinical appearance of the lesion is highly variable. There may be white or gray discoloration of the skin, and lesions may appear to be similar to those of condyloma acuminatum. The primary symptom is itching.

b. **Lichen sclerosus**

The lesion of lichen sclerosus is characterized by epithelial thinning that results in an atrophic, parchment-like appearance to the vulva and perineum. This can result in agglutination and shrinking of the labia and subsequently in stenosis of the introitus. The primary symptoms are itching and dyspareunia. This condition is most commonly encountered in prepubertal and postmenopausal patients.

c. Vulvar vestibulitis

This is an inflammatory condition of the vestibule associated with vulvodynia on insertional dyspareunia. Vulvar vestibulitis is poorly understood, and the etiology has not been established. The onset of this condition can sometimes be traced back to an episode of vulvovaginitis or some type of ablative procedure for vulvar condylomata acuminata.

3. Vulvar malignancy

a. Squamous cell carcinoma

Squamous cell carcinoma of the vulva accounts for 90% of all vulvar malignancies. It is primarily a disease of older, postmenopausal women. The most common presentation is pruritus.

b. Melanoma

Melanoma is the second most common vulvar malignancy, accounting for 5 to 10% of all vulvar malignancies. The most common presenting symptom is a vulvar mass.

4. Vulvar trauma

■ MAJOR THREAT TO LIFE

- Vulvar malignancy

■ BEDSIDE

Quick Look Test

Patients with vulvar lesions will usually not appear to be ill but may appear distressed by the amount of vulvar pain and discomfort.

Vital Signs

Vital signs are usually normal.

Selective History and Chart Review

1. What type of local symptoms, if any, does the patient have?
2. Does the patient have any systemic symptoms such as fever, malaise, or myalgias?

3. Is the patient sexually active? If so, does the patient's partner have similar symptoms?
4. Does the patient have a history of sexually transmitted diseases?

   Patients with prior sexually transmitted diseases are at greater risk of having recurrent disease. This is especially true of genital herpes and human papillomavirus infection.
5. Does the patient have a history of abnormal Pap smears?

   Changes on Pap smear such as koilocytotic atypia and multinucleated giant cell can be detected in the presence of cervical HPV and HSV infections, respectively.
6. Has the patient had a previous vulvar biopsy?

   A prior vulvar biopsy often helps in confirming the diagnosis of vulvar nonneoplastic epithelial disorder.
7. Is the patient pregnant?

   Pregnancy limits the options of antibiotic treatment in patients with vulvar lesions secondary to infection.

Selective Physical Examination (Table 35–1)

Dermatological	Secondary syphilis: maculopapular rash, especially on the palms and soles
Inguinal region	Inguinal lymphadenopathy in genital herpes simplex, syphilis, and chancroid
	Groove sign in lymphogranuloma venereum
Pelvic	
External genitalia and vagina	Genital herpes: multiple small vesicles progressing to ulcers

Table 35-1 □ DIFFERENTIAL DIAGNOSIS OF GENITAL ULCERS

Characteristic	HSV	Syphilis	Chancroid	Granuloma Inguinale	LGV
Lesion	Multiple vesicles	Single ulcer	Single or multiple ulcers	Single or multiple ulcers	Single ulcer
Depth	Shallow	Shallow	Deep	Elevated	Shallow
Induration	Absent	Hard	Soft	Hard	Absent
Adenopathy	Present	Present	Present	Absent	Present
Pain	Present	Absent	Present	Absent	Variable
Incubation	3–7 days	3 weeks	3–5 days	1–12 weeks	4–21 days

HSV = herpes simplex virus; LGV = lymphogranuloma venereum.

External genitalia
and vagina
(continued)

HPV: genital warts or condylomata acuminata appearing as flesh-colored to gray excrescences that can be broad-based or on pedicles, varying in size from a pinpoint to a large cauliflower-like lesion

Primary syphilis: chancre that is a painless, round or oval ulcer with a sharp border and a firm, button-like base that is initially glistening and later covered with a gray film

Secondary syphilis: condylomata lata that are raised, white lesions similar to genital warts

Chancroid: tender papule that ulcerates and forms a painful soft ulcer with sharp borders and a base that is covered with a yellow or gray exudate

Granuloma inguinale: painless papule or nodule that progresses to an enlarging, painless ulcer with beefy-red granulation tissue

LGV: in early LGV, painless papular or vesicular lesions that progress to ulcers with local edema; in late LGV, ulcerations become invasive and destructive, resulting in severe distortion of the normal anatomy, vaginal stenosis, and fistula formation

Molluscum contagiosum: smooth, firm, spherical papule with a diameter of 2 to 5 mm and an umbilicated center; lesions usually number 1 to 20 but can be more numerous and are found not only on the external genitalia but also on the lower abdominal wall and inner thighs

Scabies: papular erythematous rash often associated with burrows 5 to 10 mm long that have the appearance of wavy lines of dirt

Crab lice: erythema and excoriation secondary to scratching; "blue spots" may appear secondary to the crab louse bite

External genitalia and vagina *(continued)*	Squamous cell hyperplasia: gross appearance highly variable and may be affected by chronic scratching; classic lesions are well demarcated and raised with a dusky-red, white, or gray color
	Lichen sclerosus: skin of the vulva and perianal region with a crinkled, pale, parchment-like appearance; labia minora may be absent and vaginal introitus may be stenotic secondary to atrophy; fissure may be present in the natural folds of the skin
	Vulvar vestibulitis: erythema in the area of the vestibule, posteriorly between 5 o'clock and 7 o'clock at the vaginal introitus; there is often pinpoint tenderness that can be elicited with palpation of the area by a cotton-tipped applicator or finger
	Squamous cell cancer: gross appearance variable; initial lesion may be a small itchy nodule that ulcerates; alternatively, lesion may appear as a cauliflower-like growth similar to genital warts
	Melanoma: gross appearance similar to melanoma elsewhere on the body; lesions usually pigmented, raised, and may be ulcerated with bleeding; most lesions appear on the labia minora and clitoris
	Trauma: highly variable appearance that is dependent on the type of trauma; falls often associated with obvious lacerations and hematomas; trauma from sexual assault may appear more subtle with abrasions and erythema
Cervix	Genital herpes: friable and erythematous with multiple ulcers
	HPV: flat or raised coarse white lesions
	Primary syphilis: chancre similar to that found on the vulva

Cervix
(continued)

Chancroid: ulcer similar to that found on the vulva

Granuloma inguinale: ulcer similar to that found on the vulva

LGV: papule and ulcer is most commonly found on the posterior lip of the cervix

Orders

1. Prepare the patient for a pelvic examination and have materials available for vaginal smears, vulvar biopsy, dark-field smear, herpes culture, chlamydia culture, and bacterial culture.
2. Obtain a Venereal Disease Research Laboratory (VDRL) test if the patient has a painless vulvar ulcer.
3. Obtain a complete blood count (CBC) if the patient had suffered trauma or assault.

■ DIAGNOSTIC TESTING

1. **Genital herpes simplex**
   a. **Herpes culture**
      Viral isolation by tissue culture is the most sensitive and specific diagnostic test for genital herpes. Culture usually becomes positive in 1 to 4 days.
   b. **Serology for herpes simplex virus**
      Anti-HSV-1 and anti-HSV-2 antibodies can be detected and measured in the acute and convalescent phases.
   c. **Cytology smear**
      The finding on Pap smear of multinucleated giant cells is suggestive of genital HSV.
2. **Human papillomavirus**
   HPV infection can usually be diagnosed by the appearance of classic condylomata acuminata. Laboratory testing is necessary only to confirm the diagnosis when the clinical presentation is unclear.
   a. **Tissue biopsy**
      Tissue biopsy is the most sensitive and specific diagnostic test for HPV.
   b. **DNA hybridization testing**
      DNA hybridization testing can be performed for HPV subtypes 6, 11, 16, 18, 31, 33, 35, 39, 45, 51, 52, 56, 58, 59, and 68. However, up to 30% of women test positive even in the absence of any lesions.

c. **Cytology smear**

The cytological finding of koilocytotic atypia is highly suggestive of HPV infection.

3. **Syphilis**

a. **Dark-field microscopy**

Dark-field examination is the most specific diagnostic test for syphilis. It is the test of choice in the presence of a chancre, because nonspecific serology such as the VDRL may be nonreactive at this early stage. This test can be performed on lesions of primary and secondary syphilis. To obtain an adequate specimen, the following steps should be taken:

(1) Cleanse the lesion with normal saline.

(2) Abrade the lesion with a scalpel blade or sterile gauze until bleeding appears.

(3) Express serum from the lesion, and place it on a microscope slide.

(4) Place a coverslip over the specimen, and seal the edges with petroleum jelly.

b. **Nonspecific serology**

(1) VDRL test: slide flocculation test

(2) Rapid plasma reagin (RPR) test: agglutination test

Both of these tests are nonspecific antibody tests for cardiolipin antibodies that are used for the screening of syphilis. Unfortunately, both have a high rate of false-positive results. In patients with syphilis, these tests turn positive 1 to 2 weeks after the appearance of a chancre. Approximately two-thirds of patients who have primary syphilis have a positive nonspecific serology test, and 99% of patients who have secondary syphilis have a positive test. In addition to the qualitative VDRL, quantitative VDRL is sometimes helpful in making the diagnosis of syphilis and is especially useful in monitoring the therapeutic response. Most patients with a false-positive VDRL result have a titer of $<1:8$, whereas most patients with secondary syphilis have a titer of at least $1:16$. A fourfold rise in the titer is highly suggestive of acute syphilis.

4. **Chancroid**

a. **Gram stain smear**

A Gram stain smear of the exudates reveals gram-negative rods in the form of chains that appear as a "school of fish."

b. **Culture**

5. **Granuloma inguinale**

a. **Tissue smear stained with Giemsa, Leishman, or Wright stain**

No culture exists for granuloma inguinale. The diagnosis is best made by crushing a tissue specimen between two microscope slides and staining with an appropriate stain. The diagnosis is made by the demonstration of Donovan bodies, encapsulated bipolar reddish bacteria within a monocyte.

6. **Lymphogranuloma venereum**
   a. **LGV complement fixation test**
      A titer of 1:64 or higher is considered to be positive.
   b. **Microimmunofluorescence test**
      This test is more specific than the complement fixation test. A titer of 1:512 or higher is consistent with LGV.

7. **Molluscum contagiosum**
   a. **Cytological smear**
   b. **Tissue biopsy**
      The diagnosis is confirmed by the demonstration of intracytoplasmic inclusion bodies on biopsy or Pap smear of scrapings of the lesion stained with Giemsa, Gram, or Wright stain.

8. **Scabies**
   a. **Microscopic examination of skin scrapings**
      To obtain adequate skin scrapings, a fresh burrow is chosen. Mineral oil is placed on the burrow, and the top of the burrow is scraped with a sterile scalpel. The scrapings are placed on a glass slide and examined for the mite, eggs, or fecal pellets.
   b. **Burrow ink test**
      This test is painless, but there may be false-negative results. To perform the test, a fountain pen is used to cover the papule with ink. An alcohol pad is then used to wipe off the ink, and an examination is performed for a burrow with ink tracking down it forming a dark, wavy line.

9. **Pediculosis pubis or crab lice**
   Visualization with magnifying glass or microscope of the lice, larvae, or eggs.

10. **Vulvar nonneoplastic epithelial disorder or malignancy**
    a. **Vulvar biopsy**
       Although clinical history and examination is usually sufficient for making the diagnosis of vulvar vestibulitis, vulvar biopsy can be used in equivocal cases.

■ MANAGEMENT

1. **Genital herpes simplex**
   a. **Primary infection**
      (1) **Acyclovir (Zovirax)**
          (a) **400 mg PO three times per day for 7 to 10 days or until clinical resolution is attained or**

       (b) **200 mg PO five times per day for 7 to 10 days** or **until clinical resolution is attained**

    (2) **Famciclovir (Famvir) 250 mg PO three times daily for 7 to 10 days**

    (3) **Valacyclovir (Valtrex) 1 g PO twice a day for 7 to 10 days**

  b. **Recurrent infection**

    (1) **Acyclovir (Zovirax)**

       (a) **400 mg PO three times per day for 5 days** or

       (b) **800 mg PO two times per day for 5 days** or

       (c) **200 mg PO five times per day for 5 days**

    (2) **Famciclovir (Famvir) 125 mg PO twice a day for 5 days**

    (3) **Valacyclovir (Valtrex) 500 mg PO twice daily for 5 days**

  c. **Severe, hospitalized patients**

    (1) **Acyclovir (Zovirax)**

       (a) **5 to 10 mg/kg IV every 8 hours for 5 to 7 days**

  d. **Prophylaxis for recurrent infection (four or more infections per year)**

    (1) **Acyclovir (Zovirax)**

       (a) **400 mg PO two times per day** or

       (b) **200 mg PO 2 to 5 times per day**

    (2) **Famiciclovir (Famvir) 250 mg PO twice a day**

    (3) **Valacyclovir (Valtrex)**

       (a) **250 mg PO twice a day** or

       (b) **500 mg PO once a day** or

       (c) **1000 mg PO once a day**

2. **Human papillomavirus**

  a. **80 to 90% topical trichloroacetic or bichloroacetic acid**

    The acid is applied in small amounts with a cotton-tipped applicator and can be repeated weekly. Petroleum jelly can be used on adjacent normal skin to prevent spreading or running of the acid. These acids work best on mucosal warts such as those on the cervix and on the vaginal side walls but can also be used for external cutaneous warts. Most important, these acids can be used during pregnancy.

  b. **Imiquimod 5% cream (Aldara) three times a week at bedtime for a maximum of 16 weeks**

    Imiquimod is an immune-response modifier. It induces interferon-alfa and tumor necrosis factor. It also induces cell-mediated immune response to the human papillomavirus.

  c. **Podofilox (Condylox) 0.5% solution** or **podophyllin resin 10 to 25% solution in benzoin**

    The recommended use of podofilox is to apply the solution twice daily, morning and evening, for 3 consecutive days followed by a hiatus of 4 days. This weekly regimen can be repeated up to four times or until no visible warts are seen.

Podophyllin is applied to the lesions and allowed to dry. It is washed off after 3 to 4 hours, although subsequent applications can be washed off after 24 hours. Applications can be repeated once or twice weekly until the lesions have disappeared.

Because of the potential complications of myelotoxicity and neurotoxicity, these agents cannot be used in pregnancy and furthermore cannot be used in the vagina or on the cervix.

d. **Local sharp excision**

Excision with a scalpel is most appropriate for large, pedunculated lesions.

e. **Carbon dioxide laser vaporization**

Laser vaporization can be performed with colposcopic guidance to magnify small and subtle lesions. Laser vaporization is the treatment of choice for extensive disease. It can be used for internal lesions on the cervix and vaginal wall and external lesions of the vulva.

f. **Electrocauterization**

g. **Cryocautery**

Cryocautery is most appropriate for small lesions.

3. **Syphilis**

a. **Primary, secondary, or early latent syphilis**

(1) **Benzathine penicillin G 2.4 million units IM once** or
(2) **Doxycycline 100 mg PO two times per day for 2 weeks** or
(3) **Tetracycline 500 mg PO four times per day for 2 weeks** or
(4) **Erythromycin 500 mg PO four times per day for 2 weeks**

b. **Late latent syphilis or latent syphilis of undetermined duration**

(1) **Benzathine penicillin G 2.4 million units IM weekly for 3 weeks** or
(2) **Doxycycline 100 mg PO two times per day for 2 to 4 weeks** or
(3) **Tetracycline 500 mg PO four times per day for 2 to 4 weeks**

Treatment with doxycycline or tetracycline is recommended for 2 weeks if the duration of infection is <1 year. Otherwise, treatment should be for 4 weeks.

4. **Chancroid**

a. **Azithromycin 1 PO once** or
b. **Ceftriaxone 250 mg IM once** or

    c. **Erythromycin 500 mg PO four times per day for 7 days** or

    d. **Ciprofloxacin 500 mg PO two times per day for 3 days**

5. **Granuloma inguinale**

    a. **Tetracycline 500 mg PO four times per day for 21 days** or

    b. **Erythromycin 500 mg PO four times per day for 21 days**

6. **Lymphogranuloma venereum**

    a. **Doxycycline 100 mg PO two times per day for 21 days** or

    b. **Erythromycin 500 mg PO four times per day for 21 days** or

    c. **Sulfisoxazole 500 mg PO four times per day for 21 days**

7. **Molluscum contagiosum**

    a. **Sharp scraping of the lesion followed by electrocautery or application of silver nitrate, trichloroacetic acid, or carbonic acid** or

    b. **Cryocautery of the lesions**

8. **Scabies**

    Any of the following three drugs can be used. Clothing and linen should be cleaned in hot water or dry-cleaned.

    a. **Crotamiton (Eurax) 10% cream or lotion** applied as follows:

        (1) Take routine shower or bath.

        (2) Apply cream or lotion from neck down to toes.

        (3) Repeat application 24 hours later.

        (4) Take a cleansing bath 48 hours after last application.

    Crotamiton may be used in pregnant and lactating women.

    b. **Lindane (Kwell) 1% cream or lotion** applied from neck down, left on for 8 to 12 hours, then washed off.

        Because this drug does not kill the eggs, treatment should be repeated in 1 week. Lindane is not recommended for pregnant or lactating women.

    c. **Permethrin (Elimite) 5% cream** applied once on the skin from head to toes and washed off in the shower or bath in 8 to 14 hours.

        Permethrin can be used by pregnant and lactating women.

9. **Pediculosis pubis**

    a. **Lindane (Kwell) 1% cream or lotion** applied to affected area for 8 to 12 hours, then washed off.

        As an alternative, **Lindane (Kwell) 1% shampoo** applied for 4 minutes, then washed off. Lindane is not recommended for pregnant or lactating women.

    b. **Pyrethrins (A-200 Pediculicide shampoo and gel)** applied to dry hair or other affected areas for 10 minutes, then washed off.

    With either drug, repeat treatment may be necessary in 1 week if lice or eggs are still seen. Clothing and bed linen used by the patient within the past 2 days should be washed in hot water or should be dry-cleaned.

10. Squamous cell hyperplasia
    a. **Low- to medium-potency topical steroids**
       (1) **Fluocinolone acetonide 0.025% or 0.01% cream or lotion applied two or three times per day** or
       (2) **Triamcinolone acetonide 0.01% cream or lotion applied two or three times per day**
    b. **Nonmedical treatment**
       (1) Personal hygiene; keep vulva dry
       (2) Avoid irritating soaps or lotions
11. Lichen sclerosus
    a. **High-potency topical steroids**
       (1) **Clobetasol propionate (Temovate) 0.05% cream applied twice daily for 2 to 3 weeks, then once daily until there is improvement**
       (2) **Halobetasol propionate (Ultravate) 0.05% cream applied twice daily for 2 to 3 weeks, then once daily until there is improvement**
    After improvement is achieved, either cream can be applied one to three times weekly for long-term maintenance.
    b. **Nonmedical treatment**
       (1) Personal hygiene; keep vulva dry
       (2) Avoid irritating soaps or lotions
       (3) Use simple emollients such as lanolin
       (4) Vaginal dilators for stenosis of the introitus
12. **Vulvar vestibulitis**
    There is no established therapy for vestibulitis. Numerous medical regimens have been used, and surgery has also been performed on patients with intractable symptoms. Most cases improve spontaneously after several years even without therapy.
    a. **Topical steroid creams**
    b. **Topical estrogen cream: Premarin vaginal cream applied daily**
    c. **Topical 2% lidocaine gel or 5% ointment**
    d. **Antifungal therapy (see Chapter 36)**
    e. **Oral steroids**
    f. **Vulvar vestibulectomy**

36 | Vulvovaginitis

■ BACKGROUND AND DEFINITION

Normal vaginal discharge is usually white and odorless and has a pH of 3.5 to 4.2. The discharge can be copious enough to pool in the posterior vaginal fornix. Therefore, the mere presence of vaginal discharge is not necessarily indicative of a vulvovaginal infection. Furthermore, there are many bacteria that can be detected in normal patients. Table 36–1 shows some of the more commonly encountered organisms. *Lactobacillus acidophilus* is a predominant organism found in normal women. *Lactobacillus* inhibits the growth of other bacteria by adhering to vaginal epithelial cells, by producing lactic acid to maintain a normal pH, and by producing hydrogen peroxide.

Vulvovaginitis: Inflammation involving the vulva and vagina resulting in symptoms of vaginal discharge, itching, burning, dyspareunia, or foul odor

Vulvovaginitis is one of the most common gynecological problems in adult women. Most patients with vulvovaginitis have one of the following four common conditions:
1. Yeast or *Candida* vulvovaginitis caused by *Candida albicans* and other *Candida* species
2. Bacterial vaginosis caused by *Gardnerella vaginalis* and other anaerobic vaginal bacteria
3. *Trichomonas* vulvovaginitis caused by the protozoan *Trichomonas vaginalis*
4. Atrophic vaginitis.

The characteristics of these four vulvovaginal conditions are listed in Table 36–2. Up to 50% of patients with *Trichomonas* infection are asymptomatic. The evaluation of a patient with a vulvovaginal infection can be accomplished in a matter of minutes, and the treatment is often simple and effective.

Table 36–1 □ NORMAL VAGINAL FLORA

Lactobacillus acidophilus	*Gardnerella vaginalis*
Escherichia coli	*Clostridium* spp.
Bacteroides fragilis	*Enterococcus*
Staphylococcus aureus	*Candida* spp.
Group B streptococci	

Table 36-2 □ COMPARISON OF THE FOUR MOST COMMON VULVOVAGINAL INFECTIONS

Parameter	Yeast Vulvovaginitis	Bacterial Vaginosis	*Trichomonas* Vulvovaginitis	Atrophic Vaginitis
Cause	*Candida* spp.	*Gardnerella vaginalis*, mixed anaerobes	*Trichomonas vaginalis*	Estrogen deficiency
Major symptoms	Itching, burning	Malodorous, watery discharge	Itching, burning, variable	Itching, vaginal dryness, burning
Discharge	White, cottage cheese	White, skim milk	Frothy, variable	Usually absent
Odor	Absent	Present	Variable	Absent
Vulvovaginal inflammation	Present	Absent or minimal	Variable	Present
Vaginal wet smear	Hyphae, spores	"Clue cells"	Trichomonads	No organisms
"Whiff test"	Negative	Positive	Negative	Negative
Vaginal pH	Normal, 3–4	Basic, 5–6	Basic, 6–7	Basic, 6–7
Treatment	Antifungal drugs	Metronidazole	Metronidazole	Estrogen supplementation

■ CLINICAL PRESENTATION

Vaginal itching or burning
Vaginal discharge
Malodorous discharge
Dyspareunia
Vulvar or vaginal erythema

■ PHONE CALL

Questions

1. **What symptoms is the patient complaining of?**
2. **Does the patient have pelvic pain or a fever?**
    These symptoms would be suggestive of pelvic inflammatory disease (PID), which can cause abnormal discharge similar to that caused by vulvovaginitis.

Degree of Urgency

Vulvovaginal infection is rarely serious or life-threatening and the patient does not need to be seen immediately.

■ ELEVATOR THOUGHTS

What is the differential diagnosis of vulvovaginal infection?
- Cervicitis
- PID
- Normal physiological cervical discharge

■ BEDSIDE

Quick Look Test

Patients with vulvovaginal infection do not usually appear ill or distressed. If the patient appears ill, PID should be suspected.

Vital Signs

Patients with vulvovaginal infections will usually have normal vital signs. The finding of fever is suggestive of PID.

Selective History and Chart Review

1. Is the patient pregnant?

   Certain antibiotics are contraindicated in pregnancy. Furthermore, pregnancy increases the risk of yeast or *Candida* vulvovaginitis.

2. Does the patient have a history of recurrent vulvovaginal infections?

3. Does the patient have a history of any sexually transmitted diseases?

4. Is the patient taking antibiotics?

   Use of antibiotics can predispose to yeast vulvovaginitis. Between 25 and 75% of women who use antibiotics develop yeast vulvovaginitis.

5. Is the patient using oral contraceptive pills?

   The use of birth control pills increases the risk of yeast vulvovaginitis.

6. Has the patient used any agents that can cause an allergic reaction or contact dermatitis?

Selective Physical Examination

Abdominal	Soft and nontender; a tender abdomen, especially with guarding and rebound tenderness, is suggestive of PID
Pelvic	
External genitalia and vagina	Yeast vulvovaginitis: erythematous with a white, "cottage cheese"–like discharge
	Bacterial vaginosis: nonerythematous with white, watery, skim milk–like malodorous discharge
	Trichomonas vulvovaginitis: erythematous with frothy, foul-smelling discharge
	Atrophic vaginitis: pale, dry, thin vaginal epithelium
Cervix	*Trichomonas* vulvovaginitis: erythematous "flea-bitten" or "strawberry" cervix, often friable and bleeding
	PID and cervicitis: usually with mucopurulent discharge with cervical motion tenderness
Uterus and adnexa	PID: usually tender to palpation

In any case of vulvovaginitis, the pelvic examination can be normal with the absence of discharge, and therefore, confirmation of the diagnosis should depend on laboratory testing and not just pelvic examination. The clinical manifestations of *Trichomonas* vulvovaginitis are especially variable, with an estimated 10 to 50% of infected women being asymptomatic.

Orders

1. Prepare the patient for a pelvic examination, and have available materials necessary for the preparation of wet smears of the vaginal discharge with both normal saline and 10% potassium hydroxide solutions.
2. Obtain a complete blood count (CBC) with differential if the patient has signs and symptoms of PID.
3. Obtain cervical cultures for *Chlamydia trachomatis* and *Neisseria gonorrhoeae* if cervicitis or PID is suspected.

■ DIAGNOSTIC TESTING (see Table 36–2)

1. **Yeast vulvovaginitis**
   a. **Vaginal wet smear with 10% potassium hydroxide**
      Hyphae and spores are noted in approximately 50 to 70% of women with yeast vulvovaginitis.
   b. **Vaginal fungal culture**
      Vaginal cultures are rarely necessary to make the diagnosis of vulvovaginitis. Fungal cultures are indicated only in patients with symptoms of yeast vulvovaginitis with negative vaginal wet smears.
2. **Bacterial vaginosis**
   a. **Vaginal wet smear with normal saline shows "clue cells"**
      In patients with bacterial vaginosis, clue cells are vaginal epithelial cells with a stippled cell wall because of the adherence of the causative bacteria onto the cell wall. The presence of clue cells signifies a high concentration of bacteria and is a more sensitive indicator of clinical infection than cultures.
   b. **Positive "whiff test" or amine test**
      A positive whiff test or amine test is the detection of a fishy or nitrogen odor when vaginal secretions are mixed with 10% potassium hydroxide.
   c. **pH of vaginal secretions is basic with a pH value of 5 to 6**
      The pH of normal vaginal secretions is acidic with a pH value of 3 to 4. Patients with bacterial vaginosis have a more basic vaginal secretion with a pH of 5 to 6.
      Table 36–3 lists the recommended criteria that should be used to make the diagnosis of bacterial vaginosis.
3. *Trichomonas* **vulvovaginitis**
   a. **Normal saline shows motile trichomonads and abundant white blood cells**

Table 36–3 □ **DIAGNOSTIC CRITERIA FOR BACTERIAL VAGINOSIS**

At least three of the following should be present:
pH >4.5
At least 20% of epithelial cells are clue cells
Homogeneous discharge with only a few white blood cells
Positive "whiff test" or amine test

The diagnosis of this vulvovaginal infection is most easily made because of the finding of the motile *Trichomonas* protozoa on vaginal wet smear. The organism has an ovoid body and a posterior flagellum and is usually found moving in circles in a jerky fashion.

b. Trichomonads can be detected on routine cervical Pap smear in 70% of cases
c. pH of vaginal secretions is very basic with a pH of 6 to 7
d. "Strawberry cervix" caused by punctated hemorrhagic lesions of the cervix is seen in 25% of patients

■ MANAGEMENT

1. Yeast vulvovaginitis
   a. Acute infection
      (1) Antifungal medication (Table 36–4)
   b. Recurrent infection
      (1) **Clotrimazole 500 mg vaginal suppository weekly** or
      (2) **Fluconazole 150 mg tablet PO once a month** or
      (3) **Ketoconazole 200 mg tablet PO daily** or
      (4) **Ketoconazole 400 mg tablet PO daily for 5 days each month starting with menses**
      (5) **Eliminate predisposing causes**

Yeast or candidal infection is usually caused by *C. albicans*, although approximately 10% of cases are caused by non-*albicans* species such as *C. glabrata, C. tropicalis,* and *C. parapsilosis.* One or more species of *Candida* can be recovered in approximately 30% of pregnant and 15% of nonpregnant asymptomatic women. These asymptomatic patients do not require treatment. In symptomatic patients, yeast vaginitis can usually be easily and effectively treated with any of several antifungal imidazole and triazole derivatives, many of which are now available over the counter. These medications are available in the form of a vaginal cream or vaginal suppository or an oral pill. All of these antifungal agents have comparable efficacy, with cure rates greater than 90%.

Despite this high cure rate, some patients continue to have

Table 36–4 □ ANTIFUNGAL MEDICATIONS FOR ACUTE YEAST VULVOVAGINITIS

Medication	Formulation	Dose
Butoconazole		
Femstat	2% vaginal cream	5 g every night for 3 nights
Clotrimazole		
Gyne-Lotrimin	100-mg vaginal tablet	1 tablet every night for 7 nights
	1% vaginal cream	5 g every night for 7 nights
Mycelex-G	500-mg vaginal tablet	1 tablet once
Mycelex-7	100-mg vaginal insert	1 insert every night for 7 nights
	1% vaginal cream	5 g every night for 7 nights
Fluconazole		
Diflucan	150-mg oral tablet	1 tablet orally once
Miconazole		
Monistat 3	200-mg suppository	1 every night for 3 nights
Monistat 7	2% cream	5 g every night for 7 nights
	100-mg suppository	1 every night for 7 nights
Terconazole		
Terazol 3	80-mg suppository	1 every night for 3 nights
	0.8% vaginal cream	5 g every night for 3 nights
Terazol 7	0.4% vaginal cream	5 g every night for 7 nights
Tioconazole		
Vagistat-1	6.5% ointment	4.6 g once
Boric acid	600 mg in gelatin capsule	1 vaginal capsule daily for 14 days

recurrent yeast infections, and this is often frustrating to both the patients and their physicians. A patient is considered to have recurrent yeast vulvovaginitis if she has four or more episodes of yeast vulvovaginitis in a year. Possible causes of recurrent yeast infections are listed in Table 36–5. In many patients, no specific cause is found. Nevertheless, the management of recurrent yeast infections begins with the elimination of these causes where possible. Oral antifungal medication has been recommended to decrease the amount of yeast in the gastrointestinal tract. Both oral ketoconazole and fluconazole have been shown to be effective in treating patients with recurrent infections. The weekly use of a 500-mg clotrimazole vaginal suppository has also been shown to be effective.

2. **Bacterial vaginosis**
   a. **Metronidazole (Flagyl) 500 mg PO two times per day for 7 days** or
   b. **Metronidazole (Flagyl) 250 mg PO three times per day for 7 days** or

Table 36–5 □ CAUSES OF RECURRENT YEAST VULVOVAGINITIS

Diabetes mellitus
Immunosuppressed state
  Steroid treatment
  Chemotherapy administration
  Acquired immunodeficiency syndrome (AIDS)
Antibiotic therapy
Oral contraceptive pills
Pregnancy
Increased yeast colonization of the gastrointestinal tract
Infection with *Candida* spp. resistant to current antifungal drugs

---

   c. **Metronidazole (Flagyl) 2 g PO one time** or
   d. **Metronidazole 0.75% vaginal gel (MetroGel-Vaginal) 5 g (1 applicator full) intravaginally two times per day for 5 days** or
   e. **Clindamycin (Cleocin) 300 mg PO twice per day for 7 days** or
   f. **Clindamycin (Cleocin) 2% vaginal cream 5 g (1 applicator full) intravaginally every night for 7 days**
      Bacterial vaginosis has implications beyond those of a vulvo-vaginal infection. A positive correlation has been found between bacterial vaginosis and premature labor, premature rupture of membranes, chorioamnionitis, endometritis, PID, postabortal infection, and infections occurring after a variety of gynecological surgical procedures. The 7-day regimens of metronidazole have cure rates of 90 to 95%, whereas the single-dose regimen has a slightly lower cure rate of approximately 70%. Broad-spectrum antibiotics such as ampicillin, erythromycin, and doxycycline are somewhat less effective, with cure rates of 40 to 50%. Sulfonamide-containing vaginal creams are also only minimally effective.
      Metronidazole is a category B drug because of findings of carcinogenic effects on rodents. However, human studies have not shown any increase in congenital anomalies in infants born to women who used metronidazole in pregnancy. Intravaginal metronidazole may be considered because it results in peak serum concentrations <2% of the concentration of the 7-day 500-mg oral regimen. Alternatively, oral clindamycin may be used. Patients being treated with metronidazole should be warned to avoid ingestion of alcohol because of nausea and vomiting from a disulfiram reaction.
3. *Trichomonas* **vulvovaginitis**
   a. **Metronidazole (Flagyl) 2.0 g PO once** or
   b. **Metronidazole (Flagyl) 500 mg PO twice a day for 7 days**
      Trichomonas vulvovaginitis is a sexually transmitted disease,

and therefore patients should be advised to have their partners evaluated and treated if necessary. Approximately 40 to 60% of male partners of infected women harbor the organism. The oral regimens of metronidazole result in cure rates of 90 to 95%. As discussed previously, rodent studies have shown teratogenic effects of metronidazole, although no such findings have been demonstrated in humans. Unfortunately, metronidazole gel is not effective against *Trichomonas* spp. The single-dose regimen of 2 g metronidazole is recommended for pregnant women beyond the first trimester of pregnancy. Alternatively, vaginal clotrimazole can be considered, although the cure rate is only 48% and the use of clotrimazole for this indication has not yet received approval by the U.S. Food and Drug Administration.

4. **Atrophic vaginitis**
   a. **Conjugated estrogen (Premarin) vaginal cream 1 to 4 g daily initially, tapering to 1 to 3 doses every week or 3 weeks on followed by 1 week off**
   b. **Estradiol 0.01% vaginal cream 2 to 4 g daily initially, tapering to a maintenance dose of 1 g one to three times every week**

Atrophic vaginitis also responds to numerous oral regimens of estrogen replacement. In the patient with an intact uterus, estrogen replacement should usually be accompanied by progestin replacement.

APPENDICES

APPENDIX A

Guidelines, Illustrations, and Tables for Obstetrics

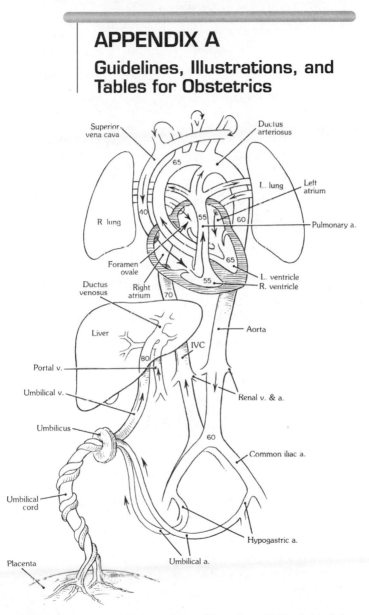

Figure A–1 □ Normal fetal circulation. (From Parer JJ: Fetal circulation. In Sciarra JJ, ed: Obstetrics and Gynecology, Vol 3, Maternal and Fetal Medicine. Hagerstown, MD, Harper & Row, 1984, p 2.)

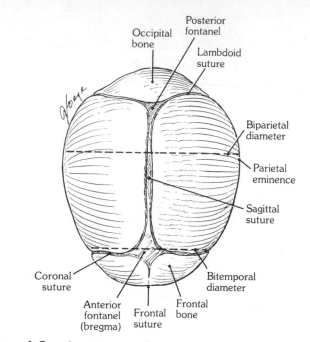

Figure A–2 □ Superior view of fetal skull and diameters. (From Hacker NF, Moore JG: Essentials of Obstetrics and Gynecology, 3rd ed. Philadelphia, WB Saunders Co, 1998, p 140.)

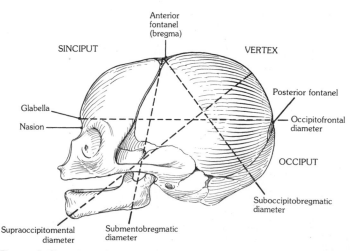

Figure A–3 □ Lateral view of fetal skull and diameters. (From Hacker NF, Moore JG: Essentials of Obstetrics and Gynecology, 3rd ed. Philadelphia, WB Saunders Co, 1998, p 141.)

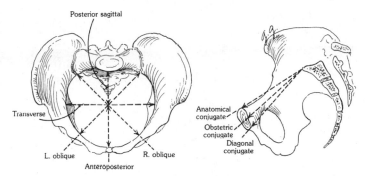

Figure A–4 □ Pelvic inlet. (From Hacker NF, Moore JG: Essentials of Obstetrics and Gynecology, 3rd ed. Philadelphia, WB Saunders Co, 1998, p 143.)

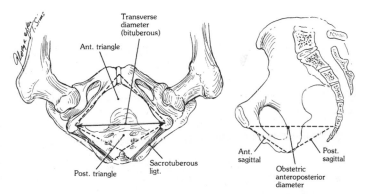

Figure A–5 □ Pelvic outlet. (From Hacker NF, Moore JG: Essentials of Obstetrics and Gynecology, 3rd ed. Philadelphia, WB Saunders Co, 1998, p 144.)

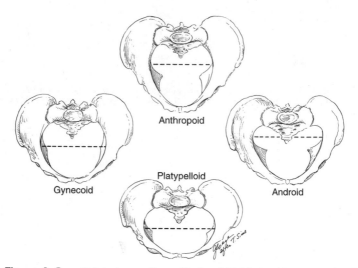

Figure A–6 □ Pelvic types. (From Hacker NF, Moore JG: Essentials of Obstetrics and Gynecology, 3rd ed. Philadelphia, WB Saunders Co, 1998, p 145.)

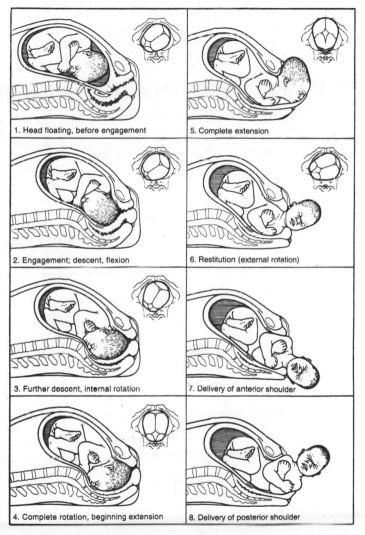

1. Head floating, before engagement

5. Complete extension

2. Engagement; descent, flexion

6. Restitution (external rotation)

3. Further descent, internal rotation

7. Delivery of anterior shoulder

4. Complete rotation, beginning extension

8. Delivery of posterior shoulder

Figure A–7 □ Movements in the mechanism of labor and delivery, left occiput anterior position. (From Cunningham FG, MacDonald PC, Gant NF, et al: Williams Obstetrics, 19th ed. Norwalk, CT, Appleton & Lange, 1993, p 364. Reproduced with permission of the McGraw-Hill Companies.)

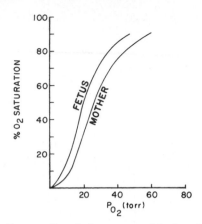

Figure A–8 □ Oxygen dissociation curves of fetal and maternal blood at pH 7.4 and 37°C. (From Hellegers AE, Schruefer JJ: Nomograms and empirical equations relating oxygen tension, percentage saturation, and pH in maternal and fetal blood. Am J Obstet Gynecol 1961;81:377.)

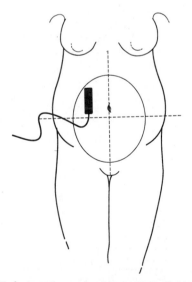

Figure A–9 □ Technique for measuring amniotic fluid index. The uterus is divided into quadrants. The transducer is held perpendicular to the floor, and the largest vertical pocket of amniotic fluid without loops of umbilical cord is measured in each quadrant and summed. (From Creasy RK, Resnik R: Maternal-Fetal Medicine: Principles and Practice, 3rd ed. Philadelphia, WB Saunders Co, 1994, p 621.)

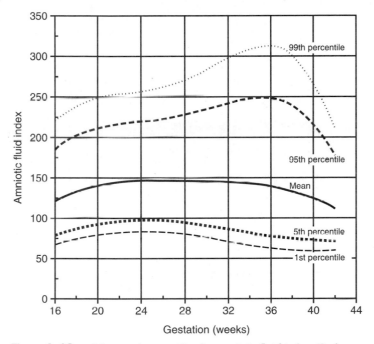

Figure A–10 □ Mean and percentiles for amniotic fluid index. (Redrawn from Moore TR, Cayle JE: Amniotic fluid index in normal human pregnancy. Am J Obstet Gynecol 1990;162:1168.)

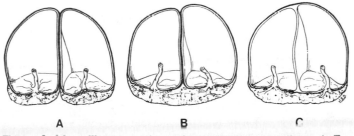

Figure A–11 □ Placenta and membranes in twin gestations. *A*, Two placentas, diamniotic, dichorionic (from either dizygotic or monozygotic twins). *B*, Single placenta, diamniotic, dichorionic (from either dizygotic or monozygotic twins). *C*, Single placenta, diamniotic, monochorionic (from monozygotic twins). (From Cunningham FG, MacDonald PC, Gant NF, et al: Williams Obstetrics, 19th ed. Norwalk, CT, Appleton & Lange, 1993, p 892. Reproduced with permission of the McGraw-Hill Companies.)

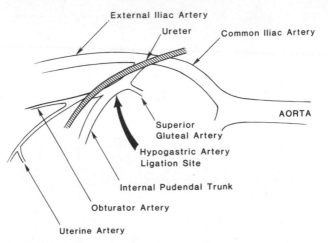

Figure A–12 □ Site of hypogastric artery ligation. (From Creasy RK, Resnik R: Maternal-Fetal Medicine: Principles and Practice, 4th ed. Philadelphia, WB Saunders Co, 1999, p 912.)

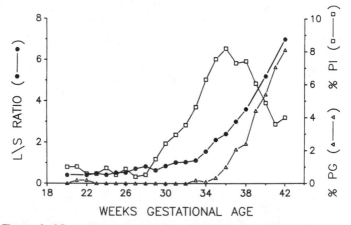

Figure A–13 □ Amniotic fluid phospholipid levels and gestational age. L/S = lecithin/sphingomyelin ratio; PG = phosphatidylglycerol; PI = phosphatidylinositol. (Data from Gluck L, et al: Am J Obstet Gynecol 1974;120:142, and Hallman M, et al: Am J Obstet Gynecol 1976;125:613, as shown in Jobe A: The developmental biology of the lung. In Fanaroff AA, Martin RJ, eds: Neonatal-Perinatal Medicine. St. Louis, Mosby-Year Book, 1992, p 792. From Creasy RK, Resnik R: Maternal-Fetal Medicine: Principles and Practice, 4th ed. Philadelphia, WB Saunders Co, 1999, p 417.)

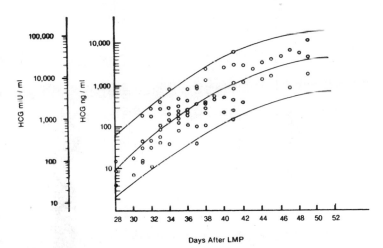

Figure A–14 □ Rise in serum hCG in normal intrauterine pregnancies. LMP = last menstrual period. (From Pittaway DE, Reish RL, Wentz AC: Doubling times of human chorionic gonadotropin increase in early viable intrauterine pregnancies. Am J Obstet Gynecol 1985;152:299.)

Table A–1 □ **COMPONENTS OF THE FETAL CIRCULATION**

Fetal Structure	From/To	Adult Remnant
Umbilical vein	Umbilicus/ductus venosus	Ligamentum teres hepatis
Ductus venosus	Umbilical vein/inferior vena cava (bypasses liver)	Ligamentum venosum
Foramen ovale	Right atrium/left atrium	Closed atrial wall
Ductus arteriosus	Pulmonary artery/descending aorta	Ligamentum arteriosum
Umbilical artery	Common iliac artery/umbilicus	Superior vesical arteries Lateral vesicoumbilical ligaments

Adapted from Main DM, Main EK: Obstetrics and Gynecology: A Pocket Reference. Chicago, Year Book, 1984, p 34.

Table A-2 □ COMMON LABORATORY VALUES IN PREGNANCY

Test	Normal Range (Nonpregnant)	Change in Pregnancy	Timing
Serum Chemistries			
Albumin	3.5–4.8 g/dl	↓ 1 g/dl	Most by 20 weeks, then gradual
Calcium (total)	9–10.3 mg/dl	↓ 10%	Gradual fall
Chloride	95–105 mEq/L	No significant change	Gradual rise
Creatinine	0.6–1.1 mg/dl	↓ 0.3 mg/dl	Most by 20 weeks
Fibrinogen	1.5–3.6 g/L	↑ 1–2 g/L	Progressive
Glucose, fasting (plasma)	65–105 mg/dl	↓ 10%	Gradual fall
Potassium (plasma)	3.5–4.5 mEq/L	↓ 0.2–0.3 mEq/L	By 20 weeks
Protein (total)	6.5–8.5 g/dl	↓ 1 g/dl	By 20 weeks, then stable
Sodium	135–145 mEq/L	↓ 2–4 mEq/L	By 20 weeks, then stable
Urea nitrogen	12–30 mg/dl	↓ 50%	First trimester
Uric acid	3.5–8 mg/dl	↓ 33%	First trimester, rise at term
Urinary Chemistries			
Creatinine	15–25 mg/kg/day (1–1.4 g/day)	No significant change	
Protein	Up to 150 mg/day	Up to 250–300 mg/day	By 20 weeks
Creatinine clearance	90–130 ml/min per 1.73 m²	↑ 40–50%	By 16 weeks

Serum Enzymatic Activities

Amylase	23–84 IU/L	↑ 50–100% Controversial
Aminotransferase		
Alanine (ALT)	5–35 mU/ml	No significant change
Aspartate (AST)	5–40 mU/ml	No significant change

Hematology

Hematocrit	36–46%	↓ 4–7% Bottoms at 30–34 weeks
Hemoglobin	12–16 g/dl	↓ 1.5–2 g/dl Bottoms at 30–34 weeks
Leukocyte count	$4.8–10.8 \times 10^3/mm^3$	↑ $3.5 \times 10^3/mm^3$ Gradual
Platelet count	$150–400 \times 10^3/mm^3$	Slight decrease

Serum Hormone Values

Cortisol (plasma)	8–21 μg/dl	↑ 20 μg/dl
Prolactin	25 ng/ml	↑ 50–400 ng/ml Gradual, peaks at term
Thyroxine, total (T$_4$)	5–11 μg/dl	↑ 5 μg/dl Early sustained
Triiodothyronine, total (T$_3$)	125–245 ng/dl	↑ 50% Early sustained

Adapted from Main DM, Main EK: Obstetrics and Gynecology: A Pocket Reference. Chicago, Year Book, 1984, p 7.

Table A–3 □ WEIGHT GAIN IN PREGNANCY

Tissues and Fluids	Increase in Weight (g) Up to			
	10 Weeks	20 Weeks	30 Weeks	40 Weeks
Fetus	5	300	1500	3400
Placenta	20	170	430	650
Amniotic fluid	30	350	750	800
Uterus	140	320	600	970
Mammary gland	45	180	360	405
Blood	100	600	1300	1250
Interstitial fluid (no edema or leg edema)	0	30	80	1680
Maternal stores	310	2050	3480	3345
Total weight gained	650	4000	8500	12,500

Adapted from Hyten F, Chamberlain G, eds: Clinical Physiology in Obstetrics. Oxford, Blackwell Scientific, 1980, p 221.

Table A–4 □ NORMAL CENTRAL HEMODYNAMIC MEASUREMENTS IN NONPREGNANT AND PREGNANT PATIENTS

Parameter	Nonpregnant	Pregnant
Cardiac output (L/min)	4.3 ± 0.9	6.2 ± 1.0
Heart rate (beats/min)	71 ± 10.0	83 ± 10.0
Systemic vascular resistance (dyne $\times$ cm $\times$ sec^{-5})	1530 ± 520	1210 ± 266
Pulmonary vascular resistance (dyne $\times$ cm $\times$ sec^{-5})	119 ± 47.0	78 ± 22
Colloid oncotic pressure (mm Hg)	20.8 ± 1.0	18.0 ± 1.5
Colloid oncotic pressure–pulmonary capillary wedge pressure (mm Hg)	14.5 ± 2.5	10.5 ± 2.7
Mean arterial pressure (mm Hg)	86.4 ± 7.5	90.3 ± 5.8
Pulmonary capillary wedge pressure (mm Hg)	6.3 ± 2.1	7.5 ± 1.8
Central venous pressure (mm Hg)	3.7 ± 2.6	3.6 ± 2.5
Left ventricular stroke work index (g $\times$ m $\times$ m^{-2})	41 ± 8	48 ± 6

From Clark SL, Cotton DB, Lee W, et al: Central hemodynamic assessments in normal term pregnancy. Am J Obstet Gynecol 1989;161:1439.

Table A-5 □ NORMAL DURATION OF THE STAGES OF LABOR

Stages of Labor	Nullipara	Multipara
First stage		
Latent phase	≤20 hr	≤14 hr
Active phase	5–8 hr	2–5 hr
Rate of dilatation	≥1.2 cm/hr	≥1.5 cm/hr
Second stage	≤2 hr	≤1 hr
Third stage	≤30 min	≤30 min

Table A-6 □ LENGTH OF PELVIC DIAMETERS

Pelvic Plane	Diameter	Average Length (cm)
Inlet	True conjugate	11.5
	Obstetric conjugate	11
	Transverse	13.5
	Oblique	12.5
	Posterior sagittal	4.5
Greatest diameter	Anteroposterior	12.75
	Transverse	12.5
Midplane	Anteroposterior	12
	Bispinous	10.5
	Posterior sagittal	4.5–5
Outlet	Anatomical anteroposterior	9.5
	Obstetric anteroposterior	11.5
	Bituberous	11
	Posterior sagittal	7.5

From Hacker NF, Moore JG: Essentials of Obstetrics and Gynecology, 3rd ed. Philadelphia, WB Saunders Co, 1998, p 143.

Table A–7 □ BIOPHYSICAL PROFILE SCORING: TECHNIQUE AND INTERPRETATION

Biophysical Variable	Normal Score	Abnormal (Score = 0)
Fetal breathing movements	At least 1 episode of FBM of at least 30 sec duration in 30 min observation	Absent FBM or no episode of ≥30 sec in 30 min
Gross body movement	At least 3 discrete body/limb movements in 30 min (episodes of active continuous movement considered as single movement)	2 or fewer episodes of body/limb movements in 30 min
Fetal tone	At least 1 episode of active extension with return to flexion of fetal limb or trunk. Opening and closing of hand considered normal tone	Either slow extension with return to partial flexion or movement of limb in full extension or absent fetal movement with fetal hand held in complete or partial deflection
Reactive FHR	At least 2 episodes of FHR acceleration of ≥15 beat/min and of at least 15 sec duration associated with fetal movement in 30 min	Less than 2 episodes of acceleration of FHR or acceleration of <15 beats/min in 30 min
Qualitative AFV*	At least 1 pocket of AF that measures at least 2 cm in 2 perpendicular planes	Either no AF pockets or pocket <2 cm in 2 perpendicular planes

FBM = fetal breathing movement; FHR = fetal heart rate; AFV = amniotic fluid volume; AF = amniotic fluid.

*Modification of the criteria for reduced amniotic fluid from <1 cm to <2 cm would seem reasonable.

From Creasy RK, Resnik R: Maternal-Fetal Medicine: Principles and Practice, 4th ed. Philadelphia, WB Saunders Co, 1999, p 322.

Table A–8 □ BIOPHYSICAL PROFILE SCORING: MANAGEMENT

Score	Interpretation	Recommended Management
10	Normal infant, low risk for chronic asphyxia	Repeat testing at weekly intervals; repeat twice weekly in diabetic patients and patients ≥42 weeks' gestation
8	Normal infant, low risk for chronic asphyxia	Repeat testing at weekly intervals; repeat twice weekly in diabetic patients and patients ≥42 weeks; oligohydramnios indication for delivery
6	Suspected chronic asphyxia	Repeat testing in 4–6 hr; deliver if oligohydramnios present
4	Suspected chronic asphyxia	If ≥36 weeks and favorable, then deliver; if ≥36 weeks and L / S <2.0, repeat test in 24 hr; if repeat score <4, deliver
0–2	Strong suspicion of chronic asphyxia	Extend testing time to 120 min; if persistent score <4, deliver, provided gestational age is sufficiently advanced to permit possible neonatal survival

L/S = amniotic fluid lecithin/sphingomyelin ratio.
From Creasy RK, Resnik R: Maternal-Fetal Medicine: Principles and Practice, 4th ed. Philadelphia, WB Saunders Co, 1999, p 322.

Table A–9 □ APGAR SCORING SYSTEM

Sign	Score		
	0	1	2
Heart rate	Absent	<100 beats / min	>100 beats / min
Respiratory effort	Absent	Slow, irregular	Good, crying
Muscle tone	Limp	Some flexion of extremities	Active motion
Reflex irritability	Absent	Grimace	Vigorous cry
Color	Pale, blue	Body pink, extremities blue	Completely pink

Table A–10 □ STEPS FOR PERFORMING AMNIOTIC FLUID "SHAKE TEST"

Materials needed	Amniotic fluid recently collected
	95% ethanol (19 parts of absolute alcohol mixed with 1 part of distilled water)
	0.9% saline
	Two 13 × 100-mm glass tubes with Teflon-lined plastic screw cap
Steps of test	1. Mix 1 ml of amniotic fluid and 1 ml of ethanol in one tube.
	2. Mix 0.5 ml of amniotic fluid, 0.5 ml of saline, and 1 ml of ethanol in the second tube.
	3. Shake both tubes for 15 seconds and place tubes upright.
	4. Wait for 15 minutes and look for a ring of bubble or foam at the air–liquid interface.
Results	Positive test: ring of bubbles is observed in both tubes
	Equivocal test: ring of bubbles is observed only in first tube
	Negative test: ring of bubbles is not observed in either tube

Table A–11 □ INTERPRETATION OF RESULTS OF DIAGNOSTIC PERITONEAL LAVAGE* AFTER BLUNT TRAUMA

Positive†
  Grossly bloody lavage fluid
  RBC count >100,000/mm³
  WBC count >175/mm³
  Amylase >175/dl
  Lavage fluid identified in Foley catheter
Indeterminate‡
  RBC count >50,000 but <100,000/mm³
  WBC count >100 but <500/mm³
  Amylase >75 but <175/dl
Negative
  RBC count <50,000/mm³
  WBC count <100/mm³
  Amylase <75/dl

RBC = red blood cell; WBC = white blood cell.
*Peritoneal lavage performed with 1 L of Ringer's lactated solution.
†Positive lavage (any one criterion) suggests need for surgical exploration.
‡Recommendations are to repeat lavage.
Modified from Rothenberger DA, Quattlesbaum FW, Zabel J, et al: Diagnostic peritoneal lavage for blunt trauma in pregnant women. Am J Obstet Gynecol 1977;129:479.

Table A–12 □ ESTIMATED OVARIAN RADIATION EXPOSURE
FROM COMMON RADIOLOGIC PROCEDURES*

Procedure	Estimated Ovarian Dose (millirad)	Average Number of Films per Examination
Chest examination		
Radiography	8	1.4
Fluoroscopy	71	
Upper GI series		
Total	558	4.4
Radiography	360	
Fluoroscopy	198	
Barium enema		
Total	805	3.5
Radiography	439	
Fluoroscopy	366	
Intravenous or retrograde pyelography	407	5.0
Abdominal radiography	289	1.7
Lumbar spine radiography	275	2.5
Pelvic radiography	41	1.5

*Ovarian dose approximates fetal exposure.
Adapted from Penfil RL, Brown ML: Genetically significant dose to the United
States population from diagnostic medical roentgenology. Radiology 1968;90:209.

Table A–13 □ SONOGRAPHIC FINDINGS IN NORMAL
FIRST-TRIMESTER PREGNANCIES

| Sonographic Finding | Gestational Age at Detection (week) | |
	Transabdominal Examination	Transvaginal Examination
Gestational sac	6	5
Yolk sac	6	5
Fetus	7	6
Fetal cardiac activity	7	6

APPENDIX B
Guidelines, Illustrations, and Tables for Gynecology

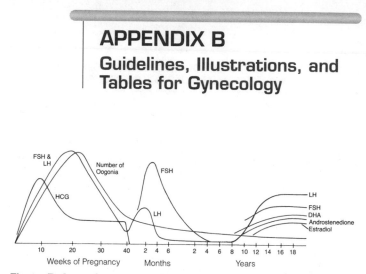

Figure B–1 □ Changes in gonadotropins and oocytes from fetal life to puberty. DHA = dehydroepiandrosterone; FSH = follicle-stimulating hormone; HCG = human chorionic gonadotropin; LH = luteinizing hormone. (From Speroff L, Glass RH, Kase NG: Neuroendocrinology. In Clinical Gynecologic Endocrinology and Infertility, 6th ed. Baltimore, Williams & Wilkins, 1999, p 193.)

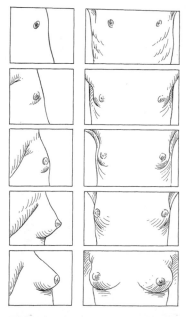

Figure B–2 □ Tanner stages of breast development. Stage 1: Preadolescent—elevation of the papilla only. Stage 2: Breast bud stage—elevation of the breast and papilla with enlargement of the areolar region. Stage 3: Further enlargement of the breast and areola without separation of their contours. Stage 4: Projection of the areola and papilla to form a secondary mound above the level of the breast. Stage 5: Mature stage—projection of the papilla only, resulting from recession of the areola to the general contour of the breast. (From Tanner M, Eveleth PB: Variability between populations in growth and development at puberty. In Bereberg SR, ed: Puberty, Biologic and Physiological Correlations. Leiden, The Netherlands, HF Stenfert Kroese, 1976, p 256.)

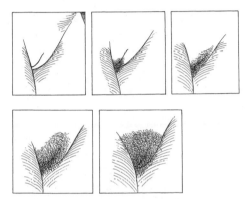

Figure B–3 □ Tanner stages of female pubic hair development. Stage 1: Preadolescent—absence of pubic hair. Stage 2: Sparse hair along the labia. Stage 3: Hair sparsely over the junction of the pubes. Hair is darker and coarser. Stage 4: Adult-type hair without spread to the medial surface of the thighs. Stage 5: Adult-type hair with spread to the medial thighs. (From Hacker NF, Moore JG: Essentials of Obstetrics and Gynecology, 3rd ed. Philadelphia, WB Saunders Co, 1998, p 571.)

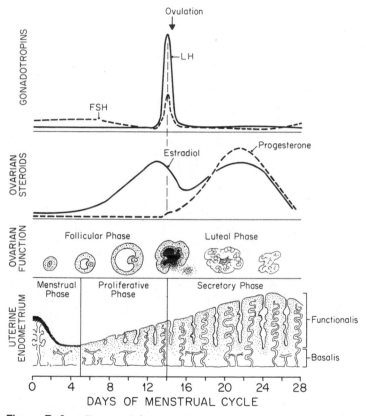

Figure B-4 □ Events of the normal menstrual cycle. FSH = follicle-stimulating hormone; LH = luteinizing hormone. (From Hacker NF, Moore JG: Essentials of Obstetrics and Gynecology, 3rd ed. Philadelphia, WB Saunders, 1998, p 61.)

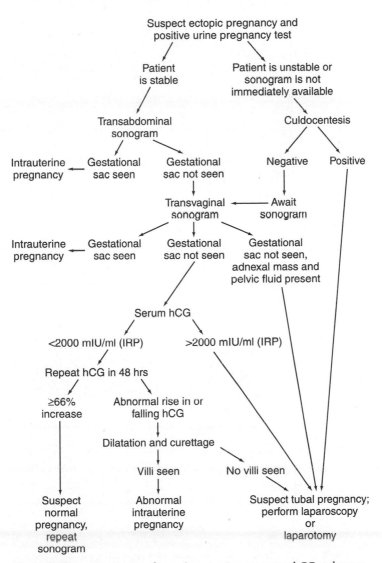

Figure B–5 □ Diagnostic scheme for ectopic pregnancy. hCG = human chorionic gonadotropin; IRP = International Reference Preparation.

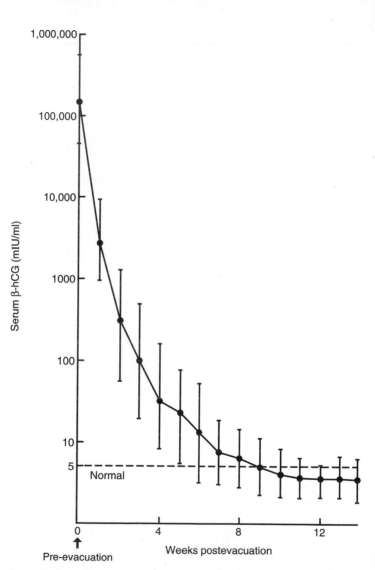

Figure B–6 □ Normal regression curve of human chorionic gonadotropin (hCG) following surgical evacuation of hydatidiform mole. (From Morrow CP, Kletzky OA, DiSaia PJ, et al: Clinical and laboratory correlates of molar pregnancy and trophoblastic disease. Am J Obstet Gynecol 1977;128:424.)

Table B–1 □ STAGES OF PUBERTAL DEVELOPMENT

Stage	Mean Age (yr)	Age Range (yr)
Thelarche (breast budding)	9.8	8–13
Adrenarche (pubic or axillary hair)	11	8–14
Peak height velocity (maximal growth)	11.5	10–14
Menarche	13	9–16
Mature pubic hair	14	12–18
Mature breasts	14.5	12–18

Table B–2 □ GONADOTROPIN AND STEROID LEVELS

Hormone	Follicular Phase	Midcycle	Luteal Phase	Postmeno-pausal
Serum FSH (mIU/ml)	5–20	10–40	5–20	>40
Serum LH (mIU/ml)	5–20	15–60	5–20	>40
Serum estradiol (pg/ml)	25–75	200–600	100–300	5–25
Serum progesterone (ng/ml)	<1	<1	5–20	<1
Serum testosterone (ng/dl)	20–80	20–80	20–80	10–40

FSH = follicle-stimulating hormone; LH = luteinizing hormone.

Table B–3 □ DIFFERENTIAL DIAGNOSIS OF THE PELVIC MASS

Source	Sonographic Characteristic	
	Cystic	Solid or Complex

Ovaries	Functional cyst
	Endometrioma
	Neoplasm
	  Benign
	  Malignant
		Neoplasm
		  Benign
		  Malignant

Fallopian tubes	Hydrosalpinx Tubo-ovarian abscess Pyosalpinx Paratubal cyst	Neoplasm Tubo-ovarian abscess Tubal pregnancy
Uterus		Intrauterine pregnancy Uterine anomaly Leiomyoma Adenomyosis Sarcoma
Bowel	Ileus	Appendiceal abscess Diverticular abscess Neoplasm Stool
Bladder and kidneys	Distended bladder	Pelvic kidney

Table B-4 □ DIFFERENTIAL DIAGNOSIS OF GENITAL ULCERS

Parameter	HSV	Syphilis	Chancroid	Granuloma Inguinale	LGV
Lesion	Multiple vesicles	Single ulcer	Single or multiple ulcers	Single or multiple ulcers	Single ulcer
Depth	Shallow	Shallow	Deep	Elevated	Shallow
Induration	Absent	Hard	Soft	Hard	Absent
Adenopathy	Present	Present	Present	Absent	Present
Pain	Present	Absent	Present	Absent	Variable
Incubation	3–7 days	3 weeks	3–5 days	1–12 weeks	4–21 days

HSV = herpes simplex virus; LGV = lymphogranuloma venereum.

Table B-5 □ COMPARISON OF THE FOUR MOST COMMON VULVOVAGINAL INFECTIONS

Parameter	Yeast Vulvaginitis	Bacterial Vaginosis	Trichomonas Vulvovaginitis	Atrophic Vaginitis
Cause	Candida species	Gardnerella vaginalis, mixed anaerobes	Trichomonas vaginalis	Estrogen deficiency
Major symptoms	Itching, burning	Malodorous, watery discharge	Itching, burning, variable	Itching, vaginal discharge, burning
Discharge	White, cottage cheese	White, skim milk	Frothy, variable	Usually absent
Odor	Absent	Present	Variable	Absent
Vulvovaginal inflammation	Present	Absent	Variable	Present
Vaginal wet smear	Hyphae, spores	"Clue cells"	Trichomonads	No organisms
"Whiff test"	Negative	Positive	Negative	Negative
Vaginal pH	Normal, 3–4	Basic, 5–6	Basic, 6–7	Basic, 6–7
Treatment	Antifungal drugs	Metronidazole	Metronidazole	Estrogen supplementation

APPENDIX C
On Call Formulary for Obstetrics and Gynecology

U.S. FOOD AND DRUG ADMINISTRATION USE-IN-PREGNANCY RATINGS

Category	Interpretation
A	**Controlled studies show no risk.** Adequate, well-controlled studies in pregnant women have failed to demonstrate risk to the fetus.
B	**No evidence of risk in humans.** Either animal findings show risk but human findings do not, or, if no adequate human studies have been done, animal findings are negative.
C	**Risk cannot be ruled out.** Human studies are lacking, and animal studies are either positive for fetal risk or also lacking. However, potential benefits may justify the potential risk.
D	**Positive evidence of risk.** Investigational or postmarketing data show risk to the fetus. Nevertheless, potential benefits may outweigh the potential risk.
X	**Contraindicated in pregnancy.** Studies in animals or humans, or investigational or postmarketing reports, have shown fetal risk that clearly outweighs any possible benefit to the patient.

USE IN BREAST-FEEDING WOMEN

Category	Interpretation
Compatible:	Use of the drug is compatible with breast feeding.
Not recommended:	Use of the drug is not recommended in breast-feeding women.
Unknown:	There are no data on either the secretion of the drug into breast milk or the effects of the drug when ingested by the infant.

Acetaminophen with codeine   *Class: Analgesic*
(Tylenol with codeine)

Category:	C
Breast feeding:	Compatible
Indications:	Mild to moderate pain
Actions:	Acetaminophen: peripherally acting analgesic; codeine: centrally acting analgesic
Side effects:	Nausea, vomiting, lightheadedness, dizziness, shortness of breath
Dose:	Acetaminophen 300 mg with codeine 15 mg (No. 2), 30 mg (No. 3), or 60 mg (No. 4). Give the number of tablets that provides 15 to 60 mg codeine PO every 4 hours.

Acyclovir (Zovirax)   *Class: Antiviral*

Category:	C
Breast feeding:	Compatible
Indications:	Treatment and prophylaxis for herpes simplex, herpes zoster, and chicken pox
Actions:	Synthetic purine nucleoside analogue inhibiting viral DNA replication
Side effects:	Nausea, vomiting, headaches
Dose:	400 mg PO 3 times per day or 200 mg PO 5 times per day for 7 to 10 days or until clinical resolution is attained for primary infection
	400 mg PO 3 times per day for 5 days or 800 mg PO 2 times per day for 5 days for recurrent infection
	400 mg PO 2 times per day or 200 mg PO 2 to 5 times per day for prophylaxis against recurrent infection
	5% ointment applied to cover all lesions every 3 hours, 6 times per day, for 7 days

Albuterol (Airet, Proventil, Ventolin)   *Class: Bronchodilator*

Category:	C
Breast feeding:	Compatible
Indications:	Treatment of bronchospasm
Actions:	Beta-sympathomimetic
Side effects:	Tremors, dizziness, nervousness, nausea, hypertension
Dose:	Bronchodilator aerosol: 2 inhalations every 4 to 6 hours
	Syrup: 1 to 2 teaspoons PO 3 to 4 times per day
	Tablets: 2 to 4 mg PO 3 to 4 times per day

Alprazolam (Xanax)   *Class: Benzodiazepine*

Category:	D
Breast feeding:	Not recommended
Indications:	Anxiety disorder
Actions:	Binding specific receptors within the central nervous system

Side effects:	Drowsiness, lightheadedness
Dose:	0.25 to 0.5 mg PO 3 times per day, maximum dose of 4 mg/day

Aminophylline   *Class: Bronchodilator*

Category:	C
Breast feeding:	Compatible
Indications:	Bronchospasm
Actions:	Relaxation of smooth muscles of the bronchi
Side effects:	Nausea, vomiting, irritability, tachycardia, arrhythmias, seizures
Dose:	Loading dose of 6 mg/kg IV followed by maintenance dose of 0.4 to 0.9 mg/kg/hr IV
	24 mg/kg PO per day in 4 divided doses

Amitriptyline (Elavil)   *Class: Tricyclic antidepressant*

Category:	D
Breast feeding:	Unknown, may be of concern
Indications:	Depression
Actions:	Unknown
Side effects:	Cardiovascular: myocardial infarction, stroke, non-specific electrocardiographic changes
	Central nervous system and neuromuscular: coma, seizure, hallucinations, delusions, confusion
	Anticholinergic: paralytic ileus, hyperpyrexia, urinary retention, constipation
	Hematological: bone marrow depression, leukopenia, thrombocytopenia
	Gastrointestinal: hepatitis
	Withdrawal symptoms
Dose:	75 to 300 mg PO per day in divided doses

Amoxicillin (Amoxil, Augmentin, Moxilin)   *Class: Antibiotic*

Category:	B
Breast feeding:	Compatible
Indications:	Treatment of infection with gram-negative organisms (*Haemophilus influenzae, Escherichia coli, Proteus mirabilis,* or *Neisseria gonorrhoeae*), gram-positive organisms (streptococci, non–penicillinase-producing staphylococci), and *Chlamydia trachomatis*
Actions:	Inhibition of cell wall synthesis
Side effects:	Nausea, vomiting, diarrhea, urticaria, erythematous maculopapular rashes
Dose:	250 to 500 mg PO 3 times per day for 7 to 10 days

Amphotericin B (Fungizone)   *Class: Antifungal agent*

Category:	B
Breast feeding:	Unknown
Indications:	Systemic fungal infection
Actions:	Interferes with cell membrane by inhibition of ergosterol

Side effects:	Fever, hypotension, tachypnea, gastrointestinal symptoms, anemia, generalized pain, elevated liver enzymes, decreased renal function tests
Dose:	Test dose of 1 mg administered IV over 20 to 30 minutes followed by a gradual increase of 5 to 10 mg/day to a final daily maintenance dose of 0.5 to 0.7 mg/kg IV

Ampicillin (Omnipen, Ampicillin)   *Class: Antibiotic*

Category:	B
Breast feeding:	Excreted into breast milk; alteration of bowel flora, candidiasis, and allergic reaction in the infant should be considered
Indications:	Treatment of infection with gram-negative organisms (*Haemophilus influenzae, Escherichia coli, Neisseria gonorrhoeae, Neisseria meningitidis, Proteus mirabilis, Salmonella* spp. or *Shigella* spp.) and gram-positive organisms (streptococci, non–penicillinase-producing staphylococci, *Bacillus anthracis, Clostridium* spp., *Corynebacterium* spp., or enterococci)
Actions:	Inhibition of cell wall synthesis
Side effects:	Gastrointestinal: nausea, vomiting, diarrhea, glossitis, stomatitis, enterocolitis, pseudomembranous colitis
Dose:	0.5 to 2.0 g IV every 6 hours 250 to 500 mg PO 4 times per day

Ampicillin and sulbactam [Unasyn]   *Class: Antibiotic*

Category:	B
Breast feeding:	Excreted into breast milk; alteration of bowel flora, candidiasis, and allergic reaction in the infant should be considered
Indications:	Treatment of gynecological infection due to beta-lactamase–producing strains of *Escherichia coli* and *Bacteroides* spp.
Actions:	Inhibition of cell wall synthesis, beta-lactamase inhibitor
Side effects:	Gastritis, stomatitis, enterocolitis
Dose:	1.5 g (1.0 g ampicillin and 0.5 g sulbactam) to 3.0 g (2.0 g ampicillin and 1.0 g sulbactam) IV every 6 hours

Astemizole [Hismanal]   *Class: Antihistamine*

Category:	C
Breast feeding:	Unknown
Indications:	Allergic rhinitis, chronic idiopathic urticaria
Actions:	Histamine H_1-receptor antagonist
Side effects:	Drowsiness, headache, fatigue, appetite increase, weight increase, nausea, nervousness, dizziness
Dose:	10 mg PO once daily

Azithromycin (Zithromax)   *Class: Antibiotic*

Category: C
Breast feeding: Excreted into breast milk; caution should be
                        excerised
Indications: Treatment of sexually transmitted diseases due to
                        Chlamydia trachomatis, Staphylococcus aureus, Strepto-
                        coccus spp., *Haemophilus influenzae,* or *Moraxella ca-*
                        tarrhalis
Actions: Macrolide antibiotic
Side effects: Nausea, diarrhea, vomiting, abdominal pain
Dose: 1 g PO once for chlamydia
                     500 mg PO on first day followed by 250 mg PO
                        per day for a total of 5 days of therapy for other
                        indications

Aztreonam (Azactam)   *Class: Antibiotic*

Category: B
Breast feeding: Compatible
Indications: Treatment of endometritis and pelvic infections
                        caused by *Escherichia coli, Klebsiella pneumoniae, En-*
                        terobacter spp., or *Proteus mirabilis*
Actions: Inhibition of cell wall synthesis
Side effects: Diarrhea, nausea, vomiting, rash
Dose: 1.0 to 2.0 g IV every 8 hours

Bromocriptine (Parlodel)   *Class: Dopamine receptor agonist*

Category: C
Breast feeding: Not recommended
Indications: Hyperprolactinemia
Actions: Dopamine receptor agonist
Side effects: Nausea, headache, dizziness, fatigue, lighthead-
                        edness, vomiting, abdominal cramps, constipation,
                        diarrhea, drowsiness, nasal congestion
Dose: 2.5 to 15 mg PO per day

Butoconazole (Femstat)   *Class: Antifungal agent*

Category: C
Breast feeding: Unknown
Indications: Vulvovaginal candidal infection
Actions: Imidazole derivative, interferes with cell membrane
                        by inhibition of ergosterol
Side effects: Vulvovaginal itching and burning
Dose: 2% vaginal cream: 5 g every night before bed for
                        3 nights

Calcium gluconate   *Class: Calcium supplement*

Category: B
Breast feeding: Compatible
Indications: Cardiac or respiratory arrest due to magnesium
                        toxicity

Actions:	Calcium replacement, increases myocardial contractility and ventricular automaticity
Side effects:	Electrocardiographic changes, arrhythmias, sensitivity to digoxin
Dose:	10% solution: administer 10 ml (1 g) IV over 3 minutes

Carbamazepine (Tegretol, Atretol)   *Class: Anticonvulsant*

Category:	C
Breast feeding:	Compatible
Indications:	Seizures, trigeminal neuralgia
Actions:	Reduction of polysynaptic responses and blockage of posttetanic potentiation
Side effects:	Aplastic anemia, agranulocytosis, dizziness, nausea, vomiting
Dose:	800 to 1200 mg PO per day

Cefixime (Suprax)   *Class: Antibiotic*

Category:	B
Breast feeding:	Excretion into breast milk is unknown; other cephalosporins are compatible
Indications:	Uncomplicated urinary tract infection caused by *Escherichia coli* or *Proteus mirabilis*
	Uncomplicated gonorrhea, gonococcal bacteremia, and arthritis
Actions:	Inhibition of cell wall synthesis
Side effects:	Diarrhea, dyspepsia, nausea, vomiting, abdominal pain
Dose:	400 mg PO once for uncomplicated gonorrhea
	200 mg 2 times per day or 400 mg per day for urinary tract infection
	400 mg PO 2 times per day for gonococcal bacteremia and arthritis

Cefoperazone (Cefobid)   *Class: Antibiotic*

Category:	B
Breast feeding:	Excreted into breast milk; caution should be exercised; other cephalosporins are compatible
Indications:	Pelvic inflammatory disease caused by *Neisseria gonorrhoeae, Escherichia coli, Clostridium* spp., *Bacteroides* spp., or group B beta-hemolytic streptococci
Actions:	Inhibition of cell wall synthesis
Side effects:	Hypersensitivity reaction, neutropenia, hepatitis, diarrhea
Dose:	0.5 to 1.0 g IV every 6 hours

Cefotaxime (Claforan)   *Class: Antibiotic*

Category:	B
Breast feeding:	Compatible
Indications:	Pelvic inflammatory disease (PID) due to *Staphylococcus* spp., *Streptococcus* spp., *Enterobacter* spp., entero-

cocci, *Klebsiella* spp., *Escherichia coli*, *Proteus mirabilis*, *Bacteroides* spp., *Clostridium* spp., *Peptococcus* spp., or *Peptostreptococcus* spp.
Gonococcal bacteremia and arthritis

Actions:	Inhibition of cell wall synthesis
Side effects:	Local inflammation at IM injection site or IV site
Dose:	1 to 2 g IM or IV every 8 hours for PID
	1 g IV every 8 hours for 2 to 3 days for gonococcal bacteremia and arthritis

Cefotetan (Cefotan) *Class: Antibiotic*

Category:	B
Breast feeding:	Excreted into breast milk; caution should be exercised; other cephalosporins are compatible
Indications:	Pelvic inflammatory disease due to *Staphylococcus* spp., *Streptococcus* spp., *Neisseria gonorrhoeae*, *Proteus mirabilis*, *Bacteroides* spp., *Peptococcus* spp., or *Peptostreptococcus* spp.
Actions:	Inhibition of cell wall synthesis
Side effects:	Nausea, diarrhea, pseudomembranous colitis, prolonged prothrombin time
Dose:	1.0 to 2.0 g IV every 12 hours

Cefoxitin (Mefoxin) *Class: Antibiotic*

Category:	B
Breast feeding:	Compatible
Indications:	Pelvic inflammatory disease due to group B streptococci, *Escherichia coli*, *Neisseria gonorrhoeae*, *Bacteroides* spp., *Clostridium* spp., *Peptococcus* spp., or *Peptostreptococcus* spp.
Actions:	Inhibition of cell wall synthesis
Side effects:	Local inflammation at IM injection site or IV site, diarrhea
Dose:	1.0 to 2.0 g IV every 6 hours

Ceftizoxime (Cefizox) *Class: Antibiotic*

Category:	B
Breast feeding:	Excreted into breast milk; caution should be exercised; other cephalosporins are compatible
Indications:	Pelvic inflammatory disease due to *Streptococcus agalactiae*, *Escherichia coli*, or *Neisseria gonorrhoeae*
	Gonococcal bacteremia and arthritis
Actions:	Inhibition of cell wall synthesis
Side effects:	Hypersensitivity reaction, elevation of liver enzymes, eosinophilia, thrombocytosis, local inflammation
Dose:	1 g IV every 8 hours

Ceftriaxone (Rocephin) *Class: Antibiotic*

Category:	B
Breast feeding:	Compatible
Indications:	Infection caused by *Neisseria gonorrhoeae*
Actions:	Inhibition of cell wall synthesis
Side effects:	Hypersensitivity reaction, elevation of liver enzymes,

eosinophilia, thrombocytosis, leukopenia, elevation of blood urea nitrogen, diarrhea, and local inflammation

Dose: 125 mg IM once for uncomplicated gonorrhea
1 g IV per day for gonococcal bacteremia and arthritis
1–2 g IV daily for gonococcal meningitis

Cephradine [Velosef]   *Class: Antibiotic*

Category:	B
Breast feeding:	Excreted into breast milk; caution should be exercised; other cephalosporins are compatible
Indications:	Bacterial vaginosis in patients allergic to penicillin
Actions:	Inhibition of cell wall synthesis
Side effects:	Nausea, vomiting, diarrhea
Dose:	500 mg PO 4 times per day for 7 days

Chloramphenicol [Chloromycetin]   *Class: Antibiotic*

Category:	C
Breast feeding:	Excreted into breast milk. Safety of breast feeding unknown; may be of concern because of the potential for idiosyncratic bone marrow suppression in the infant
Indications:	Serious infection caused by *Salmonella* spp., *Haemophilus influenzae*, *Rickettsia* spp., or other gram-negative aerobic and anaerobic bacteria
	Gonococcal meningitis
Actions:	Bacteriostatic effect due to interference with protein synthesis
Side effects:	Bone marrow depression
	"Gray syndrome," a potentially fatal toxic reaction encountered in neonates
Dose:	50 to 100 mg/kg/day in divided doses at 6-hour intervals
	4 to 6 g IV per day for at least 10 days for gonococcal meningitis

Chlorpromazine [Thorazine]   *Class: Antipsychotic*

Category:	C
Breast feeding:	Excreted into breast milk. Safety of breast feeding is unknown; may be of concern because of drowsiness and lethargy in the infant
Indications:	Psychosis, nausea, vomiting, intractable hiccups, restlessness
Actions:	Unknown, antiadrenergic and anticholinergic activity
Side effects:	Drowsiness, jaundice, hematological disorders, agranulocytosis, extrapyramidal reactions, hypotension
Dose:	10 to 25 mg PO 2 or 3 times per day
	25 mg IM, repeated in 1 hour if necessary

Cimetidine (Tagamet)   *Class: Histamine antagonist*

Category:	B
Breast feeding:	Compatible
Indications:	Peptic ulcer disease, gastrointestinal reflux
Actions:	Inhibition of gastric acid secretion induced by histamine
Side effects:	Diarrhea, headache, gynecomastia, leukopenia, thrombocytopenia, elevation of liver enzymes
Dose:	400 to 800 mg PO every night before bed
	300 mg IM or IV every 6 to 8 hours

Ciprofloxacin (Cipro)   *Class: Antibiotic*

Category:	C, contraindicated because of increased risk of major congenital malformations
Breast feeding:	Not recommended because of the risk of arthropathy and other toxicity in the infant
Indications:	Uncomplicated gonorrhea, gonococcal bacteremia, and arthritis
	Urinary tract infection and other infections caused by gram-positive or gram-negative aerobic bacteria
Actions:	Interference with enzyme DNA gyrase, which is necessary for DNA synthesis
Side effects:	Nausea, diarrhea, vomiting, abdominal discomfort, headache, restlessnesss, rash
Dose:	250 to 750 mg PO every 12 hours
	500 mg PO once for uncomplicated gonorrhea
	200 to 500 mg IV every 12 hours
	500 mg IV every 12 hours followed by 500 mg PO 2 times per day for gonococcal bacteremia and arthritis

Clindamycin (Cleocin)   *Class: Antibiotic*

Category:	B
Breast feeding:	Compatible
Indications:	Gynecological infections caused by anaerobic bacteria
	Infections caused by susceptible strains of streptococci, pneumococci, and staphylococci
	Bacterial vaginosis
Actions:	Interference with protein synthesis
Side effects:	Pseudomembranous colitis caused by *Clostridium difficile*
Dose:	300 to 600 mg IV every 6 hours or 900 mg IV every 8 hours
	150 to 450 mg PO every 6 hours
	2% vaginal cream: 5 g (1 applicator full) intravaginally every night before bed for 7 nights

Clobetasol propionate (Temovate)   *Class: Dermatological*

Category:	C
Breast feeding:	Excretion into breast milk unknown; caution should be exercised

Indications:	Dermatological conditions such as lichen sclerosus
Actions:	Topical anti-inflammatory, antipruritic, and vasoconstrictive actions
Side effects:	Local stinging and burning
Dose:	0.05% cream applied twice daily for 2 to 3 weeks

Clomiphene citrate   *Class: Ovulation stimulant*
(Clomid, Serophene)

Category:	X
Breast feeding:	Unknown
Indications:	Oligo-ovulation resulting in infertility
Actions:	Increases gonadotropins
Side effects:	Hyperstimulation of the ovaries
Dose:	50 to 100 mg PO per day for 5 days at the beginning of the menstrual cycle

Clotrimazole (Mycelex, Gyne-Lotrimin)   *Class: Antifungal agent*

Category:	C
Breast feeding:	Unknown
Indications:	*Candida* vulvovaginitis, dermatitis
Actions:	Imidazole derivative, interferes with cell membrane by inhibition of ergosterol
Side effects:	Vaginal administration: vaginal itching, irritation, cramping, headaches
	Topical administration: erythema, blistering, peeling, edema, pruritus
Dose:	100-mg vaginal tablet: 1 tablet every night before bed for 7 nights
	1% vaginal cream: 5 g every night before bed for 7 nights
	500-mg vaginal tablet: 1 tablet once
	1% lotion or cream: apply 2 times per day

Crotamiton (Eurax)   *Class: Antiparasitic*

Category:	C
Breast feeding:	Unknown
Indications:	Infection with scabies *(Sarcoptes scabiei)*
Actions:	Scabicidal and antipruritic actions
Side effects:	Allergic sensitivity and primary irritation
Dose:	10% cream or lotion applied to the skin from chin to toes. A second application is recommended 24 hours later. Bed linens and clothing should be changed the next day. A cleansing bath should be taken 48 hours after the last application.

Danazol (Danocrine)   *Class: Androgen*

Category:	X
Breast feeding:	Not recommended
Indications:	Endometriosis

Actions:	Suppression of pituitary-ovarian axis and secretion of follicle-stimulating hormone and luteinizing hormone
Side effects:	Androgen effects such as hirsutism, weight gain, and acne; postmenopausal symptoms such as vasomotor symptoms and atrophic vaginitis; hepatic dysfunction
Dose:	100 to 400 mg PO 2 times per day

Diazepam [Valium]   *Class: Benzodiazepine*

Category:	D
Breast feeding:	Unknown, may be of concern because of lethargy and weight loss in the infant
Indications:	Treatment of anxiety disorder, seizure disorder, and muscle spasms
Actions:	Acts on parts of the limbic system, the thalamus, and the hypothalamus
Side effects:	Drowsiness, fatigue, ataxia, phlebitis at injection site
Dose:	2 to 10 mg PO 3 or 4 times per day
	2 to 20 mg IM or IV

Dicloxacillin [Pathocil, Dicloxacillin]   *Class: Antibiotic*

Category:	B
Breast feeding:	Excreted into breast milk; alteration of bowel flora, candidiasis, and allergic reaction in the infant should be considered
Indications:	Infection due to penicillinase-producing staphylococci
Actions:	Inhibition of cell wall synthesis
Side effects:	Nausea, vomiting, epigastric discomfort, diarrhea, hypersensitivity reaction
Dose:	125 to 250 mg PO 4 times per day for 10 days

Digoxin [Lanoxicaps, Lanoxin]   *Class: Inotropic agent*

Category:	C
Breast feeding:	Compatible
Indications:	Heart failure, atrial fibrillation, atrial flutter, paroxysmal atrial tachycardia
Actions:	Increases myocardial contractility, slows atrioventricular (AV) conduction
Side effects:	Premature ventricular contractions, ventricular tachycardia, AV dissociation, atrial tachycardia, accelerated junctional rhythm
Dose:	Oral: 0.5 to 0.75 mg PO, then 0.125 to 0.375 mg PO every 6 to 8 hours until clinical effect is achieved, then maintenance dose of 0.125 to 0.25 mg PO every day
	IV: 0.4 to 0.6 mg IV, then 0.1 to 0.3 mg IV every 4 to 8 hours until clinical effect is achieved, then maintenance dose of 0.125 to 0.25 mg IV every day

Diphenhydramine (Benadryl)　　　　　　*Class: Antihistamine*

Category:	B
Breast feeding:	Not recommended
Indications:	Allergic reaction, motion sickness, parkinsonism
Actions:	Antihistamine, anticholinergic, and sedative effects
Side effects:	Drowsiness, dizziness, epigastric distress, thickening of bronchial secretions
Dose:	25 to 50 mg PO 3 or 4 times per day, 50 mg PO every night before bed
	10 to 50 mg IV or IM

Diphenoxylate with atropine (Lomotil)　　　*Class: Antidiarrheal*

Category:	C
Breast feeding:	Compatible
Indications:	Diarrhea
Actions:	Direct effect on circular smooth muscle of the bowel resulting in prolonged transit time
Side effects:	Numbness of the extremities, depression, euphoria, confusion, sedation, dizziness, toxic megacolon, paralytic ileus, nausea, vomiting, abdominal discomfort
Dose:	2 tablets PO 4 times per day
	10 ml PO 4 times per day

Dopamine (Intropin, Dopastat)　　　*Class: Cardiovascular agent*

Category:	C
Breast feeding:	Unknown
Indications:	Treatment of hemodynamic imbalances caused by shock, myocardial infarction, septicemia, and trauma
Actions:	Vasoactive amine with positive inotropic effects
	Increases cardiac heart rate and contractility
	Vasodilatation
Side effects:	Hypotension, ectopic heart beats, nausea, vomiting, tachycardia, anginal pain, palpitation, dyspnea, and headache
Dose:	2 to 5 μg/kg/min IV infusion with dose increased by 5-μg/kg/min increments to a maximum of 50 μg/kg/min

Doxycycline　　　　　　　　　　*Class: Antibiotic*
(Doryx, Vibramycin, Doxycycline, Monodox)

Category:	D
Breast feeding:	Compatible
Indications:	Infection caused by *Chlamydia trachomatis, Neisseria gonorrhoeae, Treponema pallidum, Mycoplasma pneumoniae, Haemophilus ducreyi*, or *Bacteroides* spp.
Actions:	Interference with protein synthesis
Side effects:	Nausea, vomiting, diarrhea, rash, rise in blood urea nitrogen, hypersensitivity reaction
Dose:	100 mg PO 2 times per day for 7 days
	100 mg IV every 12 hours

Ephedrine sulfate   *Class: Cardiovascular agent*

Category:	C
Breast feeding:	Unknown; may be of concern because of irritability and excessive crying in the infant
Indications:	Hypotension from conduction anesthesia, acute bronchospasm
Actions:	Sympathomimetic
Side effects:	Tremulousness, excitation, nervousness, palpitations, tachycardia
Dose:	25 to 50 mg IM or IV

Erythromycin   *Class: Antibiotic*
(Erythrocin, E-Mycin, ERYC, Ery-Tab, Ilosone)

Category:	B
Breast feeding:	Compatible
Indications:	Treatment of infection with *Chlamydia trachomatis, Neisseria gonorrhoeae, Treponema pallidum*, group A beta-hemolytic streptococci, *Streptococcus pneumoniae*, or *Staphylococcus aureus*
Actions:	Interference with protein synthesis
Side effects:	Nausea, vomiting, abdominal pain, diarrhea
Dose:	250 to 500 mg PO 4 times per day for 7 days
	500 to 1000 mg IV 4 times per day
	500 mg PO 4 times per day for 21 days for lymphogranuloma venereum

Estradiol (Estrace)   *Class: Hormone*

Category:	X
Breast feeding:	Compatible; suppresses milk production
Indications:	Hypoestrogenic symptoms from menopause, perimenopause, and premenopausal castration
Actions:	Estrogen replacement
Side effects:	Nausea, breast tenderness, irregular bleeding, fluid retention, enlargement of fibroid tumors of the uterus, endometrial hyperplasia, endometrial adenocarcinoma
Dose:	1 to 2 mg PO every day either continuously or cyclically
	0.01% vaginal cream: 2 to 4 g intravaginally every day for 1 to 2 weeks, then reduced gradually to a maintenance dose of 1 g 1 to 3 times per week
	Progestin should be administered to those patients who have not undergone hysterectomy, to prevent endometrial hyperplasia or adenocarcinoma

Estradiol transdermal system   *Class: Hormone*
(Estraderm, Climara, Vivelle)

Category:	X
Breast feeding:	Compatible; suppresses lactation
Indications:	Hypoestrogenic symptoms from menopause, perimenopause, and premenopausal castration
Actions:	Estrogen replacement

Side effects: Nausea, breast tenderness, irregular bleeding, fluid retention, enlargement of fibroid tumors of the uterus, endometrial hyperplasia, endometrial adenocarcinoma

Dose: 0.0375-, 0.05-, 0.075-, or 0.1-mg transdermal patch applied twice weekly

Progestin should be administered to those patients who have not undergone hysterectomy, to prevent endometrial hyperplasia or adenocarcinoma

Estrogen, conjugated (Premarin)   *Class: Hormone*

Category: X
Breast feeding: Compatible; suppresses milk production
Indications: Hypoestrogenic symptoms from menopause, perimenopause, and premenopausal castration
Actions: Estrogen replacement
Side effects: Nausea, breast tenderness, irregular bleeding, fluid retention, enlargement of fibroid tumors of the uterus, endometrial hyperplasia, endometrial adenocarcinoma
Dose: 0.3, 0.625, 0.9, or 1.25 mg PO per day either continuously or cyclically

2 to 4 g intravaginal cream per day for short-term use, tapered or discontinued every 3 to 6 months

25 mg IV every 6 to 12 hours for severe dysfunctional uterine bleeding

Progestin should be administered to those patients who are using estrogen chronically and who have not undergone hysterectomy, to prevent endometrial hyperplasia or adenocarcinoma

Estrogen, conjugated with   *Class: Hormone*
methyltestosterone (Premarin
with methyltestosterone)

Category: X
Breast feeding: Unknown
Indications: Hypoestrogenic symptoms from menopause, perimenopause, and premenopausal castration with hypoandrogenic symptoms such as decreased libido
Actions: Estrogen and androgen replacement
Side effects: Nausea, breast tenderness, irregular bleeding, fluid retention, enlargement of fibroid tumors of the uterus, endometrial hyperplasia, endometrial adenocarcinoma, hirsutism, acne
Dose: 0.625 mg estrogen with 5 mg methyltestosterone or 1.25 mg estrogen with 10 mg methyltestosterone PO per day either continuously or cyclically

Progestin should be administered to those patients who have not undergone hysterectomy, to prevent endometrial hyperplasia or adenocarcinoma

Estrogen, esterified (Estratab, Menest)   *Class: Hormone*

Category:	X
Breast feeding:	Unknown
Indications:	Hypoestrogenic symptoms from menopause, peri-menopause, and premenopausal castration
Actions:	Estrogen replacement
Side effects:	Nausea, breast tenderness, irregular bleeding, fluid retention, enlargement of fibroid tumors of the uterus, endometrial hyperplasia, endometrial adenocarcinoma
Dose:	0.3, 0.625, 0.9, or 1.25 mg PO per day either continuously or cyclically
	Progestin should be administered to those patients who have not undergone hysterectomy, to prevent endometrial hyperplasia or adenocarcinoma

Estrogen, esterified with   *Class: Hormone*
methyltestosterone (Estratest)

Category:	X
Breast feeding:	Unknown
Indications:	Hypoestrogenic symptoms from menopause, peri-menopause, and premenopausal castration with hypoandrogenic symptoms such as decreased libido
Actions:	Estrogen and androgen replacement
Side effects:	Nausea, breast tenderness, irregular bleeding, fluid retention, enlargement of fibroid tumors of the uterus, endometrial hyperplasia, endometrial adenocarcinoma, hirsutism, acne
Dose:	0.625 mg estrogen with 1.25 mg methyltestosterone or 1.25 mg estrogen with 2.5 mg methyltestosterone PO per day either continuously or cyclically
	Progestin should be administered to those patients who have not undergone hysterectomy, to prevent endometrial hyperplasia or adenocarcinoma

Estropipate (Ogen)   *Class: Hormone*

Category:	X
Breast feeding:	Unknown
Indications:	Hypoestrogenic symptoms from menopause, peri-menopause, and premenopausal castration
Actions:	Estrogen replacement
Side effects:	Nausea, breast tenderness, irregular bleeding, fluid retention, enlargement of fibroid tumors of the uterus, endometrial hyperplasia, endometrial adenocarcinoma
Dose:	0.625, 1.25, or 2.5 mg; 1 to 2 tablets PO per day either continuously or cyclically
	Progestin should be administered to those patients who have not undergone hysterectomy, to prevent endometrial hyperplasia or adenocarcinoma

Famciclovir (Famvir)   *Antiviral*

Category:	B
Breast feeding:	Unknown
Indications:	Treatment and prophylaxis for herpes simplex virus
Actions:	Transformed to penciclovir, inhibiting activity against herpes simplex virus
Side effects:	Headache, nausea, diarrhea, vomiting, fatigue, pruritus
Dose:	Primary infection: 250 mg PO 3 times per day for 7 to 10 days
	Recurrent infection: 125 mg PO 2 times per day for 5 days
	Prophylaxis: 250 mg PO 2 times per day

Fluconazole (Diflucan)   *Class: Antifungal agent*

Category:	C
Breast feeding:	Excreted into breast milk; safety unknown
Indications:	*Candida* vulvovaginitis, candidal systemic infection
Actions:	Imidazole derivative, interferes with cell membrane by inhibition of ergosterol
Side effects:	Hepatotoxicity, nausea, vomiting, headache, skin rash, abdominal pain, diarrhea
Dose:	Systemic infection: 400 mg IV on the first day, followed by 200 mg IV every day for a minimum of 3 weeks
	Vulvovaginitis: 150 mg PO once
	Recurrent vulvovaginitis: 150 mg PO once each month

Fluocinolone acetonide (Synalar)   *Class: Dermatological*

Category:	C
Breast feeding:	Unknown
Indications:	Squamous cell hyperplasia of the vulva, inflammatory and pruritic dermatoses
Actions:	Topical corticosteroid
Side effects:	Local adverse reaction
Dose:	0.025% to 0.2% cream or lotion applied 2 or 3 times per day

Fluoxetine (Prozac)   *Class: Antidepressant*

Category:	B
Breast feeding:	Excreted into breast milk; safety unknown; may be of concern because of long-term effects on neurobehavior and development
Indications:	Depression
Actions:	Inhibition of central nervous system neuronal uptake of serotonin
Side effects:	Anxiety, nervousness, insomnia, drowsiness, fatigue, gastrointestinal symptoms
Dose:	20 to 60 mg PO per day

Flurazepam (Dalmane)   *Class: Hypnotic*

Category:	D
Breast feeding:	Unknown; may be of concern
Indications:	Insomnia
Actions:	Benzodiazepine
Side effects:	Dizziness, drowsiness, lightheadedness, ataxia
Dose:	15 to 30 mg PO every night before bed

Furosemide (Lasix)   *Class: Diuretic*

Category:	C
Breast feeding:	Excreted in breast milk; caution should be exercised. Thiazide diuretics suppress lactation.
Indications:	Edema, hypertension
Actions:	Diuretic effect on distal tubule inhibiting reabsorption of sodium and chloride
Side effects:	Electrolyte depletion, hypotension, pancreatitis, jaundice
Dose:	20 to 80 mg PO or IV initial dose followed by a repeat dose or increased dose 6 to 8 hours later

Gentamicin (Garamycin)   *Class: Antibiotic*

Category:	C
Breast feeding:	Excreted into breast milk; may be of concern if bloody diarrhea develops in the infant
Indications:	Treatment of infections due to *Pseudomonas aeruginosa, Proteus* spp., *Escherichia coli, Enterobacter* spp., *Klebsiella* spp., *Serratia* spp., or *Staphylococcus* spp.
Actions:	Interference with protein synthesis
Side effects:	Renal toxicity, ototoxicity, neurotoxicity
Dose:	1.0 to 1.5 mg/kg IV every 8 hours

Halobetasol propionate (Ultravate)   *Class: Dermatological*

Category:	C
Breast feeding:	Excreted in breast milk; caution should be exercised
Indications:	Dermatological conditions such as lichen sclerosus
Actions:	Topical anti-inflammatory, antipruritic, and vasoconstrictive actions
Side effects:	Local stinging, burning, or itching
Dose:	0.05% cream applied 2 times per day for 2 to 3 weeks

Haloperidol (Haldol)   *Class: Antipsychotic*

Category:	C
Breast feeding:	Excreted into breast milk; may be of concern
Indications:	Treatment of psychosis
Actions:	Unknown
Side effects:	Tardive dyskinesia, extrapyramidal symptoms
Dose:	0.5 to 5.0 mg PO 2 or 3 times per day 2 to 5 mg IM initially for acute psychosis

Heparin   *Class: Anticoagulant*

Category: C
Breast feeding: Not excreted into breast milk; compatible with
                     breast feeding
Indications: Treatment or prevention of venous thrombosis, pul-
                     monary embolism
Actions: Synergistic activity with antithrombin III to produce
                     antithrombin effect
Side effects: Bleeding, thrombocytopenia
Dose: Prophylaxis: 5000 units SC every 8 to 12 hours
                     Treatment: 5000 to 10,000 units IV bolus followed by
                     1000 to 2000 units IV per hour with dose adjusted
                     to prolong partial thromboplastin time to 1.5 times
                     control

Hydralazine (Apresoline)   *Class: Antihypertensive*

Category: C
Breast feeding: Compatible
Indications: Hypertension
Actions: Vasodilator
Side effects: Headache, anorexia, nausea, vomiting, diarrhea, pal-
                     pitations, tachycardia, angina
Dose: 1 mg IV over 1 minute as a test dose to detect idiosyn-
                     cratic hypotension, then 5 to 25 mg IV over 2 to 4
                     minutes. After 20 minutes, if a diastolic blood pres-
                     sure of 90 to 100 mm Hg is not attained, a repeat
                     dose or lower dose can be given.
                     10 to 40 mg IM as needed
                     10 mg PO 4 times per day for first 2 to 4 days, then
                     if necessary, increase to 25 mg PO 4 times per day
                     for rest of the week. Then, if necessary, increase to
                     50 mg PO 4 times per day.

Hydrochlorothiazide (Esidrix, HydroDIURIL)   *Class: Diuretic*

Category: D
Breast feeding: Compatible; thiazide diuretics suppress lactation
Indications: Congestive heart failure, edema, hypertension
Actions: Diuretic effect on distal tubule inhibiting reabsorption
                     of sodium and chloride
Side effects: Electrolyte depletion, hypotension, pancreatitis, jaun-
                     dice
Dose: 25 to 100 mg PO every day in single or divided doses

Hydrocodone (Vicodin)   *Class: Analgesic*

Category: C
Breast feeding: Unknown
Indications: Mild to moderate pain
Actions: Centrally acting analgesic
Side effects: Lightheadedness, dizziness, sedation, nausea,
                     vomiting
Dose: 1 to 2 tablets PO every 4 to 6 hours

Hydromorphine (Dilaudid)   *Class: Analgesic*

Category:	C
Breast feeding:	Unknown
Indications:	Severe pain
Actions:	Centrally acting analgesic
Side effects:	Sedation, drowsiness
Dose:	2 to 4 mg PO every 4 to 6 hours or 1 to 2 mg IM every 4 to 6 hours

Ibuprofen (Motrin,   *Class: Nonsteroidal anti-inflammatory agent*
Nuprin, Advil)

Category:	B
Breast feeding:	Compatible
Indications:	Treatment of dysmenorrhea, mild to moderate pain
Actions:	Nonsteroidal anti-inflammatory agent
Side effects:	Gastrointestinal complaints
Dose:	600 to 800 mg 3 to 4 times per day with a maximum dosage of 3200 mg/day

Imipramine (Tofranil)   *Class: Tricyclic antidepressant*

Category:	B
Breast feeding:	Unknown; may be of concern
Indications:	Depression
Actions:	Unknown, may block norepinephrine uptake
Side effects:	Hypotension, tachycardia, palpitations, confusion, numbness, tingling, anticholinergic effects (dry mouth, disturbances of pupillary accommodation, mydriasis, constipation, blurred vision), bone marrow suppression, nausea, vomiting
Dose:	100 to 300 mg IM or PO per day in divided doses 75 to 150 mg/day initially with a maintenance dose of 50 to 150 mg/day in divided doses

Imiquimod (Aldara) **5% cream**   *Class: Immune response modifier*

Category:	B
Breast feeding:	Unknown
Indications:	Condylomata acuminata
Actions:	Induction of humoral and cell-mediated immune response
Side effects:	Local skin irritation and erythema
Dose:	Applied 3 times per week at bedtime, leaving cream on for 6 to 10 hours, for a maximum of 16 weeks

Indomethacin   *Class: Nonsteroidal anti-inflammatory agent*
(Indocin)

Category:	B
Breast feeding:	Compatible
Indications:	Arthritis
	Preterm labor
Actions:	Nonsteroidal anti-inflammatory agent
Side effects:	Gastrointestinal complaints, headache, dizziness, vertigo, somnolence, depression, tinnitus

Dose: 100-mg rectal suppository as a loading dose followed
                    by 25 mg PO every 6 hours for premature labor
                    25 to 50 mg PO 3 times per day for arthritis

Isoniazid (INH)   *Class: Antituberculosis drug*

Category: C
Breast feeding: Compatible
Indications: Active tuberculosis, prophylaxis against tuberculosis
Actions: Bactericidal
Side effects: Peripheral neuropathy, hepatitis, nausea, vomiting
Dose: 5 mg/kg to 300 mg PO per day in a single dose
                    Prophylactic dose: 300 mg PO per day for 6 to 12
                    months

Isoproterenol (Isuprel)   *Class: Cardiovascular drug*

Category: C
Breast feeding: Unknown
Indications: Heart block, cardiac arrest, bronchospasm, hypovo-
                    lemic and septic shock
Actions: Beta-sympathomimetic
Side effects: Nervousness, headache, dizziness, tachycardia, an-
                    gina, palpitations
Dose: Shock: 0.5 to 5.0 µg/min IV
                    Bronchospasm: 0.01 to 0.02 mg IV
                    Heart block and cardiac arrest: 5 µg/min IV

Ketoconazole (Nizoral)   *Class: Antifungal agent*

Category: C
Breast feeding: Unknown
Indications: Systemic fungal infection
                    Fungal dermatitis
                    Recurrent *Candida* vulvovaginitis
Actions: Inhibition of cell wall synthesis
Side effects: Reversible idiosyncratic hepatitis
Dose: 200- to 400-mg tablet PO daily
                    400-mg tablet PO for 5 days each month starting with
                    menses may also be given for recurrent *Candida*
                    vulvovaginitis
                    2% cream applied once daily

Labetalol (Normodyne, Trandate)   *Class: Antihypertensive*

Category: C
Breast feeding: Compatible
Indications: Hypertension
Actions: Beta-adrenergic blocker
Side effects: Dizziness, nausea, vomiting, fatigue, dyspepsia, par-
                    esthesias
Dose: 20-mg IV bolus dose, followed by 10 to 50 mg IV
                    every 10 minutes
                    100 to 400 mg PO 2 times per day

Leuprolide acetate (Lupron)   *Class: Hormone*

Category:	X
Breast feeding:	Unknown
Indications:	Endometriosis, uterine leiomyomata
Actions:	Gonadotropin-releasing hormone agonist with antagonist effect
Side effects:	Vasomotor symptoms, genitourinary atrophy, osteoporosis
Dose:	Lupron: 1 mg SC per day
	Lupron Depot: 3.75 to 7.5 mg SC once monthly or 11.25 mg SC every 3 months

Levothyroxine (Levothyroid,   *Class: Thyroid supplement*
Levoxine, Synthroid)

Category:	A
Breast feeding:	Excreted into breast milk; caution should be exercised
Indications:	Hypothyroidism
Actions:	Synthetic T_4
Side effects:	Hyperthyroidism
Dose:	Initial dose: 25 to 50 µg PO per day, with daily dose increased in increments of ≤25 µg every 2 to 3 weeks as needed
	Usual maintenance dose: 100 to 200 µg PO per day

Lindane (Kwell)   *Class: Antiparasitic*

Category:	B
Breast feeding:	Unknown
Indications:	Infection with scabies *(Sarcoptes scabiei)*, crab lice (pediculosis pubis)
Actions:	Scabicidal and antipruritic actions
Side effects:	Allergic sensitivity and primary irritation
Dose:	Lindane (Kwell) 1% cream or lotion applied to affected area for 8 to 12 hours, then washed off
	Lindane (Kwell) 1% shampoo applied for 4 minutes, then washed off

Lithium (Eskalith, Lithobid, Lithonate, Lithotab)   *Class: Antipsychotic*

Category:	D
Breast feeding:	Not recommended because of lithium toxicity in the infant
Indications:	Manic episodes of manic-depressive illness
Actions:	Alteration of sodium transport in nerve and muscle cells and change in the metabolism of catecholamines
Side effects:	Diarrhea, vomiting, drowsiness, muscular weakness, ataxia, blurred vision, tinnitus
Dose:	Acute mania: 600 mg PO 3 times per day
	Maintenance dose: 300 mg PO 3 or 4 times per day

Loperamide (Imodium)   *Class: Antidiarrheal*

Category:	B
Breast feeding:	Compatible
Indications:	Diarrhea
Actions:	Slowing of intestinal motility, change in water and electrolyte movement through the bowel, inhibition of peristaltic activity of the bowel
Side effects:	Hypersensitivity reactions, abdominal pain, constipation, fatigue, drowsiness
Dose:	Initial dose: 4 mg PO followed by 2 mg PO after each loose stool
	Dose not to exceed 16 mg/day

Magnesium gluconate or magnesium oxide (Magonate, Mag-Ox, Uro-Mag, Beelith)   *Class: Magnesium salt*

Category:	B
Breast feeding:	Compatible
Indications:	Magnesium supplementation
	Preterm labor
Actions:	Decreases myometrial contractility
Side effects:	None
Dose:	0.5 to 2.0 g PO every 2 to 4 hours

Magnesium sulfate   *Class: Anticonvulsant, uterine tocolytic*

Category:	B
Breast feeding:	Compatible
Indications:	Preeclampsia, eclampsia, preterm labor, uterine hypertonus
Actions:	Decreases myometrial contractility, inhibition of neuromuscular transmission and the cardiac conducting system, depression of central nervous system irritability
Side effects:	Flushing, nausea, vomiting, hypocalcemia, magnesium toxicity (somnolence, respiratory and cardiac depression)
Dose:	2.0 to 6.0 g IV over 20 minutes as a loading dose
	1.0 to 3.0 g/hr IV as the maintenance dose
	5.0 IM every 4 hours can also be used as a maintenance dose for preeclampsia

Meclizine (Antivert, Bonine)   *Class: Antihistamine*

Category:	B
Breast feeding:	Unknown
Indications:	Vertigo, motion sickness
Actions:	Blockage of H_1-histamine receptor
Side effects:	Drowsiness, dry mouth, blurred vision
Dose:	Vertigo: 25 to 100 mg PO per day in divided doses
	Motion sickness: 25 to 50 mg PO 1 hour before trip; dose can be repeated every 24 hours

Medroxyprogesterone (Provera, Depo-Provera, Amen, Cycrin) *Class: Hormone*

Category:	D
Breast feeding:	Compatible
Indications:	Hormone replacement, anovulatory bleeding, endometrial hyperplasia, contraception
Actions:	Progestin supplementation
Side effects:	Irregular bleeding, breast tenderness, amenorrhea, thromboembolic disease
Dose:	2.5 to 10 mg PO per day for 10 to 14 days each month for anovulatory bleeding or treatment of endometrial hyperplasia
	2.5 mg PO per day or 5.0 mg PO for 12 days each month for postmenopausal hormone replacement if a patient is taking estrogen replacement and has not had a hysterectomy
	Depo-Provera: 150 mg IM every 3 months for contraception

Meperidine hydrochloride (Demerol) *Class: Narcotic analgesic*

Category:	B
Breast feeding:	Compatible
Indications:	Sedation, relief of moderate to severe pain
Actions:	Agonist interacting with receptors in the brain and spinal cord
Side effects:	Respiratory depression, nausea, vomiting, hypotension, constipation, agitation, skin rash
Dose:	50 to 100 mg IM or SC every 4 hours for analgesia in labor
	50 to 150 mg PO every 3 to 4 hours

Metaproterenol (Alupent, Metaprel) *Class: Bronchodilator*

Category:	C
Breast feeding:	Unknown
Indications:	Bronchial asthma, bronchospasm, emphysema
Actions:	Beta-sympathomimetic
Side effects:	Nervousness, headache, dizziness, palpitations, gastrointestinal distress, nausea, vomiting, tremor
Dose:	Inhalation aerosol: 2 or 3 inhalations, repeated not more than every 3 to 4 hours
	Tablet: 20 mg PO 3 or 4 times per day

Methadone (Dolophine) *Class: Analgesic*

Category:	B
Breast feeding:	Compatible if mother is taking <20 mg/day
Indications:	Severe pain, treatment of narcotic addiction
Actions:	Agonist interacting with receptors in the brain and spinal cord

Side effects:	Lightheadedness, dizziness, sedation, nausea, vomiting, respiratory depression and arrest, cardiac arrest, shock
Dose:	Analgesic effect: 2.5 to 10 mg IM or SC every 3 to 4 hours
	Detoxification: Initial dose of 15 to 20 mg PO per day for 2 to 3 days for stabilization, then dose is decreased every 1 to 2 days

Methimazole [Tapazole]   *Class: Thyroid suppressant*

Category:	D
Breast feeding:	Compatible
Indications:	Hyperthyroidism
Actions:	Inhibits organification of iodine and therefore inhibits production of triiodothyronine (T_3) and thyroxine (T_4)
Side effects:	Bone marrow suppression, hepatitis, dermatitis
Dose:	20 to 30 mg PO every 12 hours

Methotrexate   *Class: Antimetabolite*

Category:	X
Breast feeding:	Not recommended because of possible immunosuppression, carcinogenic effects, and adverse effects on growth in the infant
Indications:	Treatment of tubal pregnancy, gestational trophoblastic disease
Actions:	Inhibition of folic acid synthesis
Side effects:	Bone marrow suppression, stomatitis, nausea, abdominal distress
Dose:	50 mg/m^2 IM for tubal pregnancy; dose is repeated depending on the response in serum hCG levels

Methylergonovine [Methergine]   *Class: Oxytocic*

Category:	C
Breast feeding:	Excreted into breast milk; caution should be exercised
Indications:	Postpartum atony and hemorrhaging, subinvolution of the uterus
Actions:	Ergot alkaloid that acts directly on smooth muscle of the uterus resulting in increased tone, frequency, and amplitude of uterine contractions
Side effects:	Hypertension, nausea, vomiting
Dose:	0.2 mg PO 3 or 4 times per day for maximum of 1 week
	0.2 mg IM or IV, repeated every 2 to 4 hours

Metronidazole [Flagyl, Protostat, MetroGel]   *Class: Antibiotic*

Category:	B
Breast feeding:	Excreted into breast-milk; caution should be exercised. Discontinuation of breast-feeding for 12 to 24 hours is recommended if the 2 g PO dose is used

Indications:	Trichomoniasis, bacterial vaginosis, amebiasis, pseudomembranous colitis caused by *Clostridium difficile* infection, anaerobic infection
Actions:	Interference with DNA synthesis
Side effects:	Gastrointestinal symptoms, peripheral neuropathy
Dose:	250 mg PO 3 times per day for 7 days or 500 mg PO 2 times per day for 7 days for trichomoniasis or bacterial vaginosis
	2 g PO once for trichomoniasis
	500 mg PO 3 times per day for 7 to 10 days for *C. difficile*
	Metronidazole vaginal gel 5 g (1 applicator full) intravaginally 2 times per day for 5 days

Miconazole (Monistat)   *Class: Antifungal agent*

Category:	C
Breast feeding:	Unknown
Indications:	*Candida* vulvovaginitis, dermatitis, or systemic infection
Actions:	Imidazole derivative, interferes with cell membrane by inhibition of ergosterol
Side effects:	IV administration: phlebitis, pruritus, rash, nausea, vomiting, diarrhea, anorexia, flushes
	Vaginal administration: vaginal itching, irritation, cramping, headaches
Dose:	Systemic infection: 200 to 1200 mg IV 3 times per day
	Vulvovaginitis: 200-mg suppository every night before bed for 3 nights; 100-mg suppository every night before bed for 7 nights
	2% cream 5 g every night before bed for 7 nights

Midazolam (Versed)   *Class: Benzodiazepine*

Category:	C
Breast feeding:	Unknown but may be of concern
Indications:	Conscious sedation or premedication for short diagnostic or surgical procedure
Actions:	Short-acting central nervous system depressant
Side effects:	Respiratory depression, headache, fluctuation of vital signs, hiccups, nausea, vomiting, drowsiness
Dose:	0.07 to 0.08 mg/kg IM 1 hour before procedure
	0.02 to 0.05 mg/kg IV before procedure

Misoprostol (Cytotec)   *Class: Prostaglandin analog*

Category:	X
Breast feeding:	Not recommended because of drug-induced diarrhea in the infant
Indications:	Prevention of gastric and duodenal ulcers in patients taking nonsteroidal anti-inflammatory drugs; cervical ripening; induction of labor in the second trimester for fetal demise or elective termination
Actions:	Prostaglandin E_1 analog
Side effects:	Diarrhea, abdominal pain, uterine hyperstimulation, uterine rupture

Dose: 25 to 50 μg intravaginally or PO every 3 to 6 hours for cervical ripening

200 μg intravaginally or orally every 12 hours for induction of labor

200 μg PO four times per day for prevention of ulcers

Morphine sulfate [Morphine sulfate, MS Contin, MSIR, Rescudose, Roxanol, MS/L, OMS Concentrate]   *Class: Narcotic analgesic*

Category:	C
Breast feeding:	Compatible
Indications:	Sedation, relief of moderate to severe pain
Actions:	Agonist interacting with receptors in the brain and spinal cord
Side effects:	Respiratory depression, nausea, vomiting, hypotension, dizziness, sweating, constipation, agitation, flushing, skin rash
Dose:	10 to 30 mg PO every 4 hours
	5 to 20 mg IM every 4 hours
	2.5 to 15 mg IV every 4 hours

Nafarelin acetate [Synarel]   *Class: Hormone*

Category:	X
Breast feeding:	Not recommended
Indications:	Pelvic pain and dysmenorrhea secondary to endometriosis
Actions:	Gonadotropin-releasing hormone agonist with antagonist effect
Side effects:	Vasomotor symptoms, genitourinary atrophy, osteoporosis
Dose:	200 μg intranasal spray 2 times per day (patients who do not achieve amenorrhea can be placed on 400 μg 2 times per day)

Nafcillin [Unipen]   *Class: Antibiotic*

Category:	B
Breast feeding:	Excreted into breast milk; alteration of bowel flora, candidiasis, and allergic reaction in the infant should be considered
Indications:	Treatment of infection due to penicillinase-producing staphylococci
Actions:	Inhibition of cell wall synthesis
Side effects:	Hypersensitivity reaction, transient leukopenia, thrombocytopenia, skin rash
Dose:	250 to 500 mg PO every 4 to 6 hours
	500 to 1000 mg IV every 4 hours

Naloxone [Narcan]   *Class: Narcotic antagonist*

Category:	B
Breast feeding:	Unknown
Indications:	Reversal of narcotic effects
Actions:	Competitive antagonism of narcotics
Side effects:	Nausea, vomiting, tachycardia, hypertension, tremulousness, seizures

Dose: 0.4 to 2 mg SC, IM, or IV, repeated at 2- to 3-minute intervals until a maximum dose of 10 mg has been administered

Naproxen (Naprosyn,   *Class: Nonsteroidal anti-inflammatory agent*
Anaprox, Anaprox DS)

Category:	B
Breast feeding:	Compatible
Indications:	Treatment of dysmenorrhea, mild to moderate pain
Actions:	Nonsteroidal anti-inflammatory agent
Side effects:	Gastrointestinal complaints
Dose:	Naprosyn: 250 to 500 mg PO every 6 to 8 hours with maximum dose of 1250 mg/day
	Anaprox: 275 to 550 mg PO every 6 to 8 hours with maximum dose of 1375 mg/day

Nifedipine (Adalat,   *Class: Antihypertensive, uterine tocolytic*
Procardia)

Category:	C
Breast feeding:	Compatible
Indications:	Hypertension
	Vasospastic and chronic stable angina
	Preterm labor
Actions:	Calcium channel blocker
Side effects:	Dizziness, lightheadedness, flushing, headache, weakness, nausea, muscle cramps, peripheral edema
Dose:	Hypertension: 10 to 30 mg PO 3 or 4 times per day
	Preterm labor: 10 mg PO or sublingual, repeat after 20 minutes if necessary; 10 to 20 mg every 4 to 6 hours, maintenance dose

Nitrofurantoin (Macrodantin)   *Class: Antibiotic*

Category:	B
Breast feeding:	Compatible
Indications:	Treatment of urinary tract infection
Actions:	Inactivation and alteration of bacterial ribosomal proteins and other macromolecules resulting in inhibition of protein synthesis, DNA and RNA synthesis, aerobic energy metabolism, and cell wall synthesis
Side effects:	Pulmonary hypersensitivity reactions, hepatitis, nausea, vomiting, peripheral neuropathy, dermatitis
Dose:	50 to 100 mg PO 4 times per day
	Suppressive therapy: 50 to 100 mg PO every night before bed

Nystatin (Mycostatin, Mytrex)   *Class: Antifungal agent*

Category:	B
Breast feeding:	Compatible
Indications:	*Candida* vulvovaginitis or dermatitis
Actions:	Polyene compound, binds to ergosterol causing cell membrane permeability

Side effects: Topical application: skin irritation
                Oral administration: nausea
Dose: Vaginal: 100,000 units every night before bed for 14
                days
                Oral: 200,000 to 400,000 units 4 to 5 times per day for
                14 days
                Topical: Apply 2 or 3 times every day

Ofloxacin (Floxin)   *Class: Antibiotic*

Category: C, contraindicated because of increased risk of major
                congenital malformations
Breast feeding: Not recommended because of the risk of arthropathy
                and other toxicity to the infant
Indications: Uncomplicated infection with *Neisseria gonorrhoeae* or
                Chlamydia trachomatis, gonococcal bacteremia, and
                arthritis
                Lower respiratory infection due to *Haemophilus in-
                fluenzae* or *Streptococcus pneumoniae*
                Urinary tract infection due to *Enterobacter acrogenes,
                Escherichia coli, Klebsiella pneumoniae, Proteus mira-
                bilis,* or *Pseudomonas aeruginosa*
Actions: Interference with enzyme DNA gyrase, which is nec-
                essary for DNA synthesis
Side effects: Nausea, diarrhea, vomiting, insomnia, headache, diz-
                ziness, rash
Dose: 200 to 400 mg PO or IV 2 times per day
                Chlamydia: 300 mg PO 2 times per day for 7 days
                Gonorrhea: 400 mg PO once
                400 mg IV every 12 hours followed by 400 mg PO 2
                times per day for gonococcal bacteremia and arthri-
                tis

Oxycodone (Percodan, Percocet)   *Class: Analgesic*

Category: C
Breast feeding: Excreted into breast milk; caution should be exercised
                because of risk of sedation, lethargy, and gastroin-
                testinal symptoms
Indications: Moderate to severe pain
Actions: Agonist interacting with receptors in the brain and
                spinal cord
Side effects: Lightheadedness, dizziness, sedation, nausea, vom-
                iting
Dose: 1 tablet PO every 6 hours

Oxytocin (Pitocin, Syntocinon)   *Class: Oxytocic*

Category: C
Breast feeding: Excreted into breast milk; caution should be exercised
Indications: Induction or augmentation of labor
                Treatment of uterine atony
Actions: Promotes contractility of uterine smooth muscle by
                increasing intracellular calcium

Side effects: Hypertonus, antidiuretic effect with high doses given over a prolonged period

Dose: Induction or augmentation of labor: A solution of 10 IU of oxytocin in 1000 ml of 5% dextrose and lactated Ringer's solution or 5% dextrose and 0.5 normal saline is used. Infusion is started at a rate of 0.1 ml/min or 1 mIU/min and increased until regular uterine contractions are achieved. The infusion rate is increased by 1 mIU/min every 20 to 30 minutes up to a dose of 8 mIU/min. Above this dose, the rate can be increased in increments of 2 mIU/min every 20 to 30 minutes up to a dose of 20 mIU/min

                  Treatment of uterine atony: A solution of 20 to 40 IU of oxytocin in 1000 ml of 5% dextrose and lactated Ringer's solution or 5% dextrose and 0.5 normal saline is infused at rates of 250 to 500 ml/hr

Penicillin G benzathine suspension (Bicillin)   *Class: Antibiotic*

Category: B

Breast feeding: Excreted into breast milk; alteration of bowel flora, candidiasis, and allergic reaction in the infant should be considered

Indications: Syphilis, upper respiratory infection due to streptococci, prophylactic therapy for rheumatic heart disease and acute glomerulonephritis

Actions: Inhibition of cell wall synthesis

Side effects: Hypersensitivity reactions

Dose: Primary, secondary, and latent syphilis: 2.4 million units IM once

                  Tertiary and neurosyphilis: 2.4 million units IM 1 time per week for 3 weeks

Penicillin G Procaine (Wycillin)   *Class: Antibiotic*

Category: B

Breast feeding: Excreted into breast milk; alteration of bowel flora, candidiasis, and allergic reaction in the infant should be considered

Indications: Syphilis, infection caused by *Neisseria gonorrhoeae*, *Streptococcus* spp., or *Staphylococcus* spp.

Actions: Inhibition of cell wall synthesis

Side effects: Hypersensitivity reactions

Dose: Uncomplicated gonorrhea: 4.8 million units IM divided into two doses and given in two different sites with 1 g probenecid PO given just before injection

                  Gonococcal meningitis: 10 million units IV per day for at least 10 days

                  Primary, secondary, and latent syphilis: 600,000 units IM per day for 8 days

                  Tertiary, neurosyphilis, and latent syphilis with positive cerebrospinal fluid: 600,000 units IM per day for 10 to 15 days

Penicillin V potassium [Pen-Vee K]   *Class: Antibiotic*

Category:	B
Breast feeding:	Excreted into breast milk; alteration of bowel flora, candidiasis, and allergic reaction in the infant should be considered
Indications:	Mild to moderate infection due to gram-positive bacteria such as *Staphylococcus* spp., *Streptococcus* spp., *Clostridium* spp., or *Corynebacterium* spp.
Actions:	Inhibition of cell wall synthesis
Side effects:	Nausea, vomiting, diarrhea, epigastric distress, hypersensitivity reactions
Dose:	250 to 500 mg PO 4 times per day

Pentobarbital   *Class: Anticonvulsant, hypnotic sedative*
[Nembutal]

Category:	D
Breast feeding:	Unknown
Indications:	Insomnia, preanesthetic sedation
	Seizure disorder
Actions:	Central nervous system depressant
Side effects:	Somnolence
Dose:	100- to 200-mg capsule PO for hypnosis and sedation in early labor
	150 to 200 mg IM
	100 to 500 mg IV by slow infusion not to exceed 50 mg/min

Permethrin [Elimite]   *Class: Antiparasitic*

Category:	B
Breast feeding:	Unknown; because of tumorigenic effects in animals, breast feeding should be discontinued
Indications:	Treatment of *Sarcoptes scabiei* (scabies)
Actions:	Disrupts sodium channel current by which polarization of the membrane is regulated, resulting in delayed repolarization and paralysis of the organism
Side effects:	Burning, pruritus, erythema, numbness, tingling, rash
Dose:	5% cream: massage into skin from head to toes and wash off after 8 to 14 hours

Phenazopyridine [Pyridium, Prodium]   *Class: Urinary tract agent*

Category:	B
Breast feeding:	Unknown
Indications:	Urinary tract infection
Actions:	Topical analgesic effect on mucosa of urinary tract
Side effects:	Headache, rash, pruritus, gastrointestinal symptoms, orange discoloration of the urine
Dose:	200 mg PO 3 times per day

Phenobarbital   *Class: Barbiturate*

Category:	D
Breast feeding:	Excreted into breast milk; caution should be exercised
Indications:	Sedation, anticonvulsant
Actions:	Central nervous system depressant
Side effects:	Respiratory depression, residual sedation

Dose: Sedation: 30 to 120 mg PO or IM, doses repeated as needed with maximum of 400 mg in 24 hours

Anticonvulsant effect: 60 to 200 mg PO or IM per day

Phenytoin (Dilantin)   *Class: Anticonvulsant*

Category:	D
Breast feeding:	Compatible
Indications:	Treatment and prevention of seizures
Actions:	Inhibition of spread of seizure activity in the motor cortex, possibly by promoting the efflux of sodium from neurons
Side effects:	Nystagmus, ataxia, slurred speech, mental confusion, nausea, vomiting, atrial and ventricular conduction depression, ventricular fibrillation
Dose:	Sedation: 30 to 120 mg PO or IM per day
	Anticonvulsant effect: 100 mg PO 3 or 4 times per day
	Status epilepticus: Loading dose of 10 to 15 mg/kg by slow IV infusion not to exceed 50 mg/min, followed by a maintenance dose of 100 mg PO or IV every 6 to 8 hours

Prochlorperazine (Compazine)   *Class: Antiemetic*

Category:	C
Breast feeding:	Compatible
Indications:	Nausea, vomiting, nonpsychotic anxiety
Actions:	Phenothiazine effect
Side effects:	Drowsiness, dizziness, amenorrhea, blurred vision, hypotension, tardive dyskinesia, neuroleptic malignant syndrome (hyperpyrexia, muscle rigidity, altered mental status, autonomic instability)
Dose:	Nausea: 5 to 10 mg PO 3 or 4 times per day; 5 to 10 mg IM every 3 to 4 hours; 25-mg rectal suppository 2 times per day; or 2.5 to 10 mg by slow IV infusion, not to exceed 5 mg/min
	Nonpsychotic anxiety: 5 mg PO 3 or 4 times per day; or 10 to 20 mg IM, repeated if necessary every 2 to 4 hours

Progesterone in oil   *Class: Hormone*

Category:	X
Breast feeding:	Unknown; probably compatible based on data on medroxyprogesterone
Indications:	Anovulatory or dysfunctional bleeding
Actions:	Progestin supplementation
Side effects:	Irregular bleeding, breast tenderness, amenorrhea, thromboembolic disease
Dose:	50 to 100 mg IM each month

Promethazine (Phenergan)   *Class: Antiemetic*

Category:	C
Breast feeding:	Unknown
Indications:	Nausea, vomiting, motion sickness, sedation
Actions:	Phenothiazine derivative with antihistaminic, sedative, antimotion sickness, and anticholinergic effects
Side effects:	Drowsiness, tachycardia, bradycardia, constipation, dry mouth
Dose:	Nausea: 12.5 to 25 mg PO, IM, rectally, or IV every 4 to 6 hours
	Sedation: 25 to 50 mg PO, IM, rectally, or IV for preoperative or obstetrical sedation

Propoxyphene (Darvon, Darvocet-N,   *Class: Analgesic*
Darvon-N, Darvon compound)

Category:	C
Breast feeding:	Compatible
Indications:	Mild to moderate pain
Actions:	Narcotic analgesic with central nervous system effect
Side effects:	Dizziness, sedation, nausea, vomiting
Dose:	1 tablet PO every 4 hours

Propranolol (Inderal)   *Class: Beta blocker*

Category:	C
Breast feeding:	Compatible
Indications:	Hypertension, cardiac arrhythmias, myocardial infarction, migraine headaches, tremors, hypertrophic subaortic stenosis, pheochromocytoma, thyrotoxicosis
Actions:	Beta-adrenergic receptor–blocking agent
Side effects:	Bradycardia, hypotension, congestive heart failure, lightheadedness, mental depression, nausea, vomiting, bronchospasm, hallucinations, vivid dreams
Dose:	10 to 80 mg PO 2, 3, or 4 times per day

Propylthiouracil (PTU)   *Class: Thyroid suppressant*

Category:	D
Breast feeding:	Compatible
Indications:	Hyperthyroidism
Actions:	Inhibits organification of iodine and therefore inhibits production of triiodothyronine (T_3) and thyroxine (T_4), inhibits conversion of T_4 to T_3
Side effects:	Leukopenia, skin rash
Dose:	100 to 150 mg PO every 8 hours

Prostaglandin E₂ (Prostin E2, Prepidil Gel)   *Class: Prostaglandin*

Category:	C
Breast feeding:	Unknown
Indications:	Termination of pregnancy from 12 to 20 weeks of gestation

Management of missed abortion or intrauterine fetal demise up to 28 weeks of gestation

Ripening of unfavorable cervix

Actions: Stimulation of myometrium

Induces biochemical changes in the cervix, resulting in collagen degradation

Side effects: Vomiting, diarrhea, nausea, fever, headache, chills, backache, joint pain, flushing, dizziness, arthralgia, vaginal pain, chest pain, dyspnea

Dose: Prostin E2: 20-mg vaginal suppositories inserted every 4 hours until the patient is in labor

Prepidil Gel: 0.5 mg intracervically every 6 hours for 2 or 3 doses for cervical ripening

Protamine sulfate   *Class: Heparin antagonist*

Category: C
Breast feeding: Unknown
Indications: Heparin overdose
Actions: Binds with heparin, neutralizing anticoagulant effect
Side effects: Hypotension, bradycardia, flushing, dyspnea, nausea, vomiting
Dose: Solution of 10 mg/ml given by slow IV infusion at a rate not to exceed 20 mg/min or 50 mg in a 10-minute period

Each mg of protamine will neutralize 90 to 115 units of heparin

Pyrethrins (A-200 Pediculicide   *Class: Antiparasitic* shampoo and gel)

Category: C
Breast feeding: Unknown
Indications: Treatment of pediculosis pubis or crab lice
Actions: Kills lice and eggs
Side effects: Skin irritation
Dose: Apply undiluted to dry hair. Wet entirely and leave on for 10 minutes, then wash thoroughly. Repeat treatment in 7 to 10 days.

Ranitidine (Zantac)   *Class: Histamine H_2-receptor antagonist*

Category: B
Breast feeding: Compatible
Indications: Duodenal ulcer, hypersecretory conditions, gastroesophageal reflux, esophagitis
Actions: Inhibition of histamine-induced secretion of gastric acid by binding histamine H_2-receptor sites in gastric cells
Side effects: Headache, malaise, dizziness, hepatitis, jaundice, leukopenia
Dose: Oral: 150 mg PO 2 times per day or 300 mg PO per day followed by maintenance dose: 150 mg PO every night before bed

Parenteral: 50 mg IM or IV every 6 to 8 hours

Rifampin (Rifadin)   *Class: Antibiotic*

Category:	C
Breast feeding:	Compatible
Indications:	Tuberculosis, *Neisseria meningitidis* carriers
Actions:	Inhibition of DNA-dependent RNA polymerase activity
Side effects:	Epigastric distress, nausea, vomiting, thrombocytopenia, headache, drowsiness, dizziness, hepatitis
Dose:	Tuberculosis: 600 mg PO or IV per day
	N. meningitidis: 600 mg PO or IV 2 times per day for 2 days

Ritodrine (Yutopar)   *Class: Tocolytic*

Category:	B
Breast feeding:	Unknown
Indications:	Preterm labor, uterine hypertonus
Actions:	Beta-sympathomimetic
Side effects:	Nausea, emesis, restlessness, agitation, hypotension, pulmonary edema, cardiac insufficiency, cardiac arrhythmia, myocardial ischemia, hyperglycemia, hypokalemia
Dose:	0.050 to 0.350 mg/min IV or 5 to 10 mg IM every 2 to 4 hours or 20 mg PO every 2 to 4 hours

Secobarbital (Seconal)   *Class: Sedative, hypnotic*

Category:	D
Breast feeding:	Compatible
Indications:	Insomnia, sedation prior to administration of anesthesia
Actions:	Central nervous system depresssant
Side effects:	Somnolence, confusion, agitation, respiratory depression, bradycardia, hypotension, nausea, vomiting, headache
Dose:	100 mg PO every night before bed
	200 to 300 mg PO 1 to 2 hours before procedure

Sertraline (Zoloft)   *Class: Antidepressant*

Category:	B
Breast feeding:	Unknown, may be of concern
Indications:	Depression
Actions:	Inhibition of central nervous system neuronal uptake of serotonin
Side effects:	Nausea, diarrhea, dyspepsia, tremor, dizziness, insomnia, dry mouth
Dose:	Initial dose of 50 mg PO per day followed by maintenance dose of 50 to 200 mg PO per day

Spectinomycin (Trobicin)   *Class: Antibiotic*

Category:	B
Breast feeding:	Unknown

Indications:	Uncomplicated gonorrhea, gonococcal bacteremia, and arthritis
Actions:	Inhibition of protein synthesis
Side effects:	Nausea, chills, fever, urticaria, insomnia
Dose:	2 g IM once

Sulfasalazine (Azulfidine)   *Class: Antibiotic*

Category:	B
Breast feeding:	Caution should be exercised
Indications:	Ulcerative colitis
Actions:	Anti-inflammatory effect
Side effects:	Anorexia, headache, nausea, vomiting, gastric distress
Dose:	Initial dose of 3 to 4 g PO per day in divided doses, followed by maintenance dose of 2 g PO per day in divided doses

Sulfisoxazole (Gantrisin)   *Class: Antibiotic*

Category:	C
Breast feeding:	Compatible
Indications:	Urinary tract infection due to *Escherichia coli, Klebsiella* spp., *Staphylococcus* spp., and *Proteus mirabilis*
	Meningococcal meningitis
	Acute otitis media
	Infection due to *Chlamydia trachomatis*
Actions:	Inhibition of synthesis of dihydrofolic acid
Side effects:	Hypersensitivity reactions, gastrointestinal symptoms
Dose:	500 to 1000 mg PO 4 times per day
	500 mg PO 4 times per day for 10 days for chlamydial infections

Tamoxifen (Nolvadex)   *Class: Antineoplastic*

Category:	D
Breast feeding:	Not recommended because of possible adverse effects on the infant and inhibition of lactation
Indications:	Breast cancer
Actions:	Nonsteroidal agent with antiestrogenic properties
Side effects:	Vasomotor symptoms, nausea, vomiting, irregular bleeding, vaginal discharge, endometrial hyperplasia, endometrial carcinoma
Dose:	10 to 20 mg PO 2 times per day

Terbutaline (Brethine, Bricanyl)   *Class: Bronchodilator, tocolytic*

Category:	B
Breast feeding:	Compatible
Indications:	Bronchial asthma, bronchospasm
	Preterm labor
Actions:	Beta-sympathomimetic
Side effects:	Nausea, vomiting, palpitations, tachycardia, tremors, nervousness, dizziness, headache, drowsiness, dyspnea, chest discomfort, weakness, flushing, sweating

Dose: 0.01 to 0.08 mg/min IV
0.25 to 0.50 mg IM or SC every 3 to 4 hours
2.5 to 5.0 mg PO every 2 to 4 hours
If decrease in uterine activity is not achieved in 15 to 30 minutes, a second dose can be administered

Terconazole (Terazol) *Class: Antifungal agent*

Category: C
Breast feeding: Unknown
Indications: *Candida* vulvovaginitis
Actions: Imidazole derivative, interferes with cell membrane by inhibition of ergosterol
Side effects: Vaginal itching, irritation, dysmenorrhea, headaches
Dose: Terazol 3 80-mg suppository: 1 every night before bed for 3 nights
Terazol 3 0.8% vaginal cream: 5 g every night before bed for 3 nights
Terazol 7 0.4% vaginal cream: 5 g every night before bed for 7 nights

Tetracycline (Achromycin) *Class: Antibiotic*

Category: D
Breast feeding: Compatible
Indications: Infection caused by *Chlamydia trachomatis, Neisseria gonorrhoeae, Treponema pallidum, Mycoplasma pneumoniae, Haemophilus ducreyi,* or *Bacteroides* spp.
Actions: Interference with protein synthesis
Side effects: Nausea, vomiting, diarrhea, rash, rise in blood urea nitrogen, hypersensitivity reaction
Dose: 250 to 500 mg PO 4 times per day for 10 to 14 days

Theophylline (Aerolate, Asbron, Quibron, Respbid, Theo-Dur, Theolair, Theo-X, T-Phyl, Uniphyl) *Class: Bronchodilator*

Category: C
Breast feeding: Compatible
Indications: Asthma, bronchospasm associated with bronchitis and emphysema
Actions: Relaxation of smooth muscle of the bronchi
Side effects: Nausea, vomiting, irritability, tachycardia, arrhythmias, seizures
Dose: 13 mg/kg PO per day in divided doses, not to exceed 900 mg/day

Ticarcillin and clavulanic acid (Timentin) *Class: Antibiotic*

Category: B
Breast feeding: Compatible
Indications: Infection due to beta-lactamase–producing strains of *Escherichia coli, Klebsiella pneumoniae, Staphylococcus aureus,* or *Enterobacter* spp.

Actions: Inhibition of cell wall synthesis
Side effects: Hypersensitivity reactions
Dose: 50 to 75 mg/kg IV every 6 hours

Tioconazole [Vagistat-1]   *Class: Antifungal agent*

Category: C
Breast feeding: Unknown
Indications: *Candida* vulvovaginitis
Actions: Imidazole derivative, interferes with cell membrane
                  by inhibition of ergosterol
Side effects: Vulvovaginal burning, itching
Dose: 6.5% ointment: 4.6 g inserted with prefilled applicator
                  into the vagina once

Tobramycin [Nebcin]   *Class: Antibiotic*

Category: D
Breast feeding: Caution should be exercised because of possible alter-
                  ation of bowel flora and direct effects on the infant
Indications: Treatment of infections due to *Pseudomonas aeruginosa,
                  Proteus* spp., *Escherichia coli, Enterobacter* spp., *Kleb-
                  siella* spp., *Serratia* spp., *Staphylococcus aureus, Pro-
                  videncia* spp., or *Citrobacter* spp.
Actions: Inhibition of protein synthesis
Side effects: Ototoxicity, neurotoxicity, renal toxicity
Dose: 3 mg/kg IM or IV per day in 3 divided doses every
                  8 hours
                  5 mg/kg/day may be given for life-threatening infec-
                  tion

Triamcinolone acetonide   *Class: Anti-inflammatory agent*
[Aristocort A]

Category: C
Breast feeding: Unknown
Indications: Treatment of inflammatory and pruritic manifesta-
                  tions of dermatoses
                  Treatment of squamous cell hyperplasia of the vulva
Actions: Topical corticosteroid
Side effects: Burning, itching, skin irritation, dryness
Dose: 0.01% cream or lotion applied 2 or 3 times per day

Trimethobenzamide [Tigan]   *Class: Antiemetic*

Category: C
Breast feeding: Unknown
Indications: Nausea and vomiting
Actions: Unclear, may act centrally on medulla oblongata
Side effects: Hypersensitivity reactions, Parkinson-like symptoms,
                  hypotension
Dose: Oral: 250 mg PO 3 or 4 times per day
                  Rectal suppository: 200 mg rectally 3 or 4 times per
                  day
                  Intramuscular: 200 mg IM 3 or 4 times per day

Trimethoprim and sulfamethoxazole   *Class: Antibiotic*
(Bactrim, Septra)

Category:	C
Breast feeding:	Compatible
Indications:	Urinary tract infection due to *Escherichia coli, Klebsiella* spp., *Enterobacter* spp., *Proteus mirabilis, Proteus vulgaris,* or *Morganella morganii*
	Acute otitis media, chronic bronchitis, travelers' diarrhea, shigellosis, and *Pneumocystis carinii* pneumonia
Actions:	Sulfamethoxazole: inhibition of synthesis of dihydrofolic acid
	Trimethoprim: inhibition of synthesis of tetrahydrofolic acid from dihydrofolic acid
Side effects:	Nausea, vomiting, anorexia, skin reaction, leukopenia, hepatitis
Dose:	2 tablets PO every 12 hours for 10 to 14 days
	1 double-strength (DS) tablet PO every 12 hours for 10 to 14 days
	4 teaspoons or 20 ml PO every 12 hours for 10 to 14 days
	Shigellosis and travelers' diarrhea can be treated with one of the above regimens for a total of 5 days.

Valacyclovir (Valtrex)   *Class: Antiviral*

Category:	B
Breast feeding:	Compatible
Indications:	Treatment and prophylaxis for herpes simplex virus infection
Actions:	Converted into acyclovir, which has inhibitory activity against herpes simplex virus
Side effects:	Thrombocytopenia, anemia, leukopenia, renal failure, aplastic anemia
Dose:	Primary infection: 1 g PO 2 times per day for 7 to 10 days
	Recurrent infection: 500 mg PO 2 times per day for 5 days
	Prophylaxis: 250 mg PO 2 times per day or 500 mg PO per day or 1000 mg PO per day

Vancomycin (Vancocin, Vancoled)   *Class: Antibiotic*

Category:	C
Breast feeding:	Caution should be exercised; alteration of bowel flora, allergic reaction, and other effects on the infant should be considered
Indications:	Parenteral administration: treatment of methicillin-resistant staphylococcus
	Oral administration: treatment of staphylococcal enterocolitis and pseudomembranous colitis caused by *Clostridium difficile*
Actions:	Interference with protein synthesis

Side effects:	Nephrotoxicity, ototoxicity, neutropenia
Dose:	250 to 500 mg PO 4 times per day for 10 days
	500 mg IV every 6 hours or 1000 mg IV every 12 hours

Warfarin sodium (Coumadin)   *Class: Anticoagulant*

Category:	X
Breast feeding:	Compatible
Indications:	Prophylaxis and treatment of deep vein thrombosis, pulmonary embolism, atrial fibrillation with embolization
Actions:	Inhibition of production of vitamin K–dependent clotting factors (II, VII, IX, and X)
Side effects:	Hemorrhaging, necrosis of the skin and other organs, nausea, alopecia
Dose:	Initial dose of 2 to 5 mg PO per day, followed by a maintenance dose of 2 to 10 mg PO per day with dose adjusted to prolong prothrombin time by 1.2 to 1.5 times control

INDEX

Note: Page numbers in *italic* indicate illustrations; those followed by t refer to tables.

A

Abdomen, in malpresentation, 107
Abortion, definition of, 297
  habitual, 297
  inevitable, 297, 305
  missed, 297, 306
  recurrent, 297, 298–299
  septic, 297
    diagnostic tests for, 304
    treatment of, 306–307
  spontaneous, 297–307
    causes of, 298–299
    clinical presentation of, 297
    complete blood count in, 304
    completed, 297, 306
    diagnostic tests for, 301–304, 302t, *303*, 303t
    evaluation of, 298, *299*–300
    human chorionic gonadotropin in, 301, *302*–304, *303*, 303t
    hypovolemic shock in, 299
    in multiple gestation, 121
    in Rh-negative women, 307
    incidence of, 297
    incomplete, 297, 305–306
    orders for, 300–301
    physical examination of, 300
    pregnancy test in, 301
    progesterone in, 304
    treatment of, 304–307
    ultrasonography in, 301–302, 302t
    urgency of, 298
    threatened, 297, 304–305
  vs. preterm labor, 183
Abscess, Bartholin's. See *Bartholin's abscess.*
  pelvic, 157
  tubo-ovarian, 261
    Chlamydia trachomatis in, 266

Abscess *(Continued)*
  in pelvic inflammatory disease, 261–262, 268–269
Acetaminophen, with codeine, 369
Acidemia, 33
Acidosis, 33
Acyclovir, 369
  in vulvar herpes simplex virus infection, 326
Adenomyosis, 281
Adnexa, 270
  in abnormal labor, 51
  masses of, 270. See also *Pelvic mass.*
    complications of, 274
Adrenal glands, in pregnancy, 26
Adrenarche, 9, *10*
β-Adrenergic agonists, complications of, 195–196
  contraindications to, 196
  in preterm labor, 194–196
  precautions with, 196
β-Adrenergic blockers, in molar pregnancy, 258
Alanine, in pregnancy, 353t
Albumin, in pregnancy, 352t
Albuterol, 369
Alpha-fetoprotein, in pelvic mass, 277–278
Alprazolam, 369–370
Aminophylline, 370
Aminotransferase, in pregnancy, 353t
Amitriptyline, 370
Amniocentesis, in chorioamnionitis, 173, 174t
  in preterm labor, 191–193, 193t
Amnioinfusion, in meconium aspiration syndrome, 119
  in nonreassuring fetal heart rate, 43–44
  in preterm premature rupture of membranes, 181

Amniotic fluid, culture of, in
    chorioamnionitis, 173, 174t
  in premature rupture of mem-
    branes, 168
  phospholipid levels in, *350*
    gestational age and, 175, *178*
    in preterm labor, 191–192, *192*
  shake test of, 176–177, 178t, 358t
    in preterm labor, 192–193,
    193t
Amniotic fluid embolism, 57–62
  cardiogenic shock treatment in,
    61
  cardiopulmonary resuscitation
    for, 60
  catheterization for, 60–61, 61t
  clinical presentation of, 57–58
  coagulopathy in, 61–62
  cryoprecipitate in, 62
  definition of, 57
  diagnostic tests for, 60
  differential diagnosis of, 58
  electronic fetal monitoring in, 62
  evaluation of, 59–60
  fetal asphyxia from, 58
  fresh frozen plasma in, 62
  hemodynamic abnormalities in,
    57
  intubation for, 60
  maternal threats in, 58–59
  orders for, 59
  platelets in, 62
  predisposition to, 58
  red blood cells in, 61–62
  treatment of, 60–62, 61t
Amniotic fluid index, in
    preeclampsia, 78, *79*
  in premature rupture of mem-
    branes, 173, *173*, *174*
  mean for, *349*
  measurement of, *348*
  percentiles for, *349*
Amniotomy, labor induction by, 95
Amoxicillin, 370
Amphotericin B, 370–371
Ampicillin, 371
  after cesarean section, 155
  in endometritis, 155, 156
  with sulbactam, 371
Amylase, in pregnancy, 353t
Analgesia, epidural, 48
Analgesics, in mastitis, 114
  in pelvic pain, 287
Androgen, in menopause, 15, 15t

Anemia, in multiple gestation, 123
Anovulatory bleeding, 217
Antibiotics, after cesarean section,
    155
  beta-lactamase–resistant anti-
    staphylococcal, in toxic
    shock syndrome, 313–314
  in chorioamnionitis, 177
  in endometritis, 155–156
  in mastitis, 115
  in sexual assault, 294
  in uterine subinvolution, 167
Antibody(ies), anticardiolipin, 68
  lupus anticoagulant, 68
Anticardiolipin antibody, 68
Anticonvulsants, in preeclampsia,
    80–81, 81t
Antidepressants, in postpartum
    depression, 150
Antifungal drugs, in yeast
    vulvovaginitis, 336, 336t
Antipsychotics, in postpartum
    psychosis, 150
Apgar score, 357t
Appendix, in pregnancy, *28*
Arrhythmia, fetal, 35
Arterial pressure, mean, 354t
Arthritis, gonococcal, treatment of,
    249
Aspartate, in pregnancy, 353t
Asphyxia, fetal, 33
  abnormal heart rate and, 40
  abnormal labor and, 49
  amniotic fluid embolism and,
    58
  in shoulder dystocia, 202
Astemizole, 371
Asynclitism, 102, *103*
Atropine, diphenoxylate with, 379
Autopsy, in amniotic fluid
    embolism, 60
Azithromycin, 372
  in *Chlamydia* infection, 249
  in gonorrhea, 248, 249
  in vulvar chancroid, 328
Aztreonam, 372
  in endometritis, 155–156

B

Bacteremia, gonococcal, 249
Bacteria, in mastitis, 113
  vulvovaginitis from, 331, 332t,
    367t

Bacteria *(Continued)*
    diagnosis of, 335, 335t
    treatment of, 338
Bartholin's abscess, 225–229
  catheter placement for, 228
  clinical presentation of, 225
  definition of, 225
  differential diagnosis of, 226
  evaluation of, 225, 226–227
  incision/drainage of, 228
  marsupialization for, 228–229
  orders for, 227
  organisms in, 228, 228t
  physical examination of, 227
  threats of, 226
  treatment of, 227–229, 228t
  urgency of, 225
Bartholin's cyst, 225
  excision of, 229
Bartholin's duct, abscess of. See
    Bartholin's abscess.
Bartholin's glands, 225
Bedrest, in incompetent cervix, 89
Biophysical profile scoring, 356t
  in premature rupture of mem-
      branes, 175, 176t, 177t
  management and, 357t
Birth weight, estimated, 51
Bishop score, 92–93, 93t
Bladder, mass of, 365t
Bleeding. See *Hemorrhage.*
Blood pressure, in placenta previa,
    133
  in pregnancy, 22, 212
Blood sample, fetal scalp, in
    nonreassuring fetal heart rate,
    44–45, 44t
Blood urea nitrogen, in pregnancy,
    24
Blood volume, in pregnancy, 19,
    211–212
Boric acid, in yeast vulvovaginitis,
    336t
Bradycardia, fetal, 33, *34*
Breast(s), development of, 8, 8t, *9,*
    360
  mature, 10
Breast-feeding, drugs in, 368–406
  in mastitis, 114
Breech presentation, 99
  cesarean section for, 109
  complete, 99, *99*
  double footling, *99,* 100
  factors in, 104–105

Breech presentation *(Continued)*
  frank, 99, *99*
    cesarean section for, 109, 110
    external cephalic version for,
      110
    vaginal delivery for, 109–110,
      109t
  incidence of, 102
  incomplete, 99, *99*
  mortality rate in, 102
  single footling, 99, *99*
  treatment of, 109–110, 109t
Bromocriptine, 372
Brow presentation, 100, *101*
  incidence of, 102
  treatment of, 111
Butoconazole, 372

C

Calcium, in pregnancy, 352t
  replacement therapy with, 16–17
Calcium antagonists, in preterm
    labor, 199
Calcium gluconate, 372–373
  in preeclampsia, 258
Cancer antigen-125, in pelvic
    mass, 277
Candida, in vulvovaginitis, 331,
    337, 367t
Carbamazepine, 373
Carbohydrate, metabolism of, in
    pregnancy, 25–26, 27t
Carbon dioxide, arterial partial
    pressure of, in pregnancy, 24
Cardiac output, 354t
  in pregnancy, 20
Cardiopulmonary resuscitation, in
    amniotic fluid embolism, 60
Cardiovascular system, diseases
    of, cholesterol and, 17–18
  in menopause, 17, 17–18
  in pregnancy, 20–22
Catheterization, in amniotic fluid
    embolism, 60–61, 61t
  in Bartholin's abscess, 228
Cefazolin, after cesarean section,
    155
Cefixime, 373
  in gonorrhea, 248, 249
Cefoperazone, 373
  in endometritis, 156
Cefotaxime, 373–374

Cefotetan, 374
in endometritis, 156
Cefoxitin, 374
in endometritis, 156
in pelvic inflammatory disease,
267
Ceftizoxime, 374
Ceftriaxone, 374–375
in gonorrhea, 248, 249
in sexual assault, 294
in vulvar chancroid, 328
Celestone Soluspan, in preterm
labor, 200
Cellulitis, pelvic, in metritis, 151
Central nervous system, in
multiple gestation, 122
in preeclampsia, 71
Central venous pressure, 354t
Cephalic version, external, in
frank breech presentation,
110
in transverse lie, 110–111
Cephalopelvic disproportion, 47
Cephalosporin, in endometritis,
156
in mastitis, 115
Cephradine, 375
Cervical ripening, 90
fetal threats in, 91
maternal threats in, 91
technique of, 93–95
Cervix, cerclage of, 87–88
complications of, 88, 89t
chancroid of, 323
culture of, in premature rupture
of membranes, 175
dilatation of, arrest of, 53–54
treatment of, 56
in abnormal labor, 51
protracted active phase of,
treatment of, 55
granuloma inguinale of, 323
herpes simplex virus infection
of, 323
human papillomavirus infection
of, 323
in malpresentation, 107
incompetent, 85–89
bedrest for, 89
causes of, 86
cervical cerclage for, 87–88,
89t
clinical presentation of, 85
definition of, 85

Cervix (Continued)
evaluation of, 86–87
patient characteristics in, 85
pregnancy loss from, 85, 85t
prematurity from, 86
treatment of, 87–89, 89t
ultrasonography of, 87
urgency of, 86
lacerations of, early postpartum
hemorrhage from, 159
treatment of, 165
length of, in preterm labor, 188,
189
lymphogranuloma venereum of,
323
status of, in labor induction, 92–
93, 93t
syphilis of, 323
trauma to, incompetent cervix
from, 86
Cesarean section, in arrested
cervical dilatation, 56
in breech presentation, 109, 110
in face presentation, 111
in multiple gestation, 123
in nonvertex presentation, 128
in placenta previa, 136
in placental abruption, 144
in pregnancy-associated trauma,
213–214
in preterm labor, 200
in transverse lie, 111
perimortem, in trauma, 213–214
prophylactic antibiotics after,
155
Chancroid, cervical, 323
differential diagnosis of, 366t
vulvar, 318, 321t, 322
diagnostic tests for, 325
treatment of, 328
Childhood, reproductive system
in, 8
Chlamydia infection, 244–250
clinical presentation of, 245
definition of, 244–245
diagnostic tests for, 248
evaluation of, 245–247
in pregnancy, 249–250
orders for, 247
physical examination of, 247
risk factors for, 246
threats of, 246
treatment of, 249–250
urgency of, 246

Chlamydia trachomatis, 244
  in sexual assault, 293
  in tubo-ovarian abscess, 266
Chloramphenicol, 375
  in gonorrhea, 249
Chloride, in pregnancy, 352t
Chlorpromazine, 375
  in postpartum psychosis, 150
Cholesterol, cardiovascular disease
    and, 17–18
Chorioadenoma destruens, 252
  clinical presentation of, 252, 253
Chorioamnionitis, amniocentesis
    in, 173, 174t
  antibiotics in, 177
  biophysical profile testing in,
    175, 176t, 177t
  diagnostic tests for, in prema-
    ture rupture of membranes,
    173, 174t, 176t, 177t
  in premature rupture of mem-
    branes, 170
  in preterm labor, 192–193
Choriocarcinoma, 252
  clinical presentation of, 253
  metastatic, 252, 252t
Cigarette smoking, ectopic
    pregnancy and, 232
  placental abruption and, 140
Cimetidine, 376
Ciprofloxacin, 376
  in gonorrhea, 248
  in vulvar chancroid, 328
Circulation, fetal, 343, 351t
Clavicle, fracture of, in shoulder
    dystocia, 205
Clavulanic acid, and ticarcillin,
    403–404
  in endometritis, 156
Climacteric, 13–14
Clindamycin, 376
  after cesarean section, 155
  in bacterial vulvovaginitis, 338
  in endometritis, 155
  in pelvic inflammatory disease,
    267, 268
  in septic abortion, 307
  in tubo-ovarian abscess, 268
Clobetasol propionate, 376–377
  in vulvar lichen sclerosus, 329
Clomiphene citrate, 377
Clotrimazole, 377
  in yeast vulvovaginitis, 336, 336t
Coagulation factors, in
    preeclampsia, 76

Coagulation factors *(Continued)*
  in pregnancy, 19–20
Coagulopathy, blood product
    replacement for, 165–166
  early postpartum hemorrhage
    from, 160
  in amniotic fluid embolism,
    61–62
  in toxic shock syndrome, 314
Cocaine abuse, in placental
    abruption, 140
Colloid oncotic pressure, 354t
Colloid oncotic
    pressure–pulmonary capillary
    wedge pressure, 354t
Colpotomy, in tubo-ovarian
    abscess, 268
Complete blood count, in pelvic
    mass, 277
  in pelvic pain, 286
  in spontaneous abortion, 304
Compound presentation, 100, 102
Computed tomography, in
    pregnancy-associated trauma,
    210
  of malpresentation, 108
  of pelvic mass, 276–277
  of pelvic pain, 286
Conception, endometrium in, 13,
    14
Conceptus, 13, 14
Congenital anomalies, in multiple
    gestation, 122
Corkscrew maneuver, in shoulder
    dystocia, 204, 205
Corpus luteum, cysts of, 272
Corticosteroids, in preterm labor,
    199–200
  in preterm premature rupture of
    membranes, 180
Cortisol, in pregnancy, 353t
Couvelaire uterus, in placental
    abruption, 137
Crab lice, vulvar, 319, 322
  diagnostic tests for, 326
  treatment of, 329
C-reactive protein, in
    chorioamnionitis, 175
Creatinine, in pregnancy, 352t
Creatinine clearance, in pregnancy,
    352t
Crotamiton, 377
  in vulvar scabies, 328
Cryoprecipitate, in amniotic fluid
    embolism, 62

Cryoprecipitate *(Continued)*
  in disseminated intravascular co-
      agulation, 84
  in placental abruption, 144–145
  in toxic shock syndrome, 314
Culdocentesis, in ectopic
      pregnancy, 235–236, *236*
Cyst, Bartholin's, 225
  excision of, 229
  corpus luteum, 272
  follicular, 271–272
  pelvic, 270
  rupture of, in pelvic mass, 274
  theca-lutein, 272
Cytomegalovirus infection, 68
  sexual assault and, 294

D

Danazol, 377–378
Death, fetal. See *Fetus, death of.*
Decidua basalis, 13, *14*
Decidua capsularis, 13, *14*
Decidua parietalis, 13, *14*
Delivery, breech presentation in.
      See *Breech presentation.*
  complications of, in multiple ges-
      tation, 122
  in fetal death, 66
  in multiple gestation, 122
  in postpartum depression, 147
  in preeclampsia, 76–79
  in premature rupture of mem-
      branes, 177, 179
  malpresentation in. See *Malpre-
      sentation.*
  movements in, *347*
  of previable fetus, 108
  posterior shoulder, in shoulder
      dystocia, 204–205
  preterm, in multiple gestation,
      121
  vaginal, in brow presentation,
      111
    in compound presentation,
        111
    in face presentation, 111
    in frank breech presentation,
        109–110, 109t
    in malpresentation, 7
    in placental abruption, 143–
        144
    in vertex-nonvertex presenta-
        tion, 127–128

Delivery *(Continued)*
    in vertex-vertex presentation,
        126–127, 126t, *127*
  operative, in arrested cervical
      dilatation, 56
Depression, postpartum. See
      Postpartum depression.
Diabetes mellitus, maternal, in
      shoulder dystocia, 201
Diazepam, 378
  in eclampsia, 84
Dicloxacillin, 378
  in mastitis, 115
Diethylstilbestrol, exposure to,
      incompetent cervix from, 86
Digoxin, 378
Dilatation and curettage, in
      ectopic pregnancy, 236, 237
  in molar pregnancy, 258
Dinoprostone, cervical ripening
      with, 93–95
  labor induction with, 179
Diphenhydramine, 379
Diphenoxylate, with atropine, 379
Disseminated intravascular
      coagulation, cryoprecipitate
      for, 84
  fresh frozen plasma for, 84
  platelets for, 84
  red blood cells for, 82, 84
  treatment of, in preeclampsia,
      82, 84
Domestic violence, 207
Dopamine, 379
  in cardiogenic shock, 61
  in toxic shock syndrome, 313
Doxycycline, 379
  in *Chlamydia* infection, 249
  in gonorrhea, 248
  in lymphogranuloma venereum,
      250
  in pelvic inflammatory disease,
      267
  in sexual assault, 294
  in tubo-ovarian abscess, 268
  in uterine subinvolution, 167
  in vulvar lymphogranuloma ve-
      nereum, 328
  in vulvar syphilis, 327, 328
Drugs. See also specific agent.
  in breast-feeding, 368–406
  in pregnancy, 368–406
Ductus arteriosus, 351t
Ductus venosus, 351t

Dyschezia, 281
Dysmenorrhea, 281
Dyspareunia, 281
Dystocia, 47
    shoulder. See *Shoulder dystocia.*
    ultrasonography of, 51–52

E

Eclampsia, 69
    presentation of, 72, 72t
    risk factors in, 73
    treatment of, 84
Edema, in mild preeclampsia, 70
Embolism, amniotic fluid. See
    Amniotic fluid embolism.
Embolization, angiographic, for
    leiomyomata, 279
Emotions, in menopause, 18
    in sexual assault, 295–296
Endocarditis, gonococcal, 249
Endocrine system, in pregnancy,
    25–26
Endometrioma, 272
Endometriosis, 281
Endometritis, 151, 261
    antibiotic regimens for, 155–156
    diagnostic tests for, 154–155
    evaluation of, 153
    organisms in, 151t
    physical examination of, 154
    postpartum, risk factors for,
        152–153
    sepsis in, 153
Endometrium, biopsy of, in
    uterine bleeding, 222
    in conception, 13, *14*
    in menstrual cycle, *11*
Endomyometritis, 151
Endoparametritis, 151
Ephedrine sulfate, 380
Epithelial disorders,
                nonneoplastic, vulvar,
                315, 319–320
            diagnostic tests for, 326
Erythromycin, 380
    in *Chlamydia* infection, 249, 250
    in gonorrhea, 249
    in lymphogranuloma venereum,
        250
    in mastitis, 115
    in pelvic inflammatory disease,
        268

Erythromycin *(Continued)*
    in uterine subinvolution, 167
    in vulvar chancroid, 328
    in vulvar granuloma inguinale,
        328
    in vulvar lymphogranuloma ve-
        nereum, 328
    in vulvar syphilis, 328
Estradiol, 380–381
    in atrophic vulvovaginitis, 339
    in sexual assault, 295
Estriol, salivary, in preterm labor,
    189–190
Estrogen, conjugated, 381
    with methyltestosterone, 381
    esterified, 382
        with methyltestosterone, 382
    in atrophic vulvovaginitis, 339
    in dysfunctional uterine bleed-
        ing, 224
    in menopause, 14, 15, 15t
    in sexual assault, 295
    positive feedback by, 10
    replacement therapy with, 16–17
Estropipate, 382
Extremity(ies), reduction of, in
    compound presentation, 111

F

Face presentation, 100, *101*
    incidence of, 102
    treatment of, 111
Fallopian tubes, abscess of, 261
    Chlamydia trachomatis in, 266
    in pelvic inflammatory dis-
        ease, 261–262, 268–269
    mass in, 272, 365t
Famciclovir, 383
    in vulvar herpes simplex virus
        infection, 326
Fertilization, 13
Fetal compromise, in premature
    rupture of membranes, 170
    in preterm premature rupture of
        membranes, 181
Fetal heart rate, abnormal patterns
        of, 33–45
    asphyxia from, 40
    causes of, 39–40
    clinical presentation of, 39
    diagnostic tests for, 41–42
    evaluation of, 40–41

Fetal heart rate *(Continued)*
    in malpresentation, 104
    in placenta previa, 133
    in placental abruption, 141
    management of, 42–45, 44t
  baseline, 33
  beat-to-beat variability in, 34–35, 35
  early deceleration in, *36*, 36–37
  in abnormal labor, 50
  in labor induction, 92
  in malpresentation, 106
  in meconium passage, 117
  in multiple gestation, 124
  late deceleration in, *37*, 37–38
  nonreassuring patterns of. See *Fetal heart rate, abnormal patterns of.*
  normal, with accelerations, 33, *34*
  periodic, 33–38, *34–38*
  sinusoidal, 35–36, *36*
  variable deceleration in, 38, *38*
Fetal heart rate monitoring, 41–42
  in meconium passage, 118–119
  in trauma, 210–211
Fetal scalp blood sampling, in nonreassuring fetal heart rate, 44–45, 44t
Fetal scalp stimulation test, in nonreassuring heart rate, 45
Fetus, arrhythmia in, 35
  asphyxia of, 33
    abnormal heart rate and, 40
    abnormal labor and, 49
    amniotic fluid embolism and, 58
    shoulder dystocia and, 202
  biophysical profile scoring of, 356t
    management and, 357t
  bradycardia in, 33, *34*
  brow presentation of, 100, *101*
  circulation in, *343*, 351t
  compound presentation of, 100
  death of, 63–68
    causes of, 64–65
      investigation of, 68
    characteristics associated with, 64
    clinical presentation of, 63
    definition of, 63
    delivery in, 66
    evaluation of, 65–66

Fetus *(Continued)*
    grief in, 67–68
    in multiple gestation, 128
    intrauterine, 63
    maternal risks in, 64, 65
    monitoring in, 64
    orders for, 66
    oxytocin in, 67
    prostaglandin E_2 in, 67
    treatment of, 66–68
    ultrasonography of, 66
    viability documentation in, 63
  electronic monitoring of, in amniotic fluid embolism, 62
  face presentation of, 100, *101*
  in multiple gestation, 121–123
  in placental abruption, 140
  in preeclampsia, 74
  infection of, biophysical profile testing of, 175, 176t, 177t
    premature rupture of membranes and, 170, 175, 176t, 177t
  karyotype of, 68
  lung maturity in, in labor induction, 92, 92t, 93, *94*
    lecithin-to-sphingomyelin ratio in, 93, *94*, 175
    phosphatidylglycerol in, 93, *94*, 175
    testing of, in premature rupture of membranes, 175–177, *178*, 178t
  malpresentation of. See *Malpresentation.*
  oblique lie of, 100
  previable, delivery of, 108
  radiation exposure of, in trauma, 213, 214t
  skull dimensions in, *344*
  tachycardia in, 33
  transverse lie of, 100, *100*
  trauma threats to, 208
Fever, postpartum. See *Postpartum fever.*
Fibrinogen, in pregnancy, 213, 352t
Fibroids, 270
Fluconazole, 383
  in yeast vulvovaginitis, 336, 336t
Fluocinolone acetonide, 383
  in vulvar squamous cell hyperplasia, 329
Fluoxetine, 383
Flurazepam, 384

Foam stability test, 176–177, 178t, 358t
   in preterm labor, 192, 193t
Follicle-stimulating hormone, in follicular phase, 12
   in luteal phase, 12–13
   in menopause, 15, 15t
   in sexual differentiation, 7, 7
Foramen ovale, 351t
Fracture, clavicular, in shoulder dystocia, 205
   in menopause, 16
Fresh frozen plasma, in amniotic fluid embolism, 62
   in disseminated intravascular coagulation, 84
   in placental abruption, 144
   in toxic shock syndrome, 314
Functional residual capacity, in pregnancy, 22, 23t
Furosemide, 384

G

Gallbladder, in pregnancy, 29
Gardnerella vaginalis, in vulvovaginitis, 331, 367t
Gastrointestinal tract, displacement of, in pregnancy, 212–213
   in mild preeclampsia, 71
   in pregnancy, 26, 28, 28–29, 29t, 213
   mass of, 365t
Genitalia, external, in malpresentation, 107
   in menopause, 16
   ulcers of, differential diagnosis of, 366t
Gentamicin, 384
   after cesarean section, 155
   in endometritis, 155
   in pelvic inflammatory disease, 267
   in septic abortion, 307
   in tubo-ovarian abscess, 268
Gestation, multiple. See *Multiple gestation*
Gestational age, amniotic fluid phospholipid levels and, 175, 178
   confirmation of, 92, 92t
   delivery and, in preeclampsia, 76

Gestational age *(Continued)*
   in malpresentation, 102, 104
   in multiple gestation, 124
   in placenta previa management, 135
   premature, in preeclampsia, 78–79, 79
   preterm labor and, survival rates in, 183–184, 183t
   ultrasonography of, in premature rupture of membranes, 173, 173, 174
Gestational trophoblastic neoplasia, 251–252
   classification of, 251t
Glomerular filtration rate, in pregnancy, 24, 25
Glucose, in pregnancy, 352t
Gonadotropin, changes in, 360
   in menopause, 15, 15t
   in menstrual cycle, 11, 365t
   in sexual differentiation, 7, 7
Gonadotropin-releasing hormone agonist, in leiomyomata, 279
   in pelvic pain, 288
Gonorrhea, 244–250
   clinical presentation of, 245
   definition of, 244
   diagnostic tests for, 248
   disseminated, 244
   evaluation of, 245–247
   in pregnancy, 249
   orders for, 247
   physical examination of, 247
   risk factors for, 246
   threats of, 246
   treatment of, 248–249
   urgency of, 246
Granuloma inguinale, cervical, 323
   differential diagnosis of, 366t
   vulvar, 318, 321t, 322
      diagnostic tests for, 325
      treatment of, 328
Grief, in fetal death, 67–68
Growth, in multiple gestation, 122
   maximal, 9

H

Halobetasol propionate, 384
   in vulvar lichen sclerosus, 329
Haloperidol, 384
   in postpartum psychosis, 150

hCG. See *Human chorionic gonadotropin (hCG)*.

Heart failure, left-sided, in amniotic fluid embolism, 57

Heart rate, 354t
fetal. See *Fetal heart rate*.
in pregnancy, 20, *21*, 212

Heart sounds, in pregnancy, 21, *21*

Height, peak velocity of, 9

HELLP (hemolysis, elevated liver enzymes and low platelets) syndrome, 69

Hematocrit, in pregnancy, 19, 353t

Hematologic system, in mild preeclampsia, 71
in pregnancy, 19–20

Hemodynamic measurements, in preeclampsia, 76, 80, 80t
in pregnancy, 354t
in toxic shock syndrome, 313, 314t

Hemoglobin, in pregnancy, 19, 353t

Hemorrhage, anovulatory, 217
concealed, in placental abruption, 137, *137*
fetal-maternal, in trauma, 213
in multiple gestation, 123
of pelvic mass, 274
postpartum. See *Postpartum hemorrhage*.
uterine. See *Uterus, abnormal bleeding from*.
vaginal, causes of, 132
in multiple gestation, 124
in placenta previa management, 135, 136
in pregnancy, 298
pelvic pain with, 282

Heparin, 385
in septic pelvic thrombophlebitis, 156–157

Hepatitis B virus infection, sexual assault and, 294, 295

Hepatitis B virus vaccination, 295

Herpes simplex virus infection, cervical, 323
differential diagnosis of, 366t
sexual assault and, 294
vulvar, 316, 321, 321t
diagnostic tests for, 323–324
treatment of, 326

Human chorionic gonadotropin (hCG), 13

Human chorionic gonadotropin (hCG) *(Continued)*
after hydatidiform mole evacuation, *364*
after uterine evacuation, 258, *259*, 260
in ectopic pregnancy, *234*, 234–235, 237
in molar pregnancy, 256, 257t
in pelvic mass, 277–278
in pregnancy, *351*
in spontaneous abortion, 301, 302–304, *303*, 303t
ultrasonography and, 302

Human immunodeficiency virus (HIV) infection, sexual assault and, 294

Human papillomavirus infection, cervical, 323
vulvar, 316–317
diagnostic tests for, 324
treatment of, 326–327

H-Y antigen, 7

Hydatidiform mole, 251
complete, 251
clinical presentation of, 252–253
evacuation of, human chorionic gonadotropin regression curve in, *364*
partial, 251–252
clinical presentation of, 253

Hydralazine, 385
in preeclampsia, 82, 83t

Hydrochlorothiazide, 385

Hydrocodone, 385

Hydromorphone, 386

Hydrosalpinx, 261

Hyperemesis gravidarum, in multiple gestation, 123

Hypermenorrhea, 217

Hypertension, 69–84
chronic, 69, 72
in preeclampsia, 70
clinical presentation of, 70–72
definitions in, 69–70
evaluation of, 74–75
in mild preeclampsia, 70
in placental abruption, 138, 140
in severe preeclampsia, 71
orders for, 75–76
patient characteristics in, 72–73
pregnancy-induced, 69
diagnostic tests for, 76

Hypertension *(Continued)*
  treatment of, 76–84
  treatment of, in preeclampsia, 82, 83t
  urgency of, 73
Hyperthyroidism, in molar pregnancy, 254, 258
Hypogastric artery, ligation of, 164, *164*, *350*
Hypomenorrhea, 217
Hypotension, maternal, in nonreassuring fetal heart rate, 43
Hypoxemia, 33
Hypoxia, 33
Hysterectomy, in leiomyomata, 279
  in molar pregnancy, 258
  in tubo-ovarian abscess, 269
  in uterine atony, 165
  postpartum, in placental abruption, 145
Hysteroscopy, in uterine bleeding, 223
Hysterotomy, in molar pregnancy, 258

I

Ibuprofen, 386
Imipramine, 386
Imiquimod, 386
  in vulvar human papillomavirus, 327
Implantation, 13, *14*
Indomethacin, 386–387
  complications of, 199
  contraindications to, 199
  in preterm labor, 198–199
  side effects of, 198–199
Infection. See also specific type, e.g., *Chlamydia infection.*
  fetal, biophysical profile testing of, 175, 176t, 177t
  premature rupture of membranes and, 170, 175, 176t, 177t
  uterine, postpartum fever in, 151
  vulvar, 315, 316–319
Insulin, metabolism of, in pregnancy, 25–26, 27t
Intrauterine growth restriction, in multiple gestation, 122

Intrauterine growth restriction *(Continued)*
  in severe preeclampsia, 71
  premature rupture of membranes and, 170
Intubation, in amniotic fluid embolism, 60
Iron, requirements for, in pregnancy, 20
Isoniazid, 387
Isoproterenol, 387
Itching, in vulvar lesions, 316

K

Kawasaki's disease, vs. toxic shock syndrome, 309
Ketoconazole, 387
  in yeast vulvovaginitis, 337
Kidney(s), in mild preeclampsia, 70–71
  in preeclampsia, 73–74, 76
  in pregnancy, 24–25, *25*
  mass of, 365t
Kleihauer-Betke stain, 68
  in pregnancy, 211

L

Labetalol, 387
  in preeclampsia, 82, 83t
Labor, abnormal, 46–56
  causes of, 49
  cervical dilatation in, 51
  clinical presentation of, 47
  definitions of, 47
  diagnostic testing in, 51–54
  effacement in, 51
  fetal asphyxia in, 49
  fetal heart rate in, 50
  fetal weight in, 50
  history in, 50
  internal uterine pressure monitor in, 52–54, *53*
  management of, 55–56
  orders for, 51
  pelvimetry in, 54, *54*, 54t
  physical examination in, 51
  pushing level in, 50
  station in, 51
  ultrasonography of, 51–52
  urgency in, 48

Labor (*Continued*)
    uterine contractions in, 49–50
  active phase of, 46, 46t
    protracted, 47
      treatment of, 55
  augmentation of, 90
  basic, 46–47
  cervical dilatation in, arrest of, 47, 53–54
      treatment of, 56
    protracted, 47
      treatment of, 55
  descent in, arrest of, 47
    protracted, 47
      treatment of, 55–56
  epidural analgesia in, 48
  failure to progress in, 47
  first stage of, 46, 46t
  in malpresentation, 7–8, 104, 106
  in multiple gestation, 126–128, 126t, 127, 128t
  induction of, 90–97
    clinical conditions in, 90–91
    contraindications to, 91
    definition of, 90
    diagnostic testing in, 93
    fetal heart rate in, 92
    fetal lung maturity in, 92, 92t
    fetal threats in, 91
    history in, 92, 92t
    in placental abruption, 143–144
    in premature rupture of membranes, 179
    indications for, 90–91
    maternal stability in, 92
    maternal threats in, 91
    physical examination in, 92–93, 93t
    technique of, 95–97, 96
  latent phase of, 46, 46t
    prolonged, 47, 48
      treatment of, 55
  movements in, 347
  normal curve of, 48
  preterm, 183–200
    after preterm premature rupture of membranes, 181
    amniocentesis in, 191–193, 193t
    amniotic fluid phospholipids in, 191–192, 192
    beta-adrenergic agonists in, 194–196

Labor (*Continued*)
    calcium antagonists in, 199
    cervical culture in, 191
    cervical examination in, 190
    cervical length in, 188, 189
    cesarean section in, 200
    chorioamnionitis in, 192–193
    clinical presentation of, 184
    corticosteroids in, 199–200
    definition of, 183
    delivery management in, 200
    diagnostic tests for, 188–193, 189, 192, 193t
    estriol in, 189–190
    evaluation of, 184–185, 187–188
    fibronectin enzyme immuno-assay in, 188–189
    foam stability test in, 192, 193t
    hydration in, 193–194
    incidence of, 183
    magnesium sulfate in, 197–198
    management of, 193–200, 194t
    maternal transport in, 200
    medical conditions associated with, 185–186
    membrane rupture in, 184, 190
    morbidity/mortality associated with, 186–187
    orders for, 188
    physical examination of, 188
    positioning in, 193
    premature rupture of membranes and, 169–170
    prostaglandin synthesis inhibitors in, 198–199
    shake test in, 192, 193t
    socioeconomic factors associated with, 185
    survival rates in, 183–184, 183t
    tocolytic drugs in, 194–199, 194t
    ultrasonography in, 190
    urgency of, 185
    urinalysis in, 191
    uterine monitoring in, 191
    vs. abortion, 183
  prolonged, in shoulder dystocia, 202
  second stage of, 46, 46t

Labor *(Continued)*
  stages of, 46, 46t, 355t
  third stage of, 46–47, 46t
Lacerations, vulvar, early
      postpartum hemorrhage
      from, 159
  treatment of, 165
β-Lactamase, in endometritis, 156
Lactobacillus acidophilus, vaginal,
    331
Laparoscopy, in pelvic
    inflammatory disease, 265
Laser, in vulvar human
    papillomavirus, 327
Lecithin-to-sphingomyelin ratio, in
    fetal lung maturity, 93, 94, 175
  in preterm labor, 191
Left ventricular stroke work index,
    354t
Leiomyomata, 270
  angiographic embolization of,
      279
  hysterectomy for, 279
  myomectomy for, 279–280
  treatment of, 278–280
Leptospirosis, vs. toxic shock
    syndrome, 310
Leukocyte count, in pregnancy,
    353t
Leuprolide acetate, 388
  in leiomyomata, 279
Levothyroxine, 388
Lichen sclerosus, vulvar, 319–320,
    322
  treatment of, 329
Lindane, 388
  in vulvar pediculosis pubis, 329
  in vulvar scabies, 328
Lipoprotein, high-density, 17–18
  low-density, 17–18
Listeria monocytogenes, in fetal
    death, 68
Lithium, 388
Liver, in pregnancy, 28–29, 29t
  in severe preeclampsia, 71
  rupture of, in preeclampsia, 74
Loperamide, 389
Lung(s), fetal, maturity in, in labor
    induction, 92, 92t
  hypoplasia of, in premature rup-
      ture of membranes, 170
Lupus anticoagulant antibody, 68
Luteinizing hormone, in follicular
    phase, 12

Luteinizing hormone *(Continued)*
  in luteal phase, 12–13
  in menopause, 15, 15t
  in sexual differentiation, 7, 7
Lymphogranuloma venereum,
    cervical, 323
  differential diagnosis of, 366t
  treatment of, 250
  vulvar, 318–319, 321t, 322
    diagnostic tests for, 325
    treatment of, 328

M

Macrosomia, fetal, in shoulder
    dystocia, 201
Magnesium, in nonreassuring fetal
    heart rate, 43
Magnesium gluconate, 389
Magnesium oxide, 389
Magnesium sulfate, 389
  complications of, 197–198
  contraindications to, 198
  in eclampsia, 84
  in preeclampsia, 81, 81t, 257–258
  in preterm labor, 197–198
  precautions with, 198
  side effects of, 197
Magnetic resonance imaging, in
    pelvic pain, 286
  of pelvic mass, 277
Malignancy, vulvar, 315, 320
    diagnostic tests for, 326
Malpresentation, 99–111. See also
    Breech presentation.
  asynclitism in, 102, 103
  brow presentation in, 100, 101,
      102
    incidence of, 102
    treatment of, 111
  cervix in, 107
  clinical presentation of, 102
  complications of, 105–106
  compound presentation in, 100,
      102
    treatment of, 111
  computed tomography of, 108
  definition of, 99
  diagnostic tests for, 108
  evaluation of, 102, 104, 106–107
  face presentation in, 100, 101,
      102
    treatment of, 111

Malpresentation *(Continued)*
  fetal heart rate in, 106
  labor in, 7–8, 104, 106
  membrane rupture in, 104
  oblique lie in, 100, *100*
  orders for, 108
  pelvic radiography of, 108
  physical examination of, 107–108
  transverse lie in, 100, *100*, 102
    treatment of, 110–111
  treatment of, 108–111, 109t
  ultrasonography of, 108
  urgency of, 104
Marsupialization, in Bartholin's abscess, 228–229
Mastitis, 112–119
  bacteria in, 113
  causes of, 112–113
  clinical presentation of, 112
  definition of, 112
  diagnostic tests of, 114
  endemic, 112
  epidemic, 112
  evaluation of, 113
  orders for, 114
  threats from, 113
  treatment of, 114–115
  urgency of, 112
Maternity blues, 146
McRoberts maneuver, in shoulder dystocia, 204
Meclizine, 389
Meconium, 116
  aspiration of, 116
  passage of, 116–119
    characteristics in, 117
    clinical presentation of, 116
    definition of, 116
    evaluation of, 117–118
    factors associated with, 117
    fetal heart rate in, 117
    fetal heart rate monitoring in, 118–119
    fetal risks in, 117
    orders for, 118
    treatment of, 118–119
Meconium aspiration syndrome, 116
  amnioinfusion in, 119
  oropharyngeal suctioning in, 119
  prevention of, 119
Medroxyprogesterone, 390
  in dysfunctional uterine bleeding, 224

Melanoma, vulvar, 320, 323
Membrane stripping, labor induction by, 95
Membranes, in multiple gestation, 124, *125*, *349*
  premature rupture of. See *Premature rupture of membranes (PROM).*
  rupture of, in malpresentation, 104
  in preterm labor, 184, 190
Menarche, 9
Meningitis, gonococcal, 249
Menometrorrhagia, 217
Menopause, 13–18
  cardiovascular disease in, *17*, 17–18
  emotional changes in, 18
  genital changes in, 16
  osteoporosis in, 16–17
  spontaneous, 14
  vasomotor symptoms of, 15
Menorrhagia, 217
Menstrual cycle, endometrium in, *11*
  follicular phase of, 12
  luteal phase of, 12–13
  normal, *11*, 11–13, *362*
  ovulation in, 12
Menstruation, blood loss in, 217
Meperidine hydrochloride, 390
Metaproterenol, 390
Methadone, 390–391
Methimazole, 391
  in molar pregnancy, 258
Methotrexate, 391
  contraindications to, 242
  in ectopic pregnancy, 239, 241–242
Methylergonovine, 391
  in uterine atony, 163
  in uterine subinvolution, 167
Metritis, with pelvic cellulitis, 151
Metronidazole, 391–392
  in bacterial vulvovaginitis, 338
  in pelvic inflammatory disease, 268
  in sexual assault, 294
  in *Trichomonas* vulvovaginitis, 338–339
  in tubo-ovarian abscess, 268
Metrorrhagia, 217
Miconazole, 392
  in yeast vulvovaginitis, 336t

Microorganisms, in Bartholin's
abscess, 228, 228t
in endometritis, 151t
in pelvic inflammatory disease,
261t
Midazolam, 392
Midpelvis, diameter of, 54, *54*, 54t
Misoprostol, 392–393
cervical ripening with, 93, 94, 95
in fetal death, 67
in inevitable abortion, 305
labor induction with, 179
Molar pregnancy, 251–260
chest radiography in, 257
classification of, 251t
clinical presentation of, 252–253
definition of, 251–252, 251t
diagnostic tests in, 256–257, 257t
differential diagnosis of, 254
electrocardiography in, 257
evaluation of, 254, 255
human chorionic gonadotropin
in, 256, 257t
after treatment, 258, *259*, 260
hyperthyroidism in, 254, 258
hypovolemic shock in, 254
hysterectomy in, 258
hysterotomy in, 258
invasive, 252, 252t, 253
orders for, 256
physical examination of, 255–
256
preeclampsia in, 257–258
respiratory difficulties in, 254
risk factors for, 254
suction dilatation and curettage
in, 258
threats in, 254
thyroid hormone in, 257
treatment of, 257–258, *259*, 260
ultrasonography of, 256
urgency of, 254
uterine evacuation in, 258
Molluscum contagiosum, vulvar,
319, 322
diagnostic tests for, 325
treatment of, 328
Montevideo units, in oxytocin
labor induction, 96, *96*
in uterine contraction, 53, *53*
Morphine sulfate, 393
Mucocutaneous lymph node
syndrome, vs. toxic shock
syndrome, 309

Multiple gestation, 120–129
antepartum surveillance in, 126
cesarean section in, 123
clinical presentation of, 120–121
congenital anomalies in, 122
conjoined twins in, 123
definition of, 120
delivery complications in, 122
dizygotic, 120
evaluation of, 121, 124–125, *125*
fetal complications in, 121–123
fetal compromise in, management of, 128
fetal heart rate in, 124
growth discordance in, 122
hemorrhage in, 123
hypovolemic shock in, 123
incidence of, 120
intrapartum management of,
127
intrauterine growth restriction
in, 121
labor management in, 126–128,
126t, *127*, 128t
maternal complications in, 123
membranes in, 124, *125*, *349*
monoamniotic twins in, 124, *125*
monozygotic, 120
multifetal reduction in, 128–129
neurological abnormalities in,
122
physical examination in, 124–
125
placenta in, 124, *125*, *349*
polyhydramnios in, 123
preeclampsia in, 123
prematurity in, 123
presentation in, incidence of,
126t, 128t
preterm delivery in, 121
preterm premature rupture of
membranes in, 121
spontaneous abortion in, 121
treatment of, 126–129, 126t, *127*,
128t
ultrasonography in, 125–126
umbilical cord accidents in, 122
urgency of, 121
vertex presentation in, 126–127,
126t, *127*, 128t
Myomectomy, for leiomyomata,
279–280
Myometritis, 261

N

Nafarelin acetate, 393
Nafcillin, 393
Naloxone, 393–394
Naproxen, 394
Neisseria gonorrhoeae, 244
  in sexual assault, 293
  in tubo-ovarian abscess, 266
Newborn, death of, 63
  in postpartum psychosis, 148
  reproductive system in, 8
  trauma to, shoulder dystocia
    and, 202
Nifedipine, 394
  complications of, 199
  contraindications to, 199
  in preeclampsia, 82, 83t
  in preterm labor, 199
Nitrazine test, of vaginal pH, 172
Nitrofurantoin, 394
Nonsteroidal anti-inflammatory
    drugs, in pelvic pain, 287
Nystatin, 394–395

O

Obesity, in shoulder dystocia, 201
Oblique lie, 100
Ofloxacin, 395
  in *Chlamydia* infection, 249
  in gonorrhea, 248, 249
  in pelvic inflammatory disease,
    268
Oligomenorrhea, 217
Oliguria, in preeclampsia, 82
  in severe preeclampsia, 71
Oocytes, changes in, *360*
  in childhood, 8
  in life cycle, *7*, 7–8
  in puberty, 8
Oophoritis, 261
Oral contraceptives, in
    dysfunctional uterine
    bleeding, 223
  in pelvic pain, 287–288
  in sexual assault, 295
Oropharynx, suctioning of, for
    meconium aspiration
    syndrome, 119
Osteoporosis, in menopause,
    16–17
Ovary(ies), abscess of, 261

Ovary(ies) *(Continued)*
  Chlamydia trachomatis in, 266
  in pelvic inflammatory dis-
    ease, 261–262, 268–269
  development of, 7
  follicular cysts of, 271–272
  in menstrual cycle, *11*
  mass of, 271–272, 271t, 365t
  neoplasms of, classification of,
    272, 273t
  radiation exposure to, 359t
  theca-lutein cyst of, 272
Ovulation, 12
Ovum, blighted, 297, 306
  fertilization of, 13
Oxycodone, 395
Oxygen consumption, in
    pregnancy, 22, 24
Oxygen dissociation curves, *348*
Oxygen therapy, in nonreassuring
    fetal heart rate, 42
Oxytocin, 395–396
  discontinuance of, in nonreassur-
    ing fetal heart rate, 42–43
  in abnormal labor, 55–56
  in fetal death, 67
  in uterine atony, 163
  labor induction by, 95–97, *96*
  water intoxication from, 91

P

Pain, in placental abruption, 138
  in vulvar lesions, 316
  pelvic. See *Pelvic pain.*
Pancreas, in pregnancy, 25–26, 27t
Parametritis, 261
Pediculosis pubis, vulvar, 319, 322
  diagnostic tests for, 326
  treatment of, 329
Pelvic congestion syndrome, 281
Pelvic examination, in abnormal
    labor, 51
Pelvic inflammatory disease,
    261–269
  clinical criteria for, 266
  clinical presentation of, 262
  definition of, 261
  diagnostic tests for, 265–266
  differential diagnosis of, 263
  drug regimens for, 267–268
  ectopic pregnancy and, 231
  evaluation of, 262–263, 264

Pelvic inflammatory disease
    (*Continued*)
  hospitalization in, 266–267
  laboratory tests for, 265–266
  laparoscopy of, 265
  orders for, 264
  organisms in, 261t
  physical examination of, 264
  risk factors for, 263
  sepsis from, 263
  sequelae of, 262
    incidence of, 267t
  symptoms of, 262t
  treatment of, 266–268
  tubo-ovarian abscess in, 261–262
    treatment for, 268–269
  ultrasonography of, 265
  urgency of, 263
  vs. vulvovaginitis, 333
Pelvic mass, 270–280
  cancer antigen–125 in, 277
  clinical presentation of, 270
  complete blood count in, 277
  complications of, 274
  computed tomography of, 276–277
  cystic rupture in, 274
  diagnostic tests for, 276–278
  differential diagnosis of, 271–272, 271t, 273t, 274, 365t
  evaluation of, 271, 274–275
  hemorrhage of, 274
  history of, 275
  magnetic resonance imaging of, 277
  orders for, 276
  pain in, 270–271
  physical examination of, 276
  pyelography of, 277
  torsion in, 274
  treatment of, 278
  ultrasonography of, 276
  urgency of, 271
  vital signs in, 275
Pelvic pain, 281–288
  analgesics for, 287
  causes of, 282–284
  chronic, 281–282
  clinical presentation of, 282
  complete blood count in, 286
  computed tomography of, 286
  definition of, 281–282
  diagnostic tests for, 286–287
  evaluation of, 284–285

Pelvic pain (*Continued*)
  gonadotropin-releasing factor
    agonist for, 288
  hypovolemic shock in, 284
  magnetic resonance imaging of, 286
  mass and, 270–271
  nonsteroidal anti-inflammatory
    drugs for, 287
  oral contraceptives for, 287–288
  orders for, 286
  physical examination of, 285–286
  psychological evaluation for, 288
  pyelography of, 287
  sepsis in, 284
  surgery for, 288
  treatment of, 287–288
  ultrasonography of, 286
  urgency of, 282
  vaginal bleeding in, 282
  vital signs in, 284
Pelvimetry, in abnormal labor, 54, *54*, 54t
Pelvis, abscess of, 157
  cellulitis of, in metritis, 151
  diameters of, 54, *54*, 54t, 355t
  functional cysts in, 270
  in malpresentation, 107
  inlet of, 54, *54*, 54t, *345*
  normal measurements of, 109, 109t
  outlet of, *345*
  physiological cysts in, 270
Penicillin, 396–397
  in gonorrhea, 249
  in vulvar syphilis, 327, 328
Pentobarbital, 397
  in eclampsia, 84
Perinatal mortality rate, 63
Peritoneal lavage, in trauma, 211, 212t, 358t
Permethrin, 397
  in vulvar scabies, 329
Phenazopyridine, 397
Phenobarbital, 397–398
Phenytoin, 398
Phosphatidylglycerol, in fetal lung
    maturity, 93, *94*, 175
  in preterm labor, 191
Phospholipid, amniotic fluid, *350*
  gestational age and, 175, *178*
  in preterm labor, 191–192, *192*
Phthirus pubis, in vulva, 319

Pituitary gland, in pregnancy, 26
Placenta, in multiple gestation, 124, *125*, *349*
  low-lying, 130, *131*
  manual removal of, *166*, 167
  retained, postpartum hemorrhage from, *159*, 159–160
  treatment of, 165
Placenta accreta, early postpartum hemorrhage from, *159*, 159–160
Placenta increta, *159*
Placenta percreta, *159*
Placenta previa, 130–136
  causes of, 132
  cesarean section in, 136
  clinical presentation of, 130, 132
  definition of, 130
  degrees of, 130, *131*
  digital examination in, 134–135
  evaluation of, 133
  fetal risks in, 132
  marginal, 130, *131*
  orders for, 134
  partial, 130, *131*
  physical examination in, 133–134
  prematurity in, 132
  risk factors in, 132
  total, 130, *131*
  treatment of, 135–136
  ultrasonography in, 134
  urgency of, 132
Placental abruption, 137–145
  cesarean section in, 144
  clinical presentation of, 138
  concealed hemorrhage in, 137, *137*
  cryoprecipitate in, 144–145
  definition of, 137
  evaluation of, 141
  expectant management in, 143
  factors associated with, 138, 140
  fetal threats in, 140
  fresh frozen plasma in, 144
  grading of, 138, 139t
  labor induction in, 143–144
  maternal threats in, 140
  orders for, 142
  pain in, 138
  physical examination in, 141–142
  platelets in, 144
  postpartum hysterectomy in, 145

Placental abruption (*Continued*)
  recurrence of, 140
  red blood cells in, 144
  severity of, 137–138
  treatment of, 142–145
  ultrasonography of, 142
  urgency of, 138
  uterine complications in, 137–138
  vaginal delivery in, 143–144
Platelets, in amniotic fluid embolism, 62
  in disseminated intravascular coagulation, 84
  in placental abruption, 144
  in pregnancy, 353t
  in toxic shock syndrome, 314
Podofilox, in vulvar human papillomavirus, 327
Polyhydramnios, in multiple gestation, 123
Polymenorrhea, 217
Postpartum blues, 146
  factors in, 147–148
  treatment of, 149
Postpartum depression, 146–150
  antidepressants for, 150
  clinical presentation of, 146–147
  definition of, 146
  delivery date and, 147
  diagnostic tests for, 149
  evaluation of, 147, 148–149
  factors in, 148
  medical conditions in, 148
  orders for, 149
  thyroid hormone replacement therapy in, 150
  treatment of, 149–150
  urgency of, 147
Postpartum fever, 151–157
  clinical presentation of, 152
  definition of, 151
  diagnostic tests for, 154–155
  differential diagnosis of, 152
  evaluation of, 153
  orders for, 154
  physical examination of, 154
  treatment of, 155–157
  urgency of, 152
  uterine infection and, 151
Postpartum hemorrhage, 158–167
  clinical presentation of, 158
  definition of, 158
  early, 158

Postpartum hemorrhage
  (Continued)
  causes of, *159,* 159–161, *160*
  coagulopathy and, 160
  genital tract lacerations and,
      159
  placenta accreta and, *159,*
      159–160
  uterine atony and, 159
  uterine inversion and, *160,*
      160–161
  uterine rupture and, 160
  evaluation of, 158–159
  in multiple gestation, 123
  in shoulder dystocia, 202
  late, 158
    causes of, 161
    diagnostic tests for, 163
    evaluation of, 161–162
    orders for, 162
    physical examination of, 162
    treatment of, 163–167, *164,*
        166
  urgency of, 159
Postpartum neurotic depression,
    146
Postpartum psychosis, 146, 147
  factors in, 148
  infant threats in, 148
  suicide in, 148
  treatment of, 150
Potassium, in pregnancy, 352t
Preeclampsia, 69
  amniotic fluid index in, 78, *79*
  anticonvulsant prophylaxis in,
      80–81, 81t
  coagulation studies in, 76
  complications of, 73–74
  delivery in, 76–79
  diagnostic tests for, 76
  disseminated intravascular coag-
      ulation in, treatment of, 82,
      84
  evaluation of, 74–75
  fetal threats in, 74
  fluid management in, 80
  hemodynamic measurements in,
      76, 80, 80t
  hypertension in, treatment of,
      82, 83t
  in chronic hypertension, 70
  in molar pregnancy, 257–258
  in multiple gestation, 123
  intrapartum management of, 79

Preeclampsia *(Continued)*
  intravascular volume in, 80
  liver function tests in, 76
  liver rupture in, 74
  maternal threats in, 74
  mild, delivery in, 76
    expectant management in, 78–
        79, *79*
    presentation of, 70–71
  oliguria in, treatment of, 82
  orders for, 75–76
  patient characteristics in, 72–73
  renal function in, 73–74, 76
  risk factors in, 73
  severe, delivery in, 76
    presentation of, 71
  thrombocytopenia in, 73
  treatment of, 76–84
  ultrasonography for, 76
Pregnancy, adrenal glands in, 26
  appendix in, *28*
  arterial carbon dioxide tension
      in, 24
  blood pressure in, 22, 212
  blood urea nitrogen in, 24
  blood volume in, 19, 211–212
  bowel displacement in, 212–213
  carbohydrate metabolism in, 25–
      26, 27t
  cardiac output in, 20
  cardiovascular system in, 20–22
  Chlamydia infection in, 249–250
  coagulation factors in, 19–20
  drugs in, 368–406
  ectopic, 230–243
    abdominal, 230–231
    cervical, 230
    clinical presentation of, 231
    conservative management of,
        239, *240,* 241, *241,* 242
    cornual, 230
    culdocentesis in, 235–236, *236*
    definition of, 230–231
    diagnosis of, *363*
      scheme for, 236–237, *238*
      tests for, *234,* 234–236, 235t,
          236
    dilatation and curettage in,
        236, 237
    evaluation of, 231, 232–233
    human chorionic gonadotro-
        pin in, *234,* 234–235, 237
    hypovolemic shock in, 231,
        232

Pregnancy (*Continued*)
   implantation sites for, *230*, 230–231
   incidence of, 230
   interstitial, 230
   linear salpingectomy in, 239, *241*
   methotrexate for, 239, 241–242
   nonconservative management of, 242–243, *243*
   orders for, 233
   ovarian, 230
   pelvic inflammatory disease and, 231
   physical examination of, 233
   pregnancy test in, 234, 237
   progesterone in, 235
   risk factors for, 231–232
   segmental resection of, 239, *240*
   total salpingectomy in, 242–243, *243*
   treatment of, 239, *240*, *241*, 242–243, *243*
   ultrasonography in, 235, 235t
   urgency of, 231
   vaginal bleeding in, 231
functional residual capacity in, 22, 23t
gallbladder in, 29
gastric emptying in, 28, 213
gastrointestinal system in, 26, *28*, 28–29, 29t, 213
glomerular filtration rate in, 24, *25*
gonorrhea in, 249
heart rate in, 20, *21*, 212
heart sounds in, 21, *21*
hematocrit in, 19, 353t
hematological system in, 19–20
hemodynamic measurements in, 354t
hemoglobin in, 19, 353t
human chorionic gonadotropin in, 302–303, *303*, 303t, *351*
hypercoagulable state in, 213
hypertension in, 69
   diagnostic tests for, 76
   treatment of, 76–84
inferior vena cava compression in, 212
insulin metabolism in, 25–26, 27t
iron requirements in, 20

Pregnancy (*Continued*)
   laboratory values in, 352t–353t
   liver function in, 28–29, 29t
   loss of, in second trimester, 85, 85t
   molar. See *Molar pregnancy*.
   multiple gestation in. See *Multiple gestation*.
   pancreas in, 25–26, 27t
   physiological changes of, 19–29, 211–213
   pituitary gland in, 26
   platelets in, 353t
   prevention of, in sexual assault, 294–295
   renal plasma flow in, 24, *25*
   renal system in, 24–25
   residual volume in, 22, 23t
   respiratory system in, 22, 23t, 24
   serum creatinine in, 24
   stroke volume in, 20, *21*
   systemic vascular resistance in, 22
   thyroid gland in, 26
   tidal volume in, 22, 23t
   total body oxygen consumption in, 22, 24
   toxemia of, 70
   trauma in, 207–214
      cesarean section in, 213–214
      clinical presentation of, 207
      computed tomography of, 210
      definition of, 207
      diagnostic tests for, 210–211
      evaluation of, 207–208, 209
      fetal heart rate monitoring in, 210–211
      fetal threats in, 208
      fetal-maternal hemorrhage in, 213
      hypovolemic shock in, 208
      Kleihauer-Betke stain in, 211
      life threatening, 208
      maternal threats in, 208–209
      obstetrical complications of, 208
      orders for, 210
      peritoneal lavage in, 211, 212t
      physical examination of, 209
      radiation exposure in, 213, 214t
      tetanus toxoid prophylaxis in, 213
      treatment of, 211–214, 214t

Pregnancy *(Continued)*
    ultrasonography of, 210
    urgency of, 208
    visceral injuries in, 208–209
    tubal, 230. See also *Pregnancy, ectopic.*
    ultrasonography of, at first-trimester, 359t
    milestones in, 301–302, 302t
    urinalysis in, 25
    vaginal bleeding in, 298
    weight gain in, 354t
    white blood cell count in, 19, 213
Pregnancy test, in ectopic pregnancy, 234, 237
    in sexual assault, 293
    in spontaneous abortion, 301
Premature rupture of membranes (PROM), 168–182
    amniotic fluid in, 168
    amniotic fluid index in, 173, 173, 174
    cervical culture in, 175
    chorioamnionitis from, 170
    chorioamnionitis testing in, 173, 174t, 175, 176t, 177t
    clinical presentation of, 168–169
    complications of, 169–170
    definition of, 168
    delivery in, 177, 179
    diagnostic tests for, 172–177
    evaluation of, 169, 171
    fetal compromise from, 170
    fetal infection from, 170
    fetal lung maturity testing in, 175–177, 178, 178t
    in multiple gestation, 121–122
    incidence of, 168
    intrauterine growth restriction from, 170
    latency period in, 168
    maternal threats in, 170
    membrane rupture documentation in, 172
    midtrimester, 168, 182
    orders for, 172
    physical examination of, 171–172
    preterm, 168
        in multiple gestation, 121
        management of, 179–181
    preterm labor from, 169–170
    pulmonary hypoplasia from, 170

Premature rupture of membranes (PROM) *(Continued)*
    risk factors for, 169
    term, 179
    treatment of, 177, 179–182
    ultrasonography of, 173, 173, 174
    urgency of, 169
Prematurity, in malpresentation, 106
    in multiple gestation, 123
    in placenta previa, 132
    in placental abruption, 140
    incompetent cervix and, 86
Presentation. See *Malpresentation.*
Prochlorperazine, 398
Progesterone, in dysfunctional uterine bleeding, 223–224
    in ectopic pregnancy, 235
    in luteal phase, 12–13
    in menopause, 14, 15, 15t
    in oil, 398
    in spontaneous abortion, 304
Prolactin, in pregnancy, 353t
Prolonged rupture of membranes, 168
PROM. See *Premature rupture of membranes (PROM).*
Promethazine, 399
Propoxyphene, 399
Propranolol, 399
    in molar pregnancy, 258
Propylthiouracil, 399
    in molar pregnancy, 258
Prostaglandin, cervical ripening with, 93–95
Prostaglandin E_2, 399–400
    in fetal death, 67
    in spontaneous abortion, 305, 306
    in uterine atony, 163
15-methyl Prostaglandin F_2alpha, in uterine atony, 163
Prostaglandin synthesis inhibitors, in preterm labor, 198–199
Protamine sulfate, 400
Protein, in pregnancy, 352t
Proteinuria, in severe preeclampsia, 71
Psychiatric consultation, in postpartum psychosis, 150
Psychological evaluation, in pelvic pain, 288
Psychosis, postpartum, 146, 147

Psychosis *(Continued)*
    factors in, 148
    infant threats in, 148
    suicide in, 148
    treatment of, 150
Psychotherapy, in postpartum
    depression, 149–150
Pubarche, 9, *10*
Puberty, precocious, 10
    reproductive system in, 8–10, 8t,
        9, 10
    stages of, 8–10, 8t, *9, 10*, 365t
Pubic hair, development of, *9, 10,*
    361
    mature, 9
Pulmonary capillary wedge
    pressure, 354t
Pulmonary hypoplasia, premature
    rupture of membranes and,
    170
Pulmonary vascular resistance,
    354t
Pulmonary vasculature,
    vasospasm of, in amniotic
    fluid embolism, 57
Pyelography, in pelvic pain, 287
    of pelvic mass, 277
Pyosalpinx, 261
Pyrethrins, 400
    in vulvar pediculosis pubis, 329

R

Radiation, fetal exposure to, in
    trauma, 213, 214t
    ovarian exposure to, 359t
Radiography, in molar pregnancy,
    257
    of malpresentation, 108
Ranitidine, 400
Rape, 289
    date (acquaintance), 289
    misconceptions about, 291
    spousal, 289
    statutory, 289
    trauma in, 291
Rape trauma syndrome, 290–291
Red blood cells, in amniotic fluid
    embolism, 61–62
    in disseminated intravascular co-
    agulation, 82, 84
    in placental abruption, 144
Renal function tests, in
    preeclampsia, 76

Renal plasma flow, in pregnancy,
    24, *25*
Reproductive system, 7–18
    in adulthood, 10–13, *11*
    in childhood, 8
    in neonates, 8
    in puberty, 8–10, 8t, *9, 10*
    sexual differentiation and, *7,* 7–8
Residual volume, in pregnancy,
    22, 23t
Respiratory tract, in molar
    pregnancy, 254
    in pregnancy, 22, 23t, 24
Rh immune globulin, in
    spontaneous abortion, 307
Rh isoimmunization, in trauma,
    213
Rh-negative, in spontaneous
    abortion, 307
Rifampin, 401
Ritodrine, 401
    in preterm labor, 195
Rocky Mountain spotted fever, vs.
    toxic shock syndrome,
    309–310
Rubin's maneuver, in shoulder
    dystocia, 205, *206*

S

Salpingectomy, linear, in ectopic
    pregnancy, 239, *241*
    total, in ectopic pregnancy, 242–
    243, *243*
Salpingitis, 261
Salpingo-oophorectomy, in tubo-
    ovarian abscess, 269
Scabies, vulvar, 319, 322
    diagnostic tests for, 325
    treatment of, 328–329
Scalp, fetal blood sampling from,
    in nonreassuring fetal heart
    rate, 44–45, 44t
Scarlet fever, vs. toxic shock
    syndrome, 309
Secobarbital, 401
Sepsis, in pelvic inflammatory
    disease, 263
    in postpartum endometritis, 153
Sertraline, 401
Serum creatinine, in pregnancy, 24
Sex hormones, in menstrual cycle,
    11, 365t

Sexual assault, 289–296
  antibiotics after, 294
  Chlamydia trachomatis in, 293
  clinical presentation of, 289
  definition of, 289
  diagnostic tests for, 293–294
  emotional support in, 295–296
  evaluation of, 291–292
  hepatitis B virus vaccination in,
    295
  legal evidence in, 295
  orders for, 292–293
  physical examination for, 292
  pregnancy prevention in, 294–
    295
  sexually transmitted disease in,
    294
  state of mind after, 291
  threats in, 291
  timing of, 290
  treatment of, 294–296
  urgency of, 290
Sexual differentiation, 7, 7–8
Sexually transmitted disease, in
    sexual assault, 294
Shake test, 176–177, 178t, 358t
  in preterm labor, 192, 193t
Shock, cardiogenic, in amniotic
    fluid embolism, 61
  hypovolemic, in ectopic preg-
    nancy, 232
    in molar pregnancy, 254
    in multiple gestation, 123
    in placenta previa, 132
    in pregnancy, 208
    in spontaneous abortion, 299
    uterine bleeding and, 219
  in placental abruption, 141
Shoulder, abduction of, 205, *206*
  oblique rotation of, 204, *205*
Shoulder dystocia, 201–206
  anesthesia in, 202
  asphyxia from, 202
  cephalic replacement in, 206
  clavicular fracture in, 205
  clinical presentation of, 201
  corkscrew maneuver in, 204, *205*
  definition of, 201
  diagnostic tests for, 203
  evaluation of, 203
  factors in, 201–202
  McRoberts maneuver in, 204
  neonatal trauma in, 202
  oblique shoulder rotation in,
    204, *205*

Shoulder dystocia *(Continued)*
  orders for, 203
  posterior shoulder delivery in,
    204–205
  postpartum hemorrhage in, 202
  Rubin's maneuver in, 205, *206*
  shoulder abduction in, 205, *206*
  suprapubic pressure in, 204
  treatment of, 204–206, *205, 206*
  urgency of, 201
  Woods' maneuver in, 204, *205*
  Zavanelli's maneuver in, 206
Skull, fetal, diameters of, *344*
Smoking, ectopic pregnancy and,
    232
  in placental abruption, 140
Sodium, in pregnancy, 352t
Spectinomycin, 401–402
  in gonorrhea, 248, 249
Squamous cell carcinoma, vulvar,
    320, 323
Squamous cell hyperplasia, vulvar,
    319, 322
  treatment of, 329
Staphylococcus aureus, in toxic
    shock syndrome, 308
Stillbirth, 63
Stomach, emptying of, in
    pregnancy, 28, 213
Stroke volume, in pregnancy, 20,
    21
Suctioning, in meconium
    aspiration syndrome, 119
Sulbactam, in endometritis, 156
  with ampicillin, 371
Sulfasalazine, 402
Sulfisoxazole, 402
  in vulvar lymphogranuloma ve-
    nereum, 328
Syphilis, cervical, 323
  differential diagnosis of, 366t
  vulvar, 317–318, 321, 321t, 322
    diagnostic tests for, 324–325
    treatment of, 327–328
Systemic vascular resistance, 354t
  in pregnancy, 22

T

Tachycardia, fetal, 33
Tamoxifen, 402
Terbutaline, 402–403
  in cervical cerclage, 88

Terbutaline *(Continued)*
 in nonreassuring fetal heart rate, 43
 in preterm labor, 195
Terconazole, 403
 in yeast vulvovaginitis, 336t
Testis (testes), development of, 7
Tetracycline, 403
 in pelvic inflammatory disease, 268
 in vulvar granuloma inguinale, 328
 in vulvar syphilis, 327, 328
Thelarche, 8, 8t
Theophylline, 403
Thrombocytopenia, in preeclampsia, 71, 74
Thrombophlebitis, septic pelvic, treatment of, 156–157
Thyroid function test, in fetal death, 68
Thyroid gland, in pregnancy, 26
Thyroid hormone, in molar pregnancy, 257
 in postpartum depression, 150
Thyroxine, in pregnancy, 353t
Ticarcillin, and clavulanic acid, 403–404
 in endometritis, 156
Tidal volume, in pregnancy, 22, 23t
Tioconazole, 404
 in yeast vulvovaginitis, 336t
Tobacco, ectopic pregnancy and, 232
 in placental abruption, 140
Tobramycin, 404
Tocolytic drugs, in frank breech, 110
 in nonreassuring fetal heart rate, 43
 in preterm labor, 194–199, 194t
 in preterm premature rupture of membranes, 180
Toxemia, of pregnancy, 70
Toxic shock syndrome, 308–314
 antibiotics in, 313–314
 clinical presentation of, 308–309
 coagulopathy treatment in, 314
 conditions necessary for, 308
 definition of, 308
 diagnostic tests for, 311–313
 differential diagnosis of, 309–310

Toxic shock syndrome *(Continued)*
 evaluation of, 309, 310–311
 hemodynamic monitoring in, 313, 314t
 incidence of, 308
 orders for, 311
 physical examination of, 311
 respiratory support in, 313
 Staphylococcus aureus in, 308
 threats of, 310
 treatment of, 313–314, 314t
 urgency of, 309
Transfusion, in placental abruption, 144–145
Transverse lie, 100, *100*
 cesarean section in, 111
 incidence of, 102
 treatment of, 110–111
Trauma, blunt, 207
 peritoneal lavage in, 358t
 in placental abruption, 140
 in pregnancy. See *Pregnancy, trauma in.*
 in rape, 291
 neonatal, shoulder dystocia and, 202
 penetrating, 207
 vulvar, 315, 320, 323
Triamcinolone acetonide, 404
 in vulvar squamous cell hyperplasia, 329
Trichomonas vaginalis, in sexual assault, 293
 in vulvovaginitis, 331, 332t, 335–336, 338–339, 367t
Triiodothyronine, in pregnancy, 353t
Trimethobenzamide, 404
Trimethoprim-sulfamethoxazole, 405
Tubo-ovarian abscess, 261
 Chlamydia trachomatis in, 266
 in pelvic inflammatory disease, 261–262, 268–269
Twins. See *Multiple gestation.*

U

Ultrasonography, human chorionic gonadotropin and, 302
 in first-trimester pregnancy, 359t
 in labor induction, 93
 in pelvic pain, 286

Ultrasonography *(Continued)*
  in pregnancy-associated trauma, 210
  in preterm labor, 190
  of abnormal labor, 51–52
  of ectopic pregnancy, 235, 235t
  of fetal death, 66
  of incompetent cervix, 87
  of malpresentation, 108
  of molar pregnancy, 256
  of multiple gestation, 125–126
  of pelvic inflammatory disease, 265
  of pelvic mass, 276
  of placenta previa, 134
  of placental abruption, 142
  of preeclampsia, 76
  of premature rupture of membranes, 173, 173, 174
  of spontaneous abortion, 301–302, 302t
  of uterine bleeding, 222
Umbilical artery, 351t
Umbilical cord, in multiple gestation, 122
  prolapse of, in malpresentation, 7–8
Umbilical vein, 351t
Urea nitrogen, in pregnancy, 352t
Ureaplasma urealyticum, in recurrent abortion, 299
Uric acid, in pregnancy, 352t
Urinalysis, in pregnancy, 25
Urine toxicology screen, in fetal death, 68
Uterine artery, anterior, ligation of, 163, 164
Uterotonic drugs, in uterine atony, 163
Uterus, abnormal bleeding from, 217–224
  anatomic causes of, 223
  causes of, 218–219
  clinical presentation of, 217–218
  definitions in, 217
  diagnostic tests in, 221–223
  endometrial sampling in, 222
  evaluation of, 218, 219
  hypovolemic shock in, 219
  hysteroscopy in, 223
  medical causes of, 223
  orders for, 221
  physical examination of, 221

Uterus *(Continued)*
    treatment of, 223–224
    ultrasonography in, 222
    urgency of, 218
  anovulatory bleeding from, 223–224
  atony of, early postpartum hemorrhage from, 159
    massage for, 163
    surgery for, 163–165, 164
    uterotonic drugs for, 163
  contraction of, in abnormal labor, 49–50
    in nonreassuring fetal heart rate, 42–43
    Montevideo units in, 53, 53
  Couvelaire, in placental abruption, 137
  decompression of, in placental abruption, 140
  evacuation of, human chorionic gonadotropin after, 258, 259, 260
    in molar pregnancy, 258
  growth restriction in, in multiple gestation, 122
  in severe preeclampsia, 71
  premature rupture of membranes and, 170
  in abnormal labor, 51
  in malpresentation, 107–108
  in placental abruption, 137–138
  in premature rupture of membranes, 172
  infection of, postpartum fever in, 151
  internal pressure monitoring of, in abnormal labor, 52–54, 53
  inversion of, early postpartum hemorrhage from, 160, 160–161
    treatment of, 166, 166–167
  masses of, 272, 274, 365t
  rupture of, 91
    early postpartum hemorrhage from, 160
    treatment of, 166
  subinvolution of, 167
  trauma to, 207

V

Vagina, bleeding from, causes of, 132

Vagina (*Continued*)
    in multiple gestation, 124
    in placenta previa manage-
            ment, 135, 136
    in pregnancy, 298
    pelvic pain with, 282
  discharge from, 331, 331t
  fluid of, in premature rupture of
        membranes, 172
  in malpresentation, 107
  lacerations of, early postpartum
        hemorrhage from, 159
    treatment of, 165
  Lactobacillus acidophilus in, 331
  normal flora in, 331, 331t
  pH of, in premature rupture of
        membranes, 172
  in preterm labor, 190
  secretions of, ferning of, in pre-
        term labor, 190
Valacyclovir, 405
  in vulvar herpes simplex virus
        infection, 326
Vancomycin, 405
  in mastitis, 115
Vasopressor therapy, in toxic
      shock syndrome, 313
Vena cava, inferior, in pregnancy,
      212
Venereal Disease Research
      Laboratory (VDRL) test, 68
  in sexual assault, 293
Vertex presentation, in multiple
      gestation, 126–127, 126t, *127*,
      128t
Vestibular glands, major, 225
Vestibulitis, vulvar, 320, 322–323
    treatment of, 329–330
Viscera, injuries to, in pregnancy,
      208–209
Vulva, chancroid of, 318, 321t, 322
    diagnostic tests for, 325
    treatment of, 328
  crab lice of, 319, 322
    diagnostic tests for, 326
    treatment of, 329
  granuloma inguinale of, 318,
        321t, 322
    diagnostic tests for, 325
    treatment of, 328
  herpes simplex virus infection
        of, 316, 321, 321t
    diagnostic tests for, 323–324
    treatment of, 326

Vulva (*Continued*)
  human papillomavirus infection
        of, 316–317
    diagnostic tests for, 324
    treatment of, 326–327
  infection of, 315, 316–319
  lacerations of, early postpartum
        hemorrhage from, 159
    treatment of, 165
  lesions of, 315–330
    appearance of, 321–323, 321t
    causes of, 316–320
    clinical presentation of, 315
    definition of, 315
    diagnostic tests for, 323–326
    differential diagnosis of, 321t
    evaluation of, 320–321
    itching in, 316
    orders for, 323
    pain in, 315–316
    patient age in, 315
    physical examination of, 321–
          323, 321t
    treatment of, 326–330
  lichen sclerosus of, 319–320, 322
    treatment of, 329
  lymphogranuloma venereum of,
        318–319, 321t, 322
    diagnostic tests for, 325
    treatment of, 328
  malignancies of, 315, 320
    diagnostic tests for, 326
  melanoma of, 320, 323
  molluscum contagiosum of, 319,
        322
    diagnostic tests for, 325
    treatment of, 328
  nonneoplastic epithelial disor-
        ders of, 315, 319–320
    diagnostic tests for, 326
  pediculosis pubis of, 319, 322
    diagnostic tests for, 326
    treatment of, 329
  scabies of, 319, 322
    diagnostic tests for, 325
    treatment of, 328–329
  squamous cell carcinoma of,
        320, 323
  squamous cell hyperplasia of,
        319, 322
    treatment of, 329
  syphilis of, 317–318, 321, 321t,
        322
    diagnostic tests for, 324–325

Vulva *(Continued)*
    treatment of, 327–328
   trauma of, 315, 320, 323
   ulcers of, 315–330. See also
     Vulva, lesions of.
    causes of, 316–320
    differential diagnosis of, 321t
   vestibulitis of, 320, 322–323
    treatment of, 329–330
Vulvovaginitis, 331–339
   atrophic, 331, 332t, 367t
    treatment of, 339
   bacterial, 331, 332t, 367t
    diagnosis of, 335, 335t
    treatment of, 338
   Candida in, 331, 337, 357t
   clinical presentation of, 331, 333
   definition of, 331
   diagnostic tests for, 335–336
   differential diagnosis of, 333
   evaluation of, 333–334
   Gardnerella vaginalis in, 331
   orders for, 334–335
   physical examination of, 334
   treatment of, 336–339, 336t
   Trichomonas, 331, 332t, 367t
    diagnosis of, 335–336

Vulvovaginitis *(Continued)*
    treatment of, 338–339
   types of, 367t
   urgency of, 333
   vs. pelvic inflammatory disease,
    333
   yeast, 331, 332t, 367t
    diagnosis of, 335
    recurrent, 337, 337t
    treatment of, 336–337, 336t

W

Warfarin sodium, 406
Weight gain, in pregnancy, 354t
White blood cell count, in
   pregnancy, 19, 213
Woods' maneuver, in shoulder
   dystocia, 204, *205*

Z

Zavanelli's maneuver, in shoulder
   dystocia, 206
Zona pellucida, 13